Health Promotion and Patient Education

Health Promotion and Patient Education

A professional's guide

Edited by

Patricia Webb

Department of Education
Trinity Hospice
London, UK

Stanley Thornes (Publishers) Ltd

First published by Chapman & Hall in 1994
(ISBN 0 412-41220-9)

Reprinted in 1997 by:
Stanley Thornes (Publishers) Ltd,
Ellenborough House,
Wellington Street,
Cheltenham GL50 1YW,
United Kingdom

97 98 99 00 01 / 10 9 8 7 6 5 4 3 2 1

A catalogue record for this book is available from the British Library

ISBN 0-7487-3564-X

Typeset by Best-set Typesetter Ltd, Hong Kong
Printed in Great Britain by T.J. International Ltd, Padstow, Cornwall.

Contents

Contributors

S.J. Campbell, Lecturer in Child Health Nursing, Department of Nursing Studies, Southampton University, Southampton General Hospital, Tremona Road, Shirley, Southampton S09 4XY

J. Comins, The College of Speech and Language Therapists, 7 Bath Place, Rivington Street, London EC2A 3DR

J. Dodge, Geriatric Clinical Nurse Specialist, 3649 W. Folley Street, Chandler, Arizona 85226, USA

Christine M. Dowding, Senior Lecturer, Institute of Health and Community Studies, Bournemouth University, Christchurch Road, Bournemouth Dorset BH1 3LH

K. Elliott, Programme Manager, Family and Child Health, The Health Education Authority, Hamilton House, Mabledon Place, London WC1H 9TX

D. Gould, Department of Nursing Studies, King's College, Cornwall House Annexe, Waterloo Road, London SE1 8TX

E.M. Hillan, Senior Lecturer in Nursing, Department of Nursing Studies, University of Glasgow, 68 Oakfield Avenue, Glasgow G12 8LS

B. Kay, Lecturer in Mental Handicap Nursing, Institute of Advanced Nursing Education, Royal College of Nursing, 20 Cavendish Square, London W1M 0AB

P. Knutesen, Faculty Associate, Arizona State University, 3100 Fairway Drive, Tempe, Arizona 85282, USA

G. Oliver, Director, Patient Services, Clatterbridge Centre for Oncology, Clatterbridge Road, Bebington, Wirral L63 4JY

M. Rowswell, Lecturer in Nursing, Department of Nursing Studies, King's College, Cornwall House Annexe, Waterloo Road, London SE1 8TX

J. Taylor, Senior Lecturer, Suffolk College and Suffolk and Great Yarmouth College of Nursing and Midwifery, Rope Walk, Ipswich, Suffolk IP4 1LT

P. Webb, Department of Education, Trinity Hospice, 30 Clapham Common North Side, London SW4 0RN

Preface

The idea for this book came to me when I first worked in the field of patient education – with cancer patients – in the mid-1980s. It was not until then that I fully appreciated both the need of patients for information and education and the totally inadequate provision of it.

On reflection, it became apparent to me that if those who are ill need to understand what is happening to them, then the well public also need the opportunity to access information to help them retain health and prevent illness. Where there is sound evidence that disease can be avoided or risks of it reduced by behaving in a particular way, then the very least the public deserves is to know about that evidence. After that the choice is, of course, theirs as to whether or not they act upon the knowledge.

My interest since 1986 has not waned but rather has been heightened.

This book is in three sections. Section one is an introduction to some concepts and ideas about health and illness, teaching, learning and the ethics of health promotion and patient education. In each chapter in sections two and three, a particular group of people – the young, the old, those with physical disabilities – is considered and the health promotion and patient education issues related to that group explored. Most of the authors then use case-study material to illustrate some of the principles expressed. The case-studies are usually sited at the end of the chapter except in Chapter 12, where shorter and more frequent examples are given throughout the text.

A small selection of societies and organizations is listed at the end of the book where these relate to more than just one chapter. Specific help agencies are cited within the chapters.

The authors were chosen because of their considerable current expertise and concern for their particular public or patient group.

Finally, with the best intentions, it is inevitable that something will be out of date by the time the book is published. I have made every attempt to avoid this.

I hope the book is useful to the practitioner so that the well public and patients may receive a better service from us all.

Patricia Webb
London
August 1993

PART ONE

Introduction

CHAPTER 1

The sociology of health and illness

Pat Webb

The health of any nation is to a certain extent 'everybody's business'. The health departments of the UK published a document in the middle 1970s to promote and emphasize this view: that people take more responsibility for their own and others' health (DHSS, 1976). The extent to which individuals can be responsible for their health is questionable. Political, social, cultural and economic influences in a society control the direction of health and other public service provision. The size of a nation may influence the extent to which health services can be provided fairly. Resources may be considerably stretched even in a developed Western culture where the public expectation is that any health problem can be cured or managed given the advances in knowledge and technology. Similarly, resources may be considerably stretched in a small, underdeveloped nation where resources of every kind are scarce and the health of the nation poor; where civil unrest, war and unstable politics combine to compromise the efforts of health care workers to raise the level of the nation's health to an acceptable level, reducing early mortality and eradicating diseases caused by poor public health.

Since the virtual eradication of infectious diseases in the developed world, there has been a re-examination of the role of public health strategies for today. For example, the UK considered the need to re-establish its pre-eminence in the pursuit of the public's health and began by producing the aforementioned publication (DHSS, 1976).

WHAT IS HEALTH?

Clearly, a definition of the term that applies to all ages and to those of different physical and mental ability would be helpful.

Several professional disciplines have posed the question and attempted to find an answer. Herzlich (1973) surveyed middle-class individuals in two regions of France – Paris and Normandy – asking their views of health and illness. She concluded that the majority believe 'health' to come from within the individual and therefore, controlled by them, but 'illness' was conceived as something external and mostly outside of their control. Sometimes these external factors were 'visible' such as pathological agents, whereas others were more to do with behaviour or lifestyle. Cancer and mental disorders were seen to be the result of these 'external factors'.

Health was seen as something internal and individual, closely linked with temperament and heredity. Herzlich identified three specific categories of 'health' from the public's responses, as follows:

- health in-a-vacuum – to imply a total absence of illness;
- the resource of health – the individual has the capacity to maintain good health both from physical strength and a potential to resist illness;
- equilibrium – the full realization of the individual's reserve of health.

This third category was rarely experienced, but those who discussed 'equilibrium' did so in terms of 'feeling strong', 'happiness', 'relaxation', 'having good relationships with people'. These concepts seem to be much more about the absence of disease rather than the absence of illness. People were expressing a balance, a wholeness rather than a mere absence of altered pathology.

Several other researchers have investigated different groups. Pill and Stott (1982) surveyed working-class mothers who included in their definitions of health, 'an absence of illness'. They also alluded to the notion that 'health' implied an ability to cope, and to function as other people expected.

The elderly identified three major dimensions of health in a study by Williams (1983).

- Health is the absence of illness and disease.
- Health is a measurement of strength, weakness and exhaustion.
- Health is functional fitness.

'Good health' was seen by this group as the 'strength' to overcome a chronic disease. Health was sometimes described as a loss of strength that heightened vulnerability to diseases not yet present. Functional fitness was described in terms of what a person was fit for. To be unfit for normal roles meant that you were diseased or sick.

There are limitations to interpreting the results of these studies as they relate to particular strata of society and findings cannot be applied to the population as a whole.

More recent work has been undertaken by Calnan and Johnson (1985) and D'Houtard and Field (1984) in England and France respectively. In each case the relationship between health concepts and social class has been more closely examined. Detailed analysis and discussion can be found in the original works, but one overall conclusion is that adverse social and financial circumstances seem to lead people to look at health as functional. That is, the resource and ability to be productive, to cope and to be responsible for others, particularly dependent relatives. Professional groups tended more towards attempts to prevent illness by being active, keeping fit and having checks to detect abnormalities early, so preventing serious illness. In the working-class group there was an assumption that they had little choice, but to go on working and caring for their families. Whereas in the professional group, time could be taken to 'retain health' and money was available to find this.

Clearly, there is no one definition to use from lay concepts.

VIEWS FROM THE PROFESSIONS

Professionals also disagree as to a way of defining health and illness. The World Health Organization defined health as:

a state of complete physical, mental and social well-being, rather than solely as absence of disease. (WHO Constitution, 1947)

Many see problems with this as it implies a static position rather than a dynamic situation. Critics of this definition see health as the ability to adapt continually to constantly changing demands and stimuli. The medical profession might rather use the medical model of health to emphasize that health is the absence of disease or biological disturbance.

Anderson (1984) classified the broad range of definitions used by professionals to define health, into five main areas:

- health as a product or outcome;
- health as a capacity to achieve or perform preferred goals or functions;
- health as a process where it is an ever-changing dynamic phenomenon;
- health as experienced by individuals;
- health as an attribute, such as physical fitness, or a characteristic such as 'emotions'.

Sociologists have defined health in a variety of ways. Talcott Parsons (1951) saw health as part of the social system. He proposed that health maximized the capacity of an individual to perform the functions or activities for which he or she has been socialized. More recently Parsons claimed that the maintenance of good health (in American society) could be synonymous with the notion of individual mastery and achievement and having good health is a function of that society's philosophy (Parsons, 1975).

Stacey (1976) has reviewed the many other sociological definitions of health, which include different brands of a Marxist approach – good health is based on the effective performance of normal roles.

There are few conclusions to be drawn from both professional and lay definitions of health, but the recently popular notion that health and illness are on a continuum seems certainly to be refuted by the majority. Illness is not inevitable even if certain factors are present within or impinge upon a human being. Health can still be achieved despite the existence of a chronic or life-threatening illness where long periods of quiescence are interrupted by exacerbations of the symptoms of the disease or condition.

WHO IS RESPONSIBLE FOR MAINTAINING HEALTH?

The earlier quotation of health being everybody's responsibility rather simplifies a complex situation.

The majority would claim that the provision of health care is a public responsibility – at least to a certain extent. Those countries that have developed a free market for health care have seen that such a system cannot by itself ensure a comprehensive and adaptable service for all categories of health need. This is particularly true for the very expensive long-term care required by an increasing number, at least in Western society. In addition, there are some preventative measures which cannot be the entire responsibility of any one individual in society.

Nationalized health service provision, funded from general taxation, is one way of providing a service of health care, each member of society contributing either at a standard rate or according to their means through progressive income taxation. Alternatively, there may be different levels of provision where basic or emergency care will be provided by a government, but individuals may also contribute to private health care schemes. This is becoming more popular in some European countries where overloaded national health services cannot provide an immediate or adequate service for everyone.

The issue of what constitutes an 'immediate' or 'adequate' provision of health service is not static. Changing demands and rising expectations from the public have resulted from the 'successes' or 'achievements' in health care. Higher standards of living and effective preventative measures – such as screening for some early causes so that treatment can be more effective or 'stop smoking' clinics to help reduce the risk of lung cancer or chronic respiratory disease – enable people to live longer. However, they may then experience some of the inevitable consequences of old age. New treatments never dreamt of 50 years ago now enable diseases to be treated and cured. The escalation of costs, as a result of this, is considerable, however, and is, in addition to funding research and treatment for new health problems, not possible to accurately predict and plan for. An example of this is the HIV and AIDS problem.

Irrespective of how payment is made for health care, Governments and statutory bodies have the responsibility to train professionals, build hospitals, provide services and implement health promotion and prevention programmes. Individual nations do this to a greater or lesser extent, but the responsibility is clear irrespective of whether or not it is carried out.

So, the wider public are responsible and the Government is responsible, but what of the individual?

There has been much discussion recently on the role of the individual with regard to health. For example a re-organization of health services in the UK (Government White Papers, 1989, 1991) promotes the idea of individuals taking more responsibility for their own health whilst the health professionals change their practice to accommodate this. Inevitably there is to be some shift in power and control from the professionals to the public, but adjustment to such a dramatic change will take time, and some 're-training' of both groups. The well public or patients will need to believe that their assertiveness (based partly on increased access to factual information about health) will be valued rather than discouraged. Health professionals need to increase their skills in communication and teaching, to enhance an effective health education role and to enable individuals to be more in control of their own lives. The radical nature of this change should not be minimized. There have already been problems in implementing such change where, cautious not to be too controlling, professionals have sometimes left patients without the expert help they need and for which they consulted them. These are teething troubles but nonetheless need to be acknowledged and dealt with.

There is considerable evidence that some individuals want to take more responsibility for their health, not least in the significant increase in self-help groups and voluntary organizations developed to encourage this. These may enable those very individuals to either establish their own organization of care or to use such bodies as pressure or lobbying groups to influence existing care provision. A real example of this is the proliferation of groups and organizations relating to cancer. For example, ten years ago the four major cancer charities in the UK (Imperial Cancer Research Foundation, The Cancer Research Campaign, The Marie Curie Memorial Foundation and Cancer Relief Macmillan Fund) were actively pursuing their respective functions – care or research activities. That work has increased particularly in relation to care, but there are also two new cancer-related charities (BACUP and Cancer Link) and many smaller organizations intent on improving the information needs of the consumers of health care as well as providing support and care in general. These developments have been as a result of need and initiative from the public, with support from empathetic professionals many of whom have themselves been patients and, therefore, know at first hand what that means.

The cancer field is only one example of this development. The Help for Health data base in Wessex could demonstrate many other similar examples.

Health professionals also have responsibility for maintenance of health and not just the investigation and treatment of people with disease of course. This is the case both as agents of the statutory bodies and as individuals in their own right. Every health carer has a health promotion role. In addition, there are those who are specifically trained to promote health and prevent ill-health, detect early disease and arrange referral for treatment. The issue of health promotion will be addressed in more detail later in this chapter.

MANAGING HEALTH AND ILLNESS

Having suggested some definitions of health, addressed the question of who is responsible for maintaining it and briefly touched on the business of preventing ill health, we move on now to looking in more depth at the way that societies manage the health and ill-health of their populations.

The professions

Maintenance of health and the treatment and care of those who are sick has been seen as the main remit of the health professions. The organization of professions *vis-à-vis* health care has a considerable influence on the management of health services and the controls that are exerted at a macro and micro level.

Medicine

The University Medical School of the Middle Ages laid the foundation for the development of clear criteria by which a specific group of workers could be identified as the arbiters of medical work. Medicine as a profession developed from that elite of higher learning and medicine developed official control over its work. This control over its own work began medicine's (and subsequently other professions') political character in that it had the aid of the State in establishing and maintaining the profession's superiority. Such is the pattern for the development of professions from occupational groups. It is by the interaction between formal agents or agencies of the occupational group (medicine) and officials of the State that the profession's control over its work is established, shaped and maintained.

The most treasured attribute of professions is autonomy to practise their expertise without challenge or interference by those outside of the profession. In terms of medicine, however, there are government controls exerted which do not regularly affect a 'clinical decision' directly, but rather influence the management of service and the quality controls and allocation of resources required to some extent to provide a similar service nationwide. However, that 'clinical decision' (for example that a person with irreversible renal failure needs a kidney transplant) may well be influenced by the more political and economic considerations that allow a certain number of transplantations a year in that health region; prevent the employment of a renal transplant specialist; reduce the number of beds and nurses to receive and care for such patients, and so on. There is not, therefore, entire autonomy to practise and with current economic pressures throughout the world, these issues are becoming more tangible and apparent in everyday practice. One might summarize this issue of professional autonomy by saying that the autonomy of individual practitioners exists within that socio-political space allowed for their benefit by other bodies – political and statutory mechanisms. Professional autonomy is not absolute – at least not in medicine.

Freidson (1970) argues that the degree to which medical autonomy can be enjoyed varies as relations with the State or Government vary. Doctors may have control over the technological or clinical aspects of their work, but lose it over the social and economic organization of their work. This may or may not be appropriate but it is the case.

Medicine across the world
There are variations in the way that medicine has developed and now functions worldwide. A brief comparison of these variations may be useful.

The USA In the USA medicine has considerable socio-economic and technical autonomy. Its professional association has been given control of many functions that in other countries remain with the State. Doctors have been relatively free of lay interference. There is no organized national system of health service in the USA, although a national system of financing a basic level of medical care has been established in Medicare, the agency through which basic and emergency medical care is available for any citizen. Apart from that, communities, counties and State organizations and programmes provide services peculiar to each area. Some of these overlap, some conflict and many are in competition. Health care is purchased in one way or another as a commodity and 'choice' is left to the consumer. The degree to which choice can be exerted, however, does ultimately depend on the cost of treatment and care or the available services. Most of the services are provided by private agencies for payment with reimbursement by insurance companies. There are some public agencies providing services for school children, the poor and those with notifiable infectious diseases such as tuberculosis, where without treatment the population at large may be at risk. Federal agencies provide a level of care for some ethnic or minority groups, war veterans and military personnel and their families. Public health is provided by the State, but the majority of out-patient and in-patient hospital services for the general population are provided by private organizations, with the aid of public taxes or by philanthropic or religious organizations.

Doctors belong to the American Medical Assocation (AMA), a national body that nonetheless has local community or district branches. It is these local branches that set the qualifications for local membership, although most licensed Medical Doctors (MDs) are eligible for admission. Representation on the national body is made by nomination at local level. As for most professional organizations, the AMA has responsibilities for maintaining standards of practice and, in this case, care also. It also provides the scrutiny to enable continued updating and licence to practise.

Currently, there appears to be more involvement than before of non health-professional groups in the management of health care – but not at the clinical level. Reimbursement by insurance companies is now much tighter with the introduction some years ago of Diagnostic Related Groups (DRGs) categorizing patients and illnesses in such a way as to standardize items for payment. This is seen by the majority as restrictive and unworkable as there is seldom a 'standard' patient. However, it simplifies the paperwork and has some benefits. The AIDS problem has presented the USA and many other countries with a public health problem (as well as a social and individual one) that is stretching resources and management of services considerably.

England and Wales   Shortly after World War II, the Ministry of Health took over the administrative and financial structure of health services and the National Health Service (NHS) was born. The three main areas for services have been in hospitals and specialist centres; general practices in the community; dentists, pharmacists, nursing and other community services; public health services including preventative medicine; school health services and maternal and child care.

Health services are managed by local units of regions and districts who are themselves accountable to the government.

Unlike the USA, hospitals are staffed by consultants (called specialists in the USA) with general practitioners having little access to hospital patients. Although there is now the re-development of smaller general practice units where general practitioners do have their own hospital beds, this is still unusual but may become popular again in the light of recent changes in general practice in the community.

Salaries are negotiated nationally for hospital consultants and are paid according to their grade and time worked. General practitioners are paid on a 'per capita' basis. However, these arrangements are currently being reviewed and some hospital and primary health care practices are now opting out of local control and becoming independent, self-governing Trusts. They still remain as part of the national health service, but organize and manage themselves differently.

Since the NHS was born, the British Medical Association (BMA) retained its control over the technical areas of medicine, but control over the terms of practice was negotiated with the government and embodied into law, to create a national system of organizing and paying for health services for all citizens.

Overall the UK system is one in which the State finances and organizes the administration of health services. However, the BMA in its role in the General Medical Council still controls the licensing of practitioners and strongly influences the formulation of practice through central, regional and yet more local committees.

The continent of Europe   Currently there is no standardization in the way that medicine is practised or health care managed in Europe generally. Clearly, with the introduction of the 'United Europe' in 1992, more standardization may occur. This will take time and many peculiarities will remain. Europe is wider than the European Community (EC). Although more countries from both East and West are applying for membership to the Community, that is not guaranteed, will take time, and the EC is itself an ever-changing organization where little is certain.

Given these uncertainties, there are some general statements to be made which will give some indication of the management of medicine and therefore health care in Europe.

The systems which direct and govern the delivery of health care can be said to fall into two main groups. There are those that are financed by a fee for service with reimbursement by insurance companies and those financed directly from taxation providing free care at the point of delivery. The former system includes countries such as Belgium, France, the Netherlands and Spain. The latter group, rather like the UK, includes Denmark, Italy and Ireland, although there are variations in the degree to which taxation 'covers' the cost of health care.

In all EC countries, the range of cover is comprehensive, however administered and the schemes tend to be similar in principle. Those who go to live and work in a different EC Member State than their own are entitled to be insured and receive benefits on the same terms and conditions as the nationals of that country.

Currently there is no one Directorate within the Commission dealing with health matters, but issues relating to the management of health services and professional training are dealt with in different Directorates. The training directives govern the mutual recognition of diplomas, the organization of training and the right to freedom to provide professional services in any EC country. There are Standing and Advisory Committees for the major health professions and the Standing Committee of Doctors was particularly active in the early 1970s when Professor Ralf Dahrendorf (the Commissioner then responsible for the Directorate of the Commission dealing with mutual recognition of medical qualifications) organized a 3-day public hearing in Brussels on the recognition of medical qualifications. This was a public meeting between the practising professions and the universities.

Dialogue continues on these issues and there is much to be resolved regarding the mutual recognition of training at basic and post-graduate levels. Autonomous medical practice, as described both for the USA and for England and Wales, is present to a greater or lesser extent in each of the countries of Europe with national and local professional bodies working with governments on matters of health.

Eastern Europe   At the time of writing there is much division and confusion in Eastern Europe generally and in Russia in particular. Extreme political and economic instability inevitably has an effect on health matters as well as other systems in society. Professional autonomy is a very weak, if present notion in the most East European countries. There is no independent association like the AMA or BMA to serve a a spokesman for the profession.

There may well be gradual, but distinct changes in Eastern Europe and Russia in the near future, but it would be a brave person to predict what these changes may be.

It would appear that, despite the socio-political framework of nations, professions can and do function autonomously and, although there are differences in the way health services are managed, the basic structures are not too different.

Nursing and other health professions

Nursing has come from an entirely different route than medicine. The history of nursing goes back centuries but perhaps it is as well to reflect back to that heroine of the Crimean War, Florence Nightingale, who in 1855 in London heralded the changes in nursing by establishing training schools to improve and standardize the quality of care given by this person, 'the nurse'. Despite her reputation as a nurse, Florence Nightingale was also an ardent politician and spent much time lobbying for one reform or another – not least for the army. St Thomas' Hospital, London was the first site chosen to train the first ever 'probationer' nurses for their one year course. Florence's book *Notes on Nursing; What it is and What it is not* (1859) is still regarded as clearly describing the fundamental principles of nursing practice today.

Training schools developed from that first example of St Thomas' in 1860 and the era of modern nursing began. However, this was only the English pattern where health care was carried out in the then so-called 'voluntary' hospitals where a hierarchy was established with the Matron at the apex.

In the US and Canada the model was followed of attaching most training schools to hospitals, but there were also programmes connected with universities, which were in some way attached to a hospital for other studies. The hospitals tended to provide the budget for nurse training, however, rather than independent university schools. The hospital hierarchy was through the Head or Superintendent of Nurses to the hospital Superintendent who may be a doctor or a layman.

On the continent of Europe, nurse training was either in a training school as an integral part of a hospital and owned by it, or was conducted in an educational institution absolutely independent of the hospital, and sometimes situated away from it. In Europe, the hierarchy in hospital was through a senior nurse (Head Nurse) to a medical director in charge of the hospital and a hospital director, a layman.

The general pattern established by Florence Nightingale at St Thomas' Hospital spread throughout Great Britain to some parts of the continent of Europe, Scandinavia and Holland. Australia, New Zealand and South Africa also continued this pattern until fairly recent changes in the structure of nursing education and the move towards more academic underpinning and credibility. The continent of Europe – East and West – variably followed either the English or the American system.

Differences in medicine and nursing

One of the purposes of describing both the medical and nursing structures and training is to underline the extreme differences in their development. Medicine was well-established as an academic discipline with clinical practice to follow. Nursing came from a practical occupation which subsequently acquired training established within its own discipline and complemented by teaching from doctors. Standard qualifications were required prior to gaining access to medical schools. Nurses come from every kind of educational background. Medicine practised as an autonomous profession with standards and controls exerted by professional organizations. Nursing was managed by hospital hierarchies through nursing, but sometimes with a layman or doctor at the head. Doctors govern their own practice (within certain codes and guidelines), nurses are less autonomous and have practice imposed upon them. The medical body of knowledge is well-established whereas the body of nursing knowledge is still being compiled and sometimes still cannot be defined.

Primary health care services

The practice of community physicians has been addressed to some extent in the previous section on medicine. Public health nursing (to encompass district nurses, school nurses, specialist nurses working in the community and those working in occupational or industrial nursing) varies in its pattern across the world. In several countries, universities offer post-graduate training for this work – Canada and the USA and parts of Australia and New Zealand. In other countries, special schools exist to train public health nurses, for example in Italy and France. Currently public health issues are part of every nurse's training, to a greater or lesser extent as the importance of the contribution of care is recognized from home to hospital and back home again; from the well person, to the sick and the rehabilitated back to health again.

Until recently, schools of nursing for training tended to be the norm, however they were organized or affiliated. Currently across the world there is a greater tendency to incorporate nursing programmes within diploma, graduate and post-graduate studies at universities and polytechnics. There is a general movement to give nursing a more credible academic base so that it can continue on its development as a profession. Changes in practice, and the knowledge-base required to deal with many nursing issues, have precipitated these moves. Critical thinking and decision-making have to be part of the modern nurse's skills, together with management, education, skilled practice and the ability to be articulate both verbally and on paper. Changes in the structure of health service provision require nurses to be able negotiators for funds and other resources. Patients and the well public make greater demands upon the nurse both for expertise and for care. There is a growing tendency for multidisciplinary teams to combine their expertise for more comprehensive patient care and preventative work with the public.

Across the world, some standardization has been achieved in nursing knowledge and practice. The International Council of Nurses (ICN) founded in 1899 links national nurses' associations from over 80 countries worldwide. The Council sometimes acts as a 'spokesman' to other bodies. For example, it persuaded the European Commission to reorganize a Standing Committee of Nurses in 1971, and there are regional ICN groups that meet to share common issues and problems. The European Nurses Group is one such body. Nurses also have their place in the more general health bodies such as the World Health Organization where nurses are employed to plan strategies for the future to accommodate the health needs and care requirements *vis-à-vis* health care for the future.

Nursing is gradually building up its own knowledge-base. In both Europe (European Nurse Researchers) and internationally (WHO) assistance has been given for nurses to conduct research. There is a good deal of evidence that there is appropriate progress in many fields of nursing – practice, management, education and research. Even more exciting are the consistent trends to work across disciplines and to strengthen collaboration in all disciplines in health care.

Professions allied to medicine

Little mention has been made of the many other professions allied to medicine and nursing. This is not the book to outline each of their roles or contribution but as several different disciplines have contributed to later sections – including speech and language therapists, health promotion experts, educators – some of their roles will become apparent.

What is important is the recognition that there are many different disciplines with differing expertise who are working in health care. Many are over-worked and many others are under-used. Sometimes the two situations co-exist and, until those who are under-used are afforded their rightful place, more resources will not be ploughed into the recruitment of additional staff to provide expertise in all aspects of health care.

Health education and health promotion
Reference has been made previously to issues of public health and the variability of services offered and personnel involved.

Part of maintaining the public's health is seen to be that of preventative medicine. Whilst that term usually refers to issues like legislation for health and safety issues, at a primary prevention level, screening, early diagnosis and treatment for particular high risk groups at a secondary level, some would claim that health education of the population also plays a significant part in prevention. However, what constitutes health education has always been controversial, as is determining what are the effective methods of doing the educating and how these can be evaluated.

Ewles and Simnett (1992) claim that health knowledge is a basic human right and endorse this by quoting the affirmation made at the Primary Health Care Conference in Alma Ata (World Health Organization 1978) that people have the right to be involved in both the planning and implementation of their health care, including health education.

While they further suggest that most members of the public want to understand health issues and be informed, they acknowledge that the methods used to educate for health are not always successful in that goals set may not be achieved. This may be due to a variety of factors – unrealistic goals, crude methods or whatever.

They claim that there is substantial documentation to support the notion of health education being an essential and intrinsic component of health promotion. However, the two terms are often erroneously used synonymously.

The differences in the two terms have been explained well by a variety of people. A summary of those explanations may read as follows.

> The terms health promotion and health education are not interchangeable. Health promotion covers all aspects of those activities that seek to improve the health status of individuals and communities. It, therefore includes both health education and all attempts to produce environmental and legislative change conducive to good health. Put another way, health promotion is concerned with making healthier choices easier choices.

While educating the public about risk factors and healthy lifestyles is important and may contribute to promoting health, the social and financial issues are equally important – some would say more so. Advising a mother to buy more fresh fruit and vegetables for her family, when the price of those is beyond her budget, does little to improve her health and well being. Indeed, it could be argued that it causes her more stress.

The Health Education Authority (HEA) is the government-funded body in the UK responsible for health educaton of the public.

Before 1987, when it was known as the Health Education Council (HEC), it seemed to have greater autonomy to make realistic plans from the extensive expertise it had. Since its change to a Special Health Authority, it is expected to work fully with the Department of Health on government policies such as the major projects 'Look after your Heart', vaccination campaigns and AIDS education. Health promotion officers working at local level seem to prefer more focused, local community projects, believing that the cost of mass media campaigns may not be justified. Clearly, there are disagreements that may hamper progress, but in 1989 the HEA launched its five year plan designed to improve the nation's health. The main areas of concern are all areas of sexual health, AIDS, heart disease, cancer, smoking, alcohol and family and child health programmes. It is also encouraging the involvement in health promotion of doctors, nurses, and health visitors, working in primary health care centres. Different countries approach these issues in different ways and it is not only government funding that provides these services. In many countries, voluntary organizations of one kind or another are very active in the promotion of health.

THE ROLE OF THE GOVERNMENT

There has been criticism of the way that the role of the individual in health promotion has been emphasized recently in the UK. While that role is important and some think it should be encouraged, there are assumptions made about how the public view health and what frame of reference they use.

For example, the so called medical model of disease causation and disease management is used, which underemphasizes the social and economic influences and overemphasizes the lifestyle of the individual.

Townsend and Davidson (1982) suggest that lifestyles are strongly influenced by the social and economic conditions under which people live and work. Also, that individuals are not always in a position to change their lifestyles, even if they wanted to. There are social and economic barriers in doing so that may not be easily overcome.

The government may decide to attempt to direct the health of the nation by intervening through legislation. Examples of this are the regulations in the manufacturing industry, or the controls exerted to avoid workplace hazards. A more topical and controversial issue would be that of controlling the places where the public can smoke cigarettes (Calnan, 1984).

Some members of the public support the notion that the government should be more involved in improving the health of the public by, for example, increasing the availability of health workers at times convenient to the public, or providing more comprehensive screening or counselling centres particularly for working women (Calnan, 1987). These same strata of society also want more socio-economic improvements rather than education which they apparently value less – possibly because they need more money to implement some of the recommended 'healthy lifestyles'. This would be the case with regard to nutrition for example.

Some sociologists claim that the middle and working classes have quite different sets of values regarding health, while others consider that may have been the case immediately post World War II, but is less of an issue today (Taylor-Gooby, 1986; Fitzpatrick and Scambler, 1984).

The extent to which governments or the State influence health education and promotion is bound to vary. In some countries active health promotion occurs via the radio and television during prime-time broadcasting or viewing. Such examples include instruction on protecting the skin from harmful ultraviolet sunlight in parts of Western Australia, to the more recent and powerful message regarding the HIV and AIDS problems related to sexual activity and drug abuse. Free 'air time' is rare for health issues that are not a threat to whole communities, although there is an increase in the use of videotapes in waiting areas of hospital out-patient departments and general practice surgeries. These may cover a whole range of topics, and in some cases have supporting literature to accompany them.

GETTING THE MESSAGE ACROSS

Acknowledging that whatever 'knowledge' is available to enable people to retain health or cope with illness should be shared, how should this be achieved to the best advantage for all? Is it just a matter of imparting knowledge from one group (health educators) to another (the lay public) or is it more the issue of attitude and behaviour change?

Recently, health education has become the centre of the same scrutiny as other health services. Does it work and is it worth doing? have been the questions posed. Could it be seen to be coercive and is this morally right? In addition, there are questions posed as to the economic efficiency of health promotion and health education issues. In today's world these are bound to be raised. If a given method or message works – with data to support this – should it be generally introduced irrespective of cost? Views will vary on these issues. Some will argue that enabling people to take control of their health may increase the burden on health services rather than reduce it. Detecting early disease may initially put greater strain on an over-stretched service.

An example of this is the thorny issue of breast self-examination (BSE). One piece of research in particular suggested that, providing adequate and appropriate instruction and practice was given to post menopausal woman, BSE was more sensitive in detecting small breast lumps than mammography (Pennypacker et al., 1982). At first sight, successful BSE would appear less expensive than mammography (cost being the main reason for a limited mammography service for women of all ages). However, the degree of training needed for women to perform BSE successfully was staff-intensive and needed a variety of technological learning media that resulted in it being a very costly exercise. Such an example illustrates the complex business of efficiency – effectiveness and cost.

Many authors and practitioners have addressed the marketing of health education and health promotion. There are many theories and strategies currently addressing these issues from a variety of stances. Recommended reading on such topics include Tones et al. (1990)

and Ewles and Simnett (1985). These will not be addressed in detail in this book.

CONCLUSIONS

There has been recent confusion in the terminology used to describe two separate but interlinked notions. Health promotion is a relatively new concept and it encompasses political, social and general policy issues intended to provide the context for a 'healthy society'. Economics, housing, employment and political decisions all affect a nation's health.

For the purposes of this book, health education is seen as a way to enable individuals to retain health and cope with illness through the acquisition of relevant knowledge based on sound research. That 'knowledge' to be made available to the public from those who hold it, in a way that it can be readily utilized.

Both health promotion and health education are important and can work powerfully together. More important still is the availability of 'specialist knowledge' to the layman, in such a way that it can be both understood and acted upon. However, the choice remains with him if it is only his own health that is in question. If the wider community is at risk – through an infectious disease, or passive smoking – then bigger questions of a socio-ethical nature are raised.

This book looks at some of these ethical issues and poses some of the conflicting arguments. More than that, it presents a variety of scenarios which attempt to look at sections of society, their health education needs and some ideas of how these may be met. It is essentially a practical guide for the health professional, but also hopefully will provide stimulus for further thought and discussion.

REFERENCES

Anderson, R. (1984) Health Promotion: an overview. *European Monographs in Health Education Research*, **6**, 4–119.

Calnan, M. (1984) The Politics of Health: The case of Smoking Control. *Journal of Social Policy*, **13**(3), 279–96.

Calnan, M. (1987) *Health and Illness – the Lay Perspective*, Tavistock Publications, London, pp. 87–100.

Calnan, M. and Johnson, B. (1985) Health, Health Risks and Inequalities: an exploratory study of women's perceptions. *Sociology of Health and Illness*, **7**(1), 55–75.

Department of Health and Social Security (1976) *Prevention and Health: Everybody's business*, HMSO, London.

D'Houtard, A. and Field, M.G. (1984) The Image of Health: Variations in Perceptions by Social class in a French Population. *Sociology of Health and Illness*, **6**, 30–60.

Ewles, L. and Simnett, I. (1992) *Promoting Health – a practical guide to health education*, John Wiley & Sons, Chichester.

Fitzpatrick, R. and Scambler, G. (1984) Social Class, Ethnicity and Illness, in *The Experience of Illness* (eds. R. Fitzpatrick *et al.*), Tavistock, London.

Florence Nightingale (1859) *Notes on Nursing: 1859. What it is and What it is not*, Blackie, Glasgow.

Freidson, E. (1970) *Profession of Medicine*, Dodd, Mead and Company, New York.

Government White Paper (1989) *Working for Patients*, HMSO, London.

Government White Paper (1991) *The Health of the Nation*, HMSO, London.

Herzlich, C. (1973) *Health and Illness*, Academic Press, London.

Parsons, T. (1951) *The Social System*, Free Press, Glencoe, Ill.

Parsons, T. (1975) The sick role of the Physician reconsidered. Millbank Memorial Fund Quarterly. *Health and Society*, **53**, 257–78.

Pennypacker, H.S., Goldstein, M.K. and Stein, G.H. (1982) Efficient technology of training (2) breast self-examination, in *Public Education About Cancer* (ed. P. Hobbs), UICC Technical Report Series, UICC, Geneva.

Pill, R., and Stott, N. (1982) Concepts of Illness Causation and Responsibility: Some Preliminary data from a sample of working class mothers. *Social Science and Medicine*, **16**, 13–51.

Stacey, M. (1976) *Concepts of Health and Illness*. A Working Paper on the Concepts and Their Relevance for Research. Social Science Research Council.

Taylor-Gooby, P.T. (1986) Privatisation, Power and the Welfare State. *Sociology*, **20**(2), 228–46.

Tones, K., Tilford, S. and Robinson, Y. (1990) *Health Education Effectiveness and Confusion*, Chapman & Hall, London.

Townsend, P. and Davidson, N. (1982) *Inequalities in Health*, Penguin, Harmondsworth.

Williams, R. (1983) Concepts of Health: An analysis of Lay Logic. *Sociology*, **17**, 185–204.

World Health Organization Constitution (1947) *Chronicle of the WHO*, **1**(3), 1.

CHAPTER 2

Teaching and learning about health and illness

Pat Webb

INTRODUCTION

Whether in the field of health prevention or in active health care, much has been documented in recent years regarding the need for the public or patients to be informed of and to learn about disease and the prevention, treatment and cure of illness. With recent changes in health care management in much of the Western world, the public are being encouraged to be more assertive in accessing information and, where necessary, knowledge and skills, to maintain their own health as much as possible. One could say that encouragement to achieve this has hardly been necessary, particularly with some sections of society who have themselves taken significant initiatives to find the information they need and to manage the health care systems to their advantage. Consumer groups, self-help groups and the explosion of other organizations to access health information and influence health care are all a clear indication of people wanting to retain more control of their own lives. It is also an indication that, for whatever reason, the public may not have been satisfied with the level of control and involvement they previously had.

Interest in health issues by the popular media has raised public awareness to such an extent that people in all sections of society are now seeking more information that may help them handle their own lives more adequately.

Choices are being offered for treatment of some illnesses in this fast-moving scientific world. Such choices lead the public to believe that there may be yet more knowledge and information which is not readily available to them and which they seek. It is in the nature of the human spirit to be inquisitive.

With so many successes in medical science and so much technology to detect and diagnose disease, the public now have very high expectations of health care professionals. Even when a cure is not a possibility, palliation and symptom control is, and the hospice movement in the UK is a prime example of this. Patients with advanced, incurable diseases can and still do have a reasonable quality of life with support from those experienced in palliative care. When for example, pain, dyspnoea and functional disabilities can be helped, people can retain a sense of control and self-esteem previously denied them.

This whole shift of control between the health professional and the public has resulted in both groups being more aware of information-giving, teaching and learning (particularly in the context of health care) and the power that can be exerted through knowledge. Now past is the once familiar scenario of doctor or nurse in a consulting room wielding a pen and prescription pad or treatment plan, whilst the patient sits passively compliant on the opposite side of the desk. The lack of knowledge about health and illness once rendered public or patients powerless to negotiate or question even at a basic level (Webb, 1988). Now that such negotiation and involvement is being encouraged, the public has more confidence to question and discover for themselves what may be the best decisions to keep their health or treat their disease.

A prerequisite of effective teaching and learning is the power to communicate. Much confusion results from ambiguities, semantic differentials, the problems of multi-ethnic and multicultural societies and the language difficulties inherent in them. On a simpler level, human beings can be extremely poor communicators of simple information. Many people leave out-patient clinics and doctors' surgeries totally bewildered by what was relatively straightforward information as far as the doctor or nurse is concerned. Assumptions are frequently made of a level of knowledge and understanding which is either not there or, in the anxiety of the moment, is so reduced as to be ineffective.

This chapter addresses some of these issues and poses some practical guidelines for improving information giving and teaching and learning between the public or patients and those providing health care expertise.

COMMUNICATION

Our whole world consists of being bombarded by messages intended to inform, instruct, persuade, coerce, shock or delight. The advertising industry uses techniques to achieve all of the above in order to 'sell' their product or service. For those who are fully able, with both physical and mental capacity, reaction to these communications occurs in a variety of ways. If topics or issues are of no interest to an individual, messages may not be received, irrespective of the potential power of those messages. Other things are attracting attention. For example, a message via an advertising poster designed to encourage an elderly couple to buy a retirement home is hardly likely to hold the attention of a teenager concerned with his or her fashion image. It would be absurd to suppose this is the case, unless the teenager was rather mature and had grandparents who may be looking for such a home.

This example highlights one of the issues of effective communication which is as real in matters of health care as it is in any other parts of our world. In order to attract attention, communication needs to be focused to real concerns and not diluted with extraneous information.

Messages need to be short, powerful and clear. Language must be used well to avoid ambiguities or irritation of the potential receiver of the message who may be struggling to fathom some obscure and occult meaning. In addition, one is relatively unlikely to gain the attention of those who have little vested interest in the message. The point was made in the example of the retirement home and the teenager. In the health context, one might use the example of a shocking poster exposing the hazards of intravenous drug abuse to an elderly group of people needing advice on mobility. The example is likely to be so removed from their reality as to have little if any impact for them as individuals (Wilkinson, 1991; Cleghorn, 1990; Scammell, 1990).

Cultural and ethnic values also need to be considered. Western values displayed in words, posters, information leaflets or however, will have little impact on the strict Muslim or Jewish immigrant who is hardly integrated into a new country, let alone a new culture.

THE MEDIA

What methods can be used to communicate messages – about health in particular?

One-to-one communication

Despite the many developments in communication techniques, effective talking and listening on a one-to-one basis is still very powerful. However, several matters need to be considered to ensure that even this simple way of communicating is effective.

1. Clear personal introductions must be made. It is very easy to assume that a white-coated man must be a doctor. Freedom to talk and discuss can only be realized when both parties are clearly identified. The introduction also serves to begin to get a feeling for the other person: to know whether he can be trusted for example. The social convention of shaking hands gives further data on the other person through that

contact, together with eye and other facial expressions, voice tone and general warmth or formality.

2. Use of language must be appropriate. A cue may be taken from the person consulting the health carer. If they appear anxious, nervous, shy, assertive, angry or whatever, this can be picked up early on and can act as a guide for the continued success of the consultation. Competence in language and level of education can be assumed to some extent also. It may be an initial guide to the degree of information given at the outset which may then be adapted as the conversation continues. Presumptions that correlate level of intellectual ability with language may be used as an initial guide, but not as an absolute indicator. Such an indication is unrealiable. Care needs to be taken when people have stammers, are deaf or just slow in speech. Such features are often assumed to indicate inability rather than personality traits of unavoidable disabilities.

3. Messages must be brief and clear, focused to current events and not those that may occur in the course of time.

> If you want to reduce your high blood pressure, there are two things you can do now. The first is to lose weight and the second is to take exercise. We can work out a plan to help you achieve both of these if you wish.

This is helpful, constructive information that an individual can see will give immediate results. Unhelpful advice may be 'If you want to reduce your high blood pressure, you must lose 2 stones in weight and raise your pulse rate by exercise to 160/minute three times a week'.

Not only is that last message too detailed but also there is no instruction as to how it may be achieved and over what time scale. There are many other examples that could be used to illustrate this point of course. When giving patients information about investigations needed prior to surgery they need to know what preciously is going to happen tomorrow, not the details of the 23 investigations that will be conducted over the next 3 weeks, or those that *may* be necessary in certain circumstances yet to be defined.

4. Involvement of the individual in the conversation at the outset to establish a partnership in dealing with a health education or illness issue. Such an atmosphere begins a trusting relationship where control is retained by the person seeking help rather than the one giving it.

5. A clear indication at the completion of the conversation as to what will happen next. When will you next meet, what will happen in between meetings, who else is to be seen – are all questions that need addressing before parting.

Written messages

These may be in the form of consent to treatment forms, information leaflets, instruction sheets, posters or books.

Many of the guidelines given in 'One-to-one communication' above apply, but need to be adapted to this different medium.

Language is just as important and must be clear and concise. Much has been written about the effectiveness of written information for patients (Blumberg *et al.*, 1983; Webb, 1983; Webb, 1988; Welch-McCaffrey, 1986) and controversy abounds regarding the use of reading-ease indicators, evaluation methods and so on.

All of us have experience of wordy documents which convey nothing or which convey such ambiguities as to be useless. Language must be clear, concise and unambiguous. Information must be appropriate, up-to-date and understandable. Jargon and abbreviations should not be used.

Illustrations of any kind should only be used if they enhance or explain the text (in the case of books and leaflets). When used as the main focus (for example on a poster), the text must complement and explain the picture, rather than create confusion. Unlike secular commercial advertising, subtle images will not attract attention when messages are being given about health. The first achievement is to attract the attention. The second must follow quickly to convey the message or else the opportunity is gone. If someone has to work out the possible meaning behind the message, the impact will be lost.

Finally, the medium should be attractive and easy on the eye. Colour, design, clear print, spacing, and size all play a part in this. A scrappily-produced photocopied sheet which is hardly legible will not inspire someone about to undergo a serious operation with confidence. An information booklet which lacks colour and style will not attract the attention of the reader.

Other media

A whole range of other media may be used to communicate messages of every kind. Models, television, audio or video tapes, computer programs are some that are used frequently. The same general principles of communication apply: clear messages, focused information, good-quality resources and use of the appropriate medium for the message. Sometimes booklets are preferable to videos. A poster is not an ideal way to instruct someone on the legal issues of informed consent. An audio tape is not helpful to give advice on a technique or skill where a visual demonstration is required.

In unusual circumstances, communication may best be achieved by music or the performing arts. Where there is sensory loss, emotional or mental disturbances, music, dance or drama may convey appropriate messages more powerfully. Every possible means to convey messages effectively should be used.

TEACHING AND LEARNING

While it is clear that good communication is a first step, the public or patient may need to do more than just receive information. They may need to change their behaviour, lifestyle or attitude; they may need to learn a new skill (giving themselves an injection or attending to a colostomy).

It is useful to look briefly at the way people learn and tailor these to some teaching methods. First, there are some general points to make about teaching and learning in different age groups.

Differences through the lifespan

People of different ages learn in different ways and teaching needs to be geared to this. Most of us have had some experience of children's learning and the immediate interest and ready uptake of new information children have as they explore their world. Adults do not necessarily learn so eagerly. Motivation may not be high, socialization may have dampened the spirit of enquiry and interest. Even if interest is high, ability to absorb and understand may be diminished for a variety of reasons, both emotional and physical. There may be real learning difficulties (see Chapters 11 and 14).

Small children

Small children need learning to be fun and to be related to their world. Toys, models, symbols are all useful and can be adapted to teach about health care. New information needs to be brought into the children's world using their language and context. Two examples to illustrate this may be as follows.

1. You need to teach a child to tell you about his pain because you are wanting to evaluate the effects of analgesia over time. Pain is a subjective experience and it is difficult enough to try and assess pain between two adults – patient and doctor, for example. The most appropriate method for asessing children's pain is to teach them how to use their language to communicate that pain to you, over a period of time. Comparative 'reports' will give an indication of the success of therapy.

Working in the small child's world, it is important to introduce toys, play, pictures and games. Several pain assessment charts have been designed for use with children. One commonly adapted one is a series of faces depicting sadness through to joy with all the expressions in between. Children are asked to identify which face most fits how they are feeling on any given day, or time of the day. This information is requested in the context of their pain.

Toys may be used to indicate the site of pain and degree of intensity. Using a well-worn teddy-bear to indicate pain in the leg and the kind of pain that is can be graphically illustrated by a child. They may indicate throbbing, shooting, piercing pain – just by the movements of their hands on the toy's leg.

Art has been seen to be a powerful way for children to communicate. Pictures about pain from children suffering with terminal illness have been described by Bach (1990) and Bertman (1991), amongst others. Teaching children to communicate in this way means more accurate assessment and, therefore, more precise treatment.

The child may then need to be taught how to relieve his pain. Again, toys can be used to instruct a child on how to take medication – by mouth, injection, ointment or whatever. Providing the medication for the favourite toy first produces a reality that the child can readily identify with and learn from.

All the time, the child needs to be kept informed and involved. Children like that and are insulted if they are ignored or if control is given to a parent instead. Because they are developing, children are much easier to teach and often more willing to learn than adults. This fact should be constructively exploited for mutual benefit in the context of learning in health care.

2. A second example may be in teaching a child to adapt his diet because of an allergy – more a health education issue this time. Many small children begin by being allergic to cow's milk or milk products. They may feel the effects of that allergy (sickness, stomach pains, rashes, etc.), but may need help to discuss what they can and cannot eat and drink. Often they will not have a parent or guardian available to consult at the time of eating. Simple lists of foods and fluids, used again in a play scenario with toys and art, will provide a powerful message. If a milk drink makes a doll sick, it will also make them sick, and so on. If words are still difficult for the child, pictures and symbols can be used instead as an *aide-mémoire*.

Puberty and adolescence

These are taken together with some hesitation, but general statements only are considered in this text.

Some time between the ages of 10 and 16 years, children develop the secondary sexual characteristics that establish them finally in the adult world. It is a turbulent time of biological, social and psychological change. Often individuals are not sure of whether they are still 'child' or now 'adult', as certain legal rights and responsibilities are also afforded them. During this time, secondary education comes to an end. Steep learning curves occur as more complex knowledge and skills are achieved.

It is important now for any health or patient education to be tailored to this age-group. Medicine and disease prevention is based in biological and behavioural sciences. School children may be learning such sciences as part of their school curriculum. Using the well-tested method of teaching from the known to the unknown (building on existing knowledge), health professionals can use the base of existing knowledge to teach new skills and attitudes.

The difficult area here that also moves into adolescence is the social and behavioural one. Whilst the young person may *understand* the dangers of cigarette-smoking or promiscuous sexual behaviour their actual behaviour may reflect the need to be identified socially with their peer group. This need may be much stronger than the need to avoid health problems.

Many schools have health education issues in their curricula – some may be successful and some not. Assessment of current levels of knowledge is a prerequisite before attempting to teach new facts. Gaining the child's confidence and valuing his current opinions and knowledge (treating him as an adult) will do much to strengthen the relationship required for effective learning to take place, particularly in this age-group.

Where possible, school teachers and parents should also be involved in both health and patient education. Successful teaching has been achieved when all three meet together with the child to consider the health need or problem. Confidence is then instilled in the child that he has support and that everyone has the same information and is giving the same message.

For adolescents through to adulthood (16–20 years) the changes are even more profound. Formal secondary education may be left far behind, but individuals may move on to university or college, to continue their learning. On the whole, childhood and young adulthood are times of health. Attracting these groups to issues of healthy behaviour is difficult, because attention is elsewhere – on learning to be a responsible individual in an adult world. However powerful the messages in a health education context are, unless the risks of not changing behaviour are clearly communicated messages will not be heard. Acceptance within the peer group is a high priority. Achievement in work and establishment in career is high on the agenda.

Acknowledging this openly with the individual may be all that is needed. If they hear the health professional say

I realize that you are in a competitive world where you study and career is of utmost importance (or whatever), but this too is important. If you continue to smoke at this rate, you will seriously harm your health. You will not be able to play sport because you will be short of breath. You will have frequent chest infections with time off work.

And so on.

Of course this technique will not always work, but openly acknowledging an understanding of the individual's priorities will at the very least indicate that you are aware of them. There may then be a better chance of them listening to you.

Adults

Teaching and learning in the adult world can be more rather than less difficult to achieve. However, it depends on the vested interest of the individual to learn.

The same problems exist *vis-à-vis* health issues, in that unless a person feels ill, on the whole, his focus is on enjoying life and not being preoccupied with what *might* happen to his health. Life is too short.

However, there is currently a health and fitness culture. Sport and exercise are seen by many as valuable and glamorous. Where this is the case, some health messages are easier to convey and individuals are more receptive to them. Weight loss and exercise to prevent heart disease are two examples of this. The high-profile fitness culture can be extremely expensive and out of the reach of many. In these instances, enterprise is needed to provide the same beneficial effect, but without cost. For example, where access to a fitness gymnasium is not realistic, a gradual exercise programme of walking, running, swimming, can be tailored individually with health professional and patient together.

I return to the important fact of acknowledging the individual's current situation and context – openly acknowledging it. From there, health professional and patient can move on together, understanding both the needs and the resources to meet their desired aim.

Other hindrances to teaching and learning in adulthood may be related to family life and responsibilities or to benefits and stresses associated with the single status of men and women. For families, preoccupation with the children's development, education and achievements may predominate. A man may need to alter his sedentary lifestyle to prevent obesity and reduce chances of heart attacks. However, his work may require a sedentary lifestyle and his preoccupation is to earn sufficient money to support his family. A woman may need a hysterectomy after menorrhagia from uterine fibroids, but would not want to be in hospital while her two children are studying for their examinations preparing them for university entrance. For the single person, priorities will be in different areas, but are just as important to consider.

Currently, there are many more problems associated with unemployment than is usually the case, as the economic recession continues to affect everyone's life.

It is a matter of focus and priority. Individuals may understand the health messages, but feel they are not in a position to act upon them. Alternatively, they may not appreciate the importance of the message – or understand it. Both issues need to be addressed.

The older adult

From middle to older age is yet another period in the lifespan where readjustment is constantly taking place. Teaching and learning for health will again need to be adapted for this group. For many individuals this is a period when past and present values are reassessed, and attitudes and behaviour modified accordingly. Physical resource is less and minor ailments more frequent, as the process of ageing continues. There is often multiple pathological disturbance.

When retirement from active work takes place, yet further adjustments are needed and memory and intellectual capacity are often reduced. Hearing and sight may be impaired. The possibilities for taking exercise and eating a healthy diet may be somewhat compromised.

These different ages and stages in life are reflected in some of the chapters in Part Two of this book where real illustrations are given of health promotion and health education issues across the lifespan.

THE PROCESS OF TEACHING AND LEARNING

It is not within the remit of this book to give a detailed analysis of learning theories and teaching methods. However, some practical guidelines for teaching in a health context will be discussed and some examples used to illustrate the points.

Assessment for teaching and learning

A prerequisite for effective teaching, whether of the well person or the patient, is adequate assessment. Knowing the current situation for an individual results in the best use of time and resources for the future and invariably gives much greater overall success.

Whatever the context, it is important to establish the following:

- what an individual already knows so that you can build on existing knowledge and skills;
- what an individual *needs* to learn to keep themselves well and safe;
- what an individual *wants* to know and what he prefers not to;
- what capacity an individual has to learn;
- preferred teaching methods and evaluation;
- where and when the learning takes place.

What does an individual need to know?

Taking these in turn, the first is really the setting of objectives by the 'teacher' (in this context a health professional). It begins the list of abilities or skills that make a good teacher. Others will be addressed under subsequent headings.

Once the health or patient education situation has been identified, there may be some facts to be learned or skills taught to enable the person to live safely. This 'need to know' is a requirement rather than necessarily what they think they need. It is more to do with the professional's than the patient's agenda.

A classic example of this is the newly diagnosed insulin-dependent diabetic. In order to stay alive and well, the person needs to understand:

- the meaning of symptoms that require either more sugar or more insulin;
- how to test their urine to determine dietary and insulin needs;
- how to test blood for sugar levels;
- how to select a diet that meets their energy needs;
- how to prepare and give themselves insulin;
- the importance of prompt response to infection or injury because of problems with healing.

Similar examples exist for all ages and all illnesses. In a health promotion context, factors for prevention of illness can be similarly assessed where preventative measures are known. The teacher therefore needs to set clear objectives with realistic achievable targets both for himself and the individual. Given each of the requirements listed above, each can be taken in turn over a series of teaching sessions, using as many visual aids as possible to achieve learning (for more details see 'Preferred teaching methods and evaluation' below).

Where appropriate, an *aide-mémoire* should be used, whether in the form of a leaflet, check list, patient diary or some other tool.

Building on existing knowledge

Part of the assessment is to establish the current level of knowledge before building on that to increase knowledge and understanding.

The assessment interview is now required. This need not be a lengthy, complicated process, but part of the overall assessment of the individual whether in a health or patient context. Good communication and questioning skills are needed to determine the level of knowledge. A good opening question might be

> What do you think is wrong with you?/what do you think you need to do to prevent heart disease?

Once you have an initial response, subsequent questions will reveal more specific detail. Open questions or open focused questions, as illustrated respectively above, allow the individual freedom to say what they wish. Directed and closed questions enable precision and factual answers. An example of a closed question is

> You say that you only drink socially. What do you mean by 'socially'? How many glasses of what kind of alcohol per day or week?

You may then want to follow on with yet more specific questions to elicit more information.

Once you have established a level of knowledge and understanding, you have a baseline to move forwards.

A similar situation occurs with skills. If you want to determine ability to test urine, ask the person to do it while you watch and to explain why he is doing it as he goes along.

Building on existing knowledge and skills has two benefits. One is to know for yourself how much further you have to go. The second is to give confidence to the person that they are not entirely ignorant. Both are important.

What people want to know

Individuals have a right to information about their health, but there are people who prefer not to know too much detail. Such preferences also need to be honoured. The difficulty is to know what information and learning is required and what is not.

The easiest way around this problem is just to ask, feeding in your own agenda as indicated in the first part of this section – where information and teaching to stay alive and well are required. Apart from this, different degrees or levels of teaching can be negotiated with the individual and agreement reached. They should, however, be made aware of the implications of selective teaching and learning. It may be necessary to start at one level and to frequently check the need to alter this as time goes by. People change their minds and their learning needs alter. In the case of a patient with an established illness, he may want more control as time goes on and earlier learning needs may well be superseded by different ones.

Preferred teaching methods and evaluation

The general rule of thumb here is that there are many different ways to make teaching (and therefore learning) effective.

Each of us from our own experience of education will know which teachers and which ways of teaching were most effective for us. Most of us would conclude that wherever our own involvement in learning occurred, the message was more likely to be received and remain.

Clearly, in health and patient education there is only a minimal role for some teaching methods – the lecture, visits to organizations to collect data and compilation of a dossier would all be unusual. The most usual would be one-to-one teaching tailored to individual needs following a needs assessment (as described above). This would then be augmented with leaflets or booklets (giving the same message) or an audio-visual presentation. Such a scenario can now be seen in some doctors' practices and in out-patient and in-patient areas of hospitals. General principles given via a common medium – booklet or audio-visual aid – and then a more personal session arranged between doctor/nurse and individuals seems to be the best combination.

The advantages of this are that immediate feedback can be given by both parties to avoid confusion and ambiguity. General information can be given effectively and powerfully via a videotape, specially prepared leaflet or similar, individual information in a one-to-one session.

Other teaching methods may be used in specific circumstances. Informal lectures or talks may be given to homogeneous groups prior to more individualized teaching. This is fairly common now with self-help groups who invite health professionals to address them on particular topics; health education centres that hold 'Quit Smoking' classes or weight reduction classes and so on.

In addition, occasionally more interactive methods are used – role-play, games, simulation, debates, discussions and sculpting. Many of these are unusual in the health care context, but some of these methods are reflected in the chapters in Parts Two and Three of this book. Specific skills are needed by teachers and should be acquired before embarking upon these methods.

Where possible, supportive material should be used for all teaching sessions – books, posters, leaflets, flipcharts, models, audio-visuals, computer-assisted learning and so on. The Health Education Authority, visual-aid agencies and many of the individual charities have examples of all of these. It is worth checking the Charities' Directory and enquire about resources produced by the relevant organizations before embarking on producing one of your own. It may save you time and money. However, there may be nothing that meets your particular need. Thorough investigation of an appropriate medium for a particular teaching session then needs to be made before embarking on what can turn out to be a time-consuming and costly exercise. However, it can also be seen as an *investment* in time and money for future work.

The most important points about the activity of teaching are preparation and evaluation. You must be clear how you are going to deliver your message, otherwise the learner will be confused. You must have some way of determining its 'success' – and what you mean by that.

Clearly, there is not space in a book such as this for too much detail on either preparation or evaluation. However, some very simple and general guidelines may be useful as a check-list. Other texts are quoted later which give more detail.

GUIDELINES FOR PREPARATION AND EVALUATION

- Be clear what message(s) you want to convey. State and quantify your objectives.
- Divide your session into introduction, main content, conclusion, action.
- Be sure to include the time factor in your stated objectives to the individual. For example,

    I want to tell you about the 'Quit Smoking' course. The course lasts for 10 weeks. The first three weeks concentrate on your planning your own schedule with one of the course teachers. You will then be given specific goals to achieve each week after that. These will be specific and achievable goals. You may plan to reduce cigarette smoking from 10 to two per day, or not to smoke after one meal or whatever.

- Plan to back up all the verbal communication with as much visual material as you can (as discussed above).
- In your conclusion, build in ways of evaluating your teaching. Formulate some questions to check that what you plan to say is received unambiguously. One way to do this is to ask the individual to give you his understanding of the teaching that has just occurred or to ask him to demonstrate the skill you have just taught.
- Be sure you have clear ideas yourself of how you will proceed over time. It may be that you plan four or five teaching sessions over a given period, each with specific objectives and evaluation.

There are good examples of public and patient teaching methods available from those agencies already mentioned, including the Health

Education Authority and Health Promotion Units for England, Scotland, Wales and Northern Ireland and a host of charities and voluntary organizations who have developed their own materials and ideas. (The Ulster Cancer Foundation has produced particularly good materials on nurses stopping smoking – see Lazenbatt and McEwen, 1991; the BMA and Imperial Cancer Research Foundation (ICRF) have produced a general booklet on stopping smoking for use throughout Europe – see BMA, 1989; Action on Smoking and Health (ASH) and many others have similar resources for this topic.) Commercial companies and the pharmaceutical industry also produce educational materials.

More practical details about planning and evaluating teaching can be found in other health promotion books, such as Ewles and Simnett (1992) and Coutts and Hardy (1985).

THE LOCATION AND MOTIVATION FOR LEARNING

Some mention has already been made regarding the motivation of individuals to learn about health and illness. When you feel well, giving time and thought to the possibility of not doing so, for many, seems to waste time; for others, it is an investment in time to prevent ill health.

To some extent, patients with existing disease or health disruption may be more motivated than the well member of the public. However, if teaching and learning means that an individual has to make additional visits to a health centre or hospital, he may not want to spend that extra time focusing on his illness when he has some ordinary living to do as well.

Individual reaction to the need for teaching and learning is given in some of the chapters in Parts Two and Three. The role of the health professionals is to be as realistic and practical as possible, acknowledging the needs and circumstances of the individual and their social milieu. It is also necessary to be very flexible and practical in approach. There is no point developing highly sophisticated methods of teaching if the intended audience cannot understand them or take the time to exploit them. The teaching has to take into account the peculiarities of a given client or patient group, the age-range, ability, economic and psychosocial advantage and limitations and a host of other factors, to make the activity worthwhile.

It is also important to consider the avantages and disadvantages of teaching for the health professional, who does not have unlimited resources in terms of time and finance. While it is impossible to adequately demonstrate the cost-effectiveness of teaching for health there must be some sound indicators to illustrate the benefits of doing so.

WHERE TO DO THE TEACHING?

Nothing has yet been mentioned about the place where teaching occurs and the general context of teaching about health and illness.

Most teaching will be either in a health centre clinic or hospital. Sometimes it will be in one individual's home, nursing home, hospice or similar institution.

The very fact of illness or health being the focus of teaching presents the first hurdle to overcome. Health professionals are seen as powerful people with a specific body of knowledge that is not the privilege of the majority. This immediately creates a social distance between them and the lay public. Overcoming this is one of the first steps in the communication process to balance the relationship more into one of negotiation and partnership. Until this is resolved, there will be problems in motivating people to become involved in the teaching/learning process – no matter where it is done.

It may be worth considering the place of teaching, in the light of this fact. People may feel more motivated to travel to a particular place and take part in a specific course or teaching session. Alternatively, if the teaching is part of a home visit by a general practitioner, nurse or health visitor, that may be better for some. Where such flexibility is possible, it should be exploited.

Wherever the teaching is to take place, consideration must be given to the location. For example, talking about the sensitive issue of sperm-banking to a young man about to undergo treatment for testicular cancer or lymphoma is not best achieved in the corner of an out-patient waiting area of a clinic. Time and privacy are prime requirements. Addressing a group of middle-aged women on the relative benefits of hormone replacement therapy (HRT) could best be achieved in a small meeting room fitted for teaching, where audio-visual aids can easily be used and general information given. Specific one-to-one issues will then be dealt with on an individual basis subsequently.

Teaching a mother and child together about insulin-dependent diabetes may be achieved at their home where other siblings, grandparents or whoever can be brought in at the appropriate points of the teaching.

Thought must be given during preparation to the best location for teaching to take place.

CONCLUSIONS

General principles only can be addressed in a chapter on these issues. Some real examples, illustrating the points, will be found in the chapters of Parts Two and Three of this book.

What is important to stress is the need for flexibililty, enterprise and expertise in this area. Health professionals need to inform and educate the public about issues of health and illness – it is part of their role, to enable individuals to take more control and responsibility for their health. Initially, this may be a costly exercise, but it can be seen as a long-term investment. However, in today's world of economic stringency, clearly identified objectives need to be stated and the costs calculated. Teaching the public and patients can be very cost effective. Existing resources for teaching may be used rather than new materials made. If it can also be demonstrated that such exercises influence life quality and contribute to the prevention of illness then it is even more worthwhile.

REFERENCES

Bach, S. (1990) *Life Paints its own Span*, Daimon Verlag, Einsieldon, Switzerland.

Bertman, S. (1991) *Facing Death*, Hemisphere Publishing Corporation.

Blumberg, B.D., Kearns, P.R. and Lewis, M.I. (1983) Adult Cancer Patient Education: An Overview. *Journal of Psychosocial Oncology*, **1**(2).

BMA and ICRF (1989) *Help Your Patient Stop*. Available from the British Medical Association, Tavistock Square, London WC1H 9JP, UK.

Cleghorn, R. (1990) Whose Life is it Anyway? British Association of Cancer United Patients – BACUP – newsletter summary 1990. 3 Bath Place, Rivington Street, London EC2A 3JR, UK.

Coutts, L.C. and Hardy, L.K. (1985) *Teaching for Health*, Churchill Livingstone, Edinburgh.

Ewles, L. and Simnett, I. (1992) *Promoting Health*, John Wiley & Sons Ltd, Chichester.

Freidson, E. (1970) *Profession of Medicine*, Dodd, Mead and Co., New York.

Lazenbatt, A. and McEwen, A. (1991) An Evaluation of the Ulster Cancer Foundation's Nurses Smoking Package and its Impact on Student Nurses. *Journal of Advanced Nursing*, **16**, 1428–38.

Scammell, B. (1990) Communicating about Patients' Care. *Nursing Times*, **86**(15), 32–4.

Webb, C. (1983) Teaching for Recovery from Surgery, in *Oncology for Nurses and Health Care Professionals* Vol. 2 (ed. R. Tiffany), Harper & Row/ Beaconsfield.

Webb, P.A. (1988) Teaching Patients and Relatives, in *Oncology for Nurses and Health Care Professionals* Vol. 2 (ed. R. Tiffany), Harper & Row/ Beaconsfield.

Wilkinson, S. (1991) Factors which influence how nurses communicate with cancer pationts. *Journal of Advanced Nursing*, **16**(6), 677–88.

CHAPTER 3

Some ethical issues in health and patient education

Pat Webb

In the introductory chapters of this book, some general principles of health promotion and patient education have been addressed. In Parts Two and Three specific issues will be raised to cover a range of health care settings and topics. For those of us working in the field it is often difficult to stand back and look objectively at the philosophical and ethical issues that are part of this practice. We have a moral conscience, but how is this used to help us make decisions about the politics of health care, use and allocation of resources and issues like choice, compliance, confidentiality, autonomy and consent?

Before going on to look at the application of principles of health and patient education to the work setting, this chapter will pose some ideas for thought and discussion concerning ethical issues (moral dilemmas) that are becoming an ever-increasing part of our everyday work challenge.

Some definitions of terms are required for the purposes of this chapter.

HEALTH PROMOTION

In recent years, confusion has been caused by the introduction of the term **health promotion** when previously **health education** alone was used. Some health professionals see no distinction between the two – to promote healthy ideals and lifestyles one may need to pursue educational activities. Others see the two as in some way related, but that they encompass different philosophies and therefore objectives. Yet others see the role of health promotion as a resurgence of the preventative **public health** of post-war days.

The simplest explanation could be that health promotion aims to encourage healthy people to stay healthy. In this context, it consists of societal and individual rules and values which promote behaviour conducive to health. Those employed in health promotion programmes are promulgators of these ideas having established philosophies and strategies underpinned by theory. Health education is part of this process – whenever the need to educate is required. Such education may be through other health professionals to the public and patients or it may be directly from a health education or promotion unit, industry, school or whatever.

The term health promotion apparently began in the 1970s. At the same time, there was much talk about re-orientating the notion of illness to the norm – health (illness being a deviation of that norm).

Several people have reviewed the literature on health promotion in Europe, including Tones (1985), Baric (1985) and Anderson (1984). Literature is also available for the USA (US Department of Health and Human Sciences, 1980) and at an international level (WHO, 1986). The World Health Organization adopts the perspective noted above that health promotion programmes are designed to promote health and that health education will be an integral part of that activity.

The promotion of health is not seen as the exclusive property of health professionals, but rather the combination of all aspects of life and society that promote the 'state of mental, physical and social wellbeing' (WHO, 1978) rather than just an absence of illness. It is, therefore, much broader than educating for health and includes a wider range of services and personnel within its remit. One can see why some believe it to be in the realms of the previous discipline of public health. Earlier this century the way to sustain a healthy nation was to provide a clean environment, good drainage, water and other public services (including a health service). Now, there are new threats to the environment, including pollution, toxic waste, noise, over-crowding, and the effects of all these on the individual. Whilst infectious diseases have been virtually eradicated newer diseases have taken over. This, together with the increasing politics of health care and the resources to provide a health service, has led to the health promotion movement. Health policy units seek to implement changes in society through legislation, fiscal and economic measures and clearly have the issues of health promotion on their agenda.

In summary, one could say that health promotion consists of legal, fiscal and environmental issues which are concerned with the achievement of health and the prevention of ill-health.

HEALTH EDUCATION

Health education has also had a stormy history. There are basically three models of health education: a **politically biased** model; a **preven-**

tative model; and a model which encourages the individual to take initiative and responsibility – an **individual** model.

Taking each of these of turn, a political model is concerned with the achievement of social and environmental change through political action. It is more a collective social activity than an individual one although it uses the notion that individuals should take more responsibility for their own health and actions than they have done traditionally.

A prevention model would be seen as the most traditional and orthodox. It encourages individuals to adopt 'healthy lifestyles' and behaviours which will prevent disease at all three levels – primary, secondary and tertiary. Some have said that this model is in itself unethical, as it ignores the fact that individual action can only ever be part of the solution to remaining healthy (Vuori, 1980). The underlying political, social and economic problems should not be ignored. Some individuals are relatively powerless in their attempts to achieve health, particularly the economically disadvantaged.

The so-called individual model is based on an American health educational ideal (SOPHE, 1976) to encourage and promote informed choice. Some of its components would be consistent only with the public health strategies and policies of North America where health care is a commodity purchased at the time of use. Parts of it would be difficult to implement in a European context – for example in the UK. However, it is alluded to frequently in European and UK health education literature. Given the increase of self-help throughout Europe, it may become more popular than even before. There are some similarities with this and the previously mentioned 'prevention' model.

Some writers adopt a more pragmatic approach – not such a philosophical or theoretical one. Ewles and Simnett (1992) state their stance clearly that health knowledge is a basic human right and if education for health is required to obtain this knowledge, then all means should be taken to do it. This notion is endorsed by the now well-referenced Report on the Primary Health Care Conference, Alma Ata (WHO, 1978). Ewles and Simnett (1992) go on to say that, without knowledge, people cannot make healthy choices about their own lifestyles or be equipped for political and social lobbying to change things for society generally.

They promote five approaches to health education: the medical approach; the behaviour change approach; the educational approach; the client-directed approach; and the social change approach (Ewles and Simnett, 1992). Some of these clearly overlap with the three mentioned previously, and they are mostly self-explanatory. Whereas the medical approach seeks to eliminate medically defined disease and disability, the behaviour change approach concentrates more on persuasive behaviour – change of strategies. The educational approach ensures that people understand why they are doing what they are doing; the client-centred approach is entirely directed by the individual – the initiative is his. Finally, the social change model goes back to the notion of health promotion again to include issues outside of the purely educational ones by being involved in social action.

PATIENT EDUCATION

Depending upon the model you follow, patient education can be seen as very much a part of health education. It addresses those who already have an established disease and therefore take on the role 'patient' for a period of time. It may be temporary or long-term with intermittent periods of ill-health and wellness. Patient education is sometimes called tertiary health education.

How does it differ from other health education settings? The main differences are the attitudinal and motivational ones (as discussed in Chapter 2). The focus on health issues usually becomes sharper once disease is established. What was a possibility has become a reality. In many cases this increases the motivation of the individual to learn about this condition, or at the very least be informed.

There are other differences also. Some would say that patients are more vulnerable as a result of their illness and, therefore, tend to be more dependent and passive towards health professionals. This varies enormously. The degree of dependency and passivity often fluctuates throughout the course of illness. It is not a static situation. It seems entirely appropriate that there will be times when patients feel so ill that they have to depend on others – one might say they are almost at another's mercy. Certainly this would be the case in an acute emergency when even consent for treatment may not be possible. Those with chronic illness may be totally unable to take decisions about their health during the acute exacerbations of illness.

However, following diagnosis and at times throughout the treatment programme, patients and their families can become partners with health professionals to address their health needs together. There is now a growing body of research to demonstrate the value of informing and teaching patients. Some projects demonstrate reduction of distressing symptoms as a result of giving information (Webb, 1983; Webb, 1988a; Wilson-Barnett, 1983), while others are more concerned with patient autonomy and control – the development of coping strategies (Bowen *et al.*, 1961; Levine *et al.*, 1979). Blumberg *et al.* (1983) published a very useful overview of adult cancer patient education, with a particular focus on chronic illness.

Barriers to patient education include the fact that many doctors, nurses and others are traditionally ill-prepared to teach (Schoenrich,

1976; Redman, 1971) or what they do teach is poorly understood and no checks or evaluations are built into the patient education pro-grammes, the professionals rather just assuming that all is well (Stanley *et al.*, 1984). Another barrier may be that conflicting information is often given because some standardization of material is not planned (Powell and Winslow, 1973; Somers, 1976). Perhaps even more import-ant in the context of this chapter, patient education has traditionally had a low priority for budgeting purposes as it is often seen as a luxury rather than a necessity (Nordberg and King, 1976). However, one could argue that giving insufficient information increases non-compliance with medical treatment and care resulting in additional pathology and possible readmission to hospital (Ausburn, 1981; Ley, 1988). This in turn increases costs. Keeping patients well-informed and in control can be very cost-effective as well as beneficial for their quality of life.

SOME ETHICAL CONSIDERATIONS

Just by reading through these definitions, ethical principles and ethical dilemmas emerge. Issues like choice (justice/fairness), compliance, control (autonomy), improving care through information-giving and education rather than doing harm (beneficence/non-maleficence/truth-telling). Some of these will be addressed in the general section fol-lowing but, as is the case with ethical issues, absolute resolution of problems is not the aim, but rather healthy debate and discussion to enable informed decisions and personal or group conclusions.

JUSTICE AND FAIRNESS

In 1989 two Government papers were published in the UK to address the needs both of the well public and patients *vis-à-vis* health (HM Government, 1989a,b). These two documents supported the notion of individuals being responsible for their own health. Support would be offered from nursing, medicine and social services working with each other and the individual and family for a strategically planned service.

In 1991 a Government consultative paper was circulated, entitled 'The Health of the Nation' (1991), aimed to raise the debate for current and future needs of citizens in England. Included amongst the stated objectives was the identification of main health needs; securing the best possible use of available resources to meet those needs; promoting good health and preventing disease: these objectives to have at least an equal focus as the treatment of established disease. Also, there must be a recognition that health is determined by a whole range of influences, including psycho-social, political and economic ones. Further, in this document, there is reflected a concern that everyone should have the best possible information in order to understand both their own and other influences on health. People should be more involved in decisions *vis-à-vis* their health and illness, both as individuals and through the influence of local, voluntary and statutory organizations.

If health promotion and patient education can be linked to the stated requirement for everyone to have sufficient information, then the system does indeed seem just and fair. Perhaps the Government has got it right after all. How does it work in practice though? In July 1992 the final paper on the Health of the Nation was agreed and ratified by the UK Government and their ideas have been finally realized.

There seems to be an assumption that a democratic society automatically gives people power because it gives them choice and autonomy. Those of us who live in a democracy know that there are still the powerful and the dependent; that is almost entirely due to economics and opportunity, even though it may not seem so at first sight. There are also leaders in a democratic society. Citizens have a vote, but they are often ambivalent as to whom to support because they are not in tune with the total party policy – just parts of it. That leads to them voting for another party, or not voting at all.

In the UK as elsewhere across Europe, each country's policies are now being complicated by European issues. While the notion of subsidiarity (the right of each nation to decide on local, national issues) is acknowledged, many people are sceptical about adherence to it and what may be termed a 'national' or 'European' issue. Elsewhere in the world, countries have different structures from those of Europe, but still there are conflicting issues and values, whether in a democracy or not.

There are other conflicts which have an impact on the notion of justice and fairness. 'Allegiance' is an interesting concept and the motivation for it.

For example, an English person may have a national pride, support local institutions (which may or may not conflict with national ones) and have allegiances to 'causes' or 'groups' all of which may conflict with each other. Someone may believe in the philosophy of a nationalized health service, but be outraged at the apparent unfairness of adequate resources in large cities and inadequate facilities in suburban or rural settings. An individual may be an active supporter of feminist or homosexual communities at national level, but feel aggrieved when loyalty to these may channel resources away from other more local health issues, for example.

In many parts of the world, these situations are further compounded by the complexities of our communities. Ethnic groups abound and in so many ways enrich society. Some ethnic groups are newly settled and still follow all their own traditions and lifestyle, speak little of the national language and find national politics and everyday life so very confusing. Second and third generations may be so nationalized as to be effectively that nation's citizens. Sometimes there are considerable conflicts between these two groups, originally of the same ethnic background.

Returning to the theme of 'justice' therefore, it can be seen that to be fair to everyone in all circumstances is not achievable in the reality of our politico-economic structures today. Even if there were adequate resources for everyone, it is clear that human beings are not so keen to always share them.

There is certainly a strong movement in Western Europe and parts of North America for personal 'empowerment'. Often this is linked to the notion of free societies, democracies or whatever, but there are problems with this as I have indicated above. That people are in theory free to choose to live as they wish does not necessarily correlate with individual power. They may live in a democratic society, but they may be educationally or economically disadvantaged within it. Even if they are not disadvantaged in these ways, Governments may not produce the policies that they themselves wish to support. The choice then is to go and live elsewhere (where there will be new problems) or to remain and acknowledge that in a society no individual can have their own way all of the time. One person's needs and rights are bound to conflict with another's. There can only be an intention to please as many of the people as possible, most of the time.

How does all of this relate to the health and patient education debate?

Some of the ideologies discussed above relate directly to the health arena. The notion that because an individual is given choice and can take responsibility that he will inevitably use these to his advantage is naïve. Some studies on patterns of health-related behaviour in conditions of economic adversity, for example, clearly demonstrate that even if information and choice is given, people do not want to change their behaviour; they have more urgent agendas (Graham, 1984).

That individuals want to be empowered and take responsibility for their health and prevention of illness may not be a correct assumption. It rather depends on their ideas of the causation of illness and where health rates in their list of priorities for living. When well, illness seldom features as an important issue for the majority, even though there is now a trend among the advantaged to attempt to keep well. Exercise, prudent diet, non-stressful lifestyle and regular medical check-ups are some of the steps people take to prevent illness. Pill and Stott (1982) have produced some interesting arguments about the UK Government's propaganda that illness prevention is everybody's business; that it is mainly the responsibility of the individual to keep well and not the Government's. In very general terms, their main conclusions were that if you were advantaged and could access all those resources that may help you retain health, then choice was exercised. If you were disadvantaged (socially and economically) then the avail-ability of choice is rather academic – because you do not have the power and resources to exercise it.

Given the circular arguments above, perhaps the answer is a part-nership between those in power (Governments and their policies) and the consumers of services provided. In part this could be seen as an answer to inequalities in health prevention, illness management and care (Mitchell, 1984) and there have been some success stories where consumers, statutory health bodies and voluntary organizations have joined together to act upon real threats to health.

Inevitably, the issue of cigarette smoking is bound to be one of the topics chosen. It is *par excellence* the story of a habit that. is avoidable and that, if exercised, leads to compromised health or early death. Health professionals worked with health authorities through the UK voluntary organization, ASH (Action on Smoking and Health) to pro-mote non-smoking policies for health authorities in the UK (as opposed to smoking policies – a shift of emphasis) (Olsen *et al.*, 1981). Also, the Group Against Smoking in Public (GASP) is a compaigning group of lay and professional people based in the west of England. They have chosen a different arena for a similar problem. Their activities led to an increase in the provision of no-smoking areas in local restaurants and the severe curtailment of tobacco product sponsorship of sports and cultural events (Naidoo, 1983). Yet another example but one which affected the whole of society was the Campaign for Lead-Free Air (CLEAR) whose aim was to influence legislation to control the levels of lead in petrol (Wilson, 1984).

These are just a few examples of what can be achieved by the combined effects of statutory (Government) authority, individuals and a voluntary organization of which there are many, particularly in the UK. There is a growing trend for this to happen in many areas of illness prevention and health care. It enables those who are disad-vantaged to gain access to more of the services in theory, because the agencies are known for producing information and literature that is usually free of charge. If knowledge (or at least information) shifts the balance of power, then at least that can be achieved through the involvement of these agencies or organizations.

PUBLIC EXPECTATIONS

Part of the reason for rising costs in health care and management is to do with the expectations people have in today's highly technical world where there is, in theory, an answer for every problem. So much has been achieved to cure or control disease that a few years ago would not have been possible, that now the expectations are high for every aspect of health management. This even traces back to prevention and health education. People now may think that they do not have to worry too much about illness (therefore, do not need to heed health education messages) because there will always be a cure, even if illness occurs as a result of a habit, addiction or whatever. The contemporary example of this that has rather backfired is the disease AIDS. Initially, anyone other than homosexuals or drug abusers felt protected from this illness and did not heed the warnings to protect themselves. Even those who were in high-risk groups somehow seemed to think that a cure would become available so quickly that there was no need for alarm. The story has been one of individuals not necessarily taking care, to protect the common good – a utilitarian philosophical principle. Spread of HIV and subsequent AIDS has been present throughout the community and not just in those two presumed high-risk groups mentioned above.

Thinking about the ethics of health and patient education, the focus has been mostly on what 'good' can be done for people and little has been said about 'harm' – the notions of beneficence and non-maleficence, which are part of our ethical framework for working as health professionals.

In the health education context, some would argue that persuading or coercing people to change habits or lifestyles is not necessarily doing them good at all. Perhaps the best-quoted and most controversial area is that of breast self-examination for early detection of cancer.

It has long been promoted, with both statutory and voluntary organizations producing information and instructions to enable women to learn how to examine their breasts properly. It has been debated that for some women this has become a rather unhealthy preoccupation, with little evidence that early cancers are found as a result of it. Others would say that women do find early breast lumps and that doing so, providing they go to their doctor early, will give them a better chance of cure. However, the 'results' are not convincing either way. The incidence of breast cancer is high in Western society and, despite these efforts on behalf of health educators and others, the mortality rate is not dropping. There are a small percentage of women who appear to have psychological problems as a result of examining their own breasts. Either they do so too often for fear they will miss detecting a lump, or they feel guilty if a cancer is diagnosed – and they were unable to detect it early on. There are now moves more to breast awareness than merely detecting lumps, but the issues for 'doing harm' are the same.

The power of the media should not be underestimated; it can be powerfully good or powerfully bad. National newspaper headlines can do more to encourage or distress the population than anything else.

Editorial bias can change the intended message so easily and can cause inappropriate alarm or delight.

Many of us will be well aware of the impact caused by the reporting of a 'breakthrough in medical science'. The doctors' surgeries and out-patient clinics for the particular specialty are centres of confusion and alarm the following day. This has been frequently the case in relation to cancer treatments, amongst other specialties.

It can also be the case for health education messages though. Again, in the cancer context, the report suggesting that breast screening by mammography for a particular age group of women could reduce deaths significantly has not entirely been realized. Certainly mammography is far better at detecting early breast cancer than some other diagnostic methods, but whether or not the fact of mammography reducing cancer deaths is true is quite another story. Also, one wonders what kind of message was received by the women outside of the age group recommended for mammography. If it is good at detecting breast lumps in older women why cannot it be used for younger women as well?

A second example could be that related to the immunization of babies and small children against the diseases that once killed – whooping cough, poliomyelitis, diphtheria and measles. While the majority of health professionals would encourage continued immunization pro-grammes for children that save so many lives, parents of those few whose children who have suffered brain damage from the effects of immunization have a different story to tell. The point of stating the argument here is not to highlight the pros and cons of immunization *per se*, but to reflect upon responsible and irresponsible media coverage of these facts. Sadly, those whose education and information levels are low tend to read the more irresponsible publishing in newspapers. The whole story can so easily become distorted and bad choices will then be made.

Mass media involvement in health education is a two-edged sword. If carried out responsibly, it can be a very powerful way of achieving much good. If used purely for commercial marketing or irresponsibly for sensationalism to 'sell' a television programme or newspaper, then it can have very negative and counter-productive effects. Communi-cation can be misinterpreted even when two individuals are looking at each other and holding a conversation. It can have much worse effects if there is no direct contact between the sender and the receiver of the messages; it is more likely that incorrect messages are received, as there is no way to check back with the communicator directly.

This section has attempted to raise some issues about justice and fairness in health education and patient education. It has addressed some of the issues of unfair allocation of resources; the advantaged and disadvantaged and the shifts of power between these two groups; the persuasive and coercive practices of governments and others *vis-à-vis* health education; the well public's attitudes to illness and the reluctance to focus on it when they are well; the public's expectations of health care and the costs involved in that. Fundamental to this section has been the discussion related to the individual taking responsibility for his own health and whether or not this is feasible, let alone fair, considering the many aspects of health that may be outside the control of the individual.

AUTONOMY

Part of being just and fair of course includes the notion of autonomy – the right to self-determination or government, but there are more specific issues related to health and patient education and the notion of autonomy.

In the previous section, most of the attention was given to the well public and their freedom or not to entirely govern the way that they live and to choose lifestyles conducive to health.

Autonomy can be even more difficult for patients either because they are outside of their own territory, as in-patients or frequent out-patients in hospitals or because they are vulnerable and dependent on health professionals to such an extent that complete independence is untenable. This may also be the case if they are regularly attending their general practitioner's surgery.

Some of the ethical issues which arise may also apply to the well public, but for the purposes of illustration and debate I will refer to patients most of the time.

Information-giving and truth-telling

Controversies surrounding these issues abound. Much literature has been written regarding the rights and wrongs of giving little or more information to patients at any stage of illness, from prevention through to terminal care. Factual information about admission to hospital and before and during diagnostic tests has been researched (Elms and Leonard, 1966; Johnson *et al.*, 1973; Wilson-Barnett, 1977).

Information-giving prior to and following surgery has been demonstrated as beneficial in reducing anxiety (Hayward, 1975; Boore, 1979). Cancer patients have been the focus of several studies regarding levels of information, because of the fear evoked by that disease and the resulting denial of its presence. Health professionals tended not to use 'cancer' to describe that illness for fear that patients would be overwhelmed by the thought and fact of having the disease. Morris *et al.* (1977) found that 33% of the cancer patients they studied were dissatisfied with the information they received compared with only 13% of patients with non-cancer disease. Wiltshaw (1985) recorded the dissatisfaction of ovarian cancer patients with the levels of information they received. The founder of one of the most successful recent cancer organizations, BACUP (British Association for Cancer United Patients) was a doctor who herself eventually died from ovarian cancer. It was her dissatisfaction with the information given that led to the establishment of this national cancer information charity.

There is much more in the literature to support the fact that health professionals hold their own information and are bad at sharing it with those who consult them for help, than there is to support the opposite notion.

Given that knowledge is power, there is an immediate imbalance of power between patient and health professional, as a result of this 'owning' of information by the professionals (Webb, 1988b, p. 88).

Part of the information-giving process is truth-telling. Again, the particular focus for this has been cancer work, where to tell the truth about serious illness was often perceived to be a very negative and unkind thing to do. Yet the contract between patient and doctor or patient and nurse should be one of trust where mutual truth-telling is practised. If patients do not give clear facts to the health professional, mis-diagnosis at the very least is a possibility.

The ethical issues, therefore, arise as to how autonomous patients and the well public can reasonably be, and how beneficial that is to both parties.

In the previously quoted UK Government document, 'Working for Patients' (a White Paper claiming it put the needs of patients first in re-planning the health service), much is made of patient autonomy (1989). One of the key changes proposed was,

> to make the Health Service more responsive to the needs of patients, as much power and responsibility as possible will be delegated to local level

and from the foreword to this document by the then Prime Minister,

> We aim to extend patient choice, to delegate responsibility to where the services are provided to secure the best value for money.

Part of that re-structuring of the UK health service (which acts as an interesting illustration of some of these issues) includes a complete overhaul of general practice (primary health care).

Some years ago, Wood (1984) looked at patient participation in general practice. The idea was that a group of patients, as representative as possible for all patients registered within the practice, should meet together regularly with doctors and other practice staff in the interests of improving communication and information-giving. A National Association of Patient Participation Groups was formed in 1978 from the first seven of these patient groups. Those numbers reached well over 50 by the mid 1980s. The groups are held in both city conurbations and rural areas and cover all social classes.

These groups were on the whole concerned with learning how general practices worked (from the inside) and attempts were made to agree changes between general practitioners and patients where that was desirable. In theory, information-giving was improved and patients minimized the 'social distance' (Webb, 1988a) between health professional and member of the public. Some of the achievements recorded by Wood (1984) were the introduction of a female general practitioner into a practice in response to women's requests; forging links between the statutory and voluntary organizations within health care (often not given time, by busy general practitioners) and generally increasing the understanding of these two groups – patients and GPs.

Currently, there are more moves to increase the power of patients in primary health care, with the introduction of general practices applying for their own NHS budgets for a defined range of hospital services. Also, the Government's intention as part of this change, to 'put the patient first', has meant the inclusion of patients in establishing their own health status and needs, on an individual basis. Many practices are asking patients to attend regularly for health checks, and are using baseline data gathered by interview and entered by a pro forma onto a computer database. Patients within the practice – whether currently ill or not – are given the opportunity to seek advice about lifestyles, health risks, hereditary or familial illnesses and so on. They are also able to take advantage of any national screening services more easily – mostly because they are made aware of them and can access them more readily.

These changes at primary health care level *vis-à-vis* information-giving and truth-telling are also present within the hospital system. Many more hospitals are now considering patient information needs and establishing strategies for their voice to be heard. Some have established patient education services with a member of staff (often a senior nurse) directing those activities and producing written and other resources (video, audio tape, etc.) to better inform and teach patients. Self-help groups are being established in some hospital settings to augment those (previously discussed in Chapter 2) within the community and voluntary sector.

More recent research and literature reviewing of general practice, by Steele *et al.* (1987), in some ways endorses previous findings, but with some reservation. In general, they concluded that there was not strong support for total patient participation in their health care and the information to achieve that, but rather a more individual approach. In each case, it is necessary for the health professional to determine the actual needs and wants of the patient and those close to them. This is best achieved by skilled assessment to determine levels of current information and knowledge and what more is required to enable that person to feel in control and be as autonomous as they wish to be. The communication skills needed to elicit such information have been well published and publicized. Two examples are in Webb (1988a) and Macleod-Clark and Sims (1988), related to cancer. This illness group is a useful illustration for these skills because of the additional impact of that disease as opposed to many others. If communication works in such a setting, the same skills can be powerful with other illness settings.

Compliance

Part of being autonomous relates to compliance with suggested solutions to health problems – or indeed to preventative programmes. Earlier in this chapter, mention was made of the need for *both* patient and health professional to be active in a partnership and in giving adequate information to the other.

Having acquired advice regarding health care, patients sometimes do not comply with it and do not, therefore, improve their health. This seems to be changing. For example, 10 years ago a study on hypertensive patients complying with treatment revealed that less than 20% took medication as prescribed (Apostolides *et al.*, 1974). Newer studies (Birket *et al.*, 1986) showed a compliance rate of up to 70%. This may be due to people being better informed of the dangers of persistent hypertension or it may be part of a general trend, in some areas, for more active participation in health. It could be that medication has improved, with less unpleasant side-effects of treatment, so that patients felt more able to take it.

There are many other examples quoted in current health education literature. This issue of compliance is an important one in terms of ethical considerations. It is balanced with the business of coercion or persuasion and getting the balance right is difficult. A question may be posed to ask how much pressure should be put upon the middle-aged, obese, high-fat diet, smoking, male patient, with five children to support. Certainly health professionals may try to persuade such a person to re-order his life and in so doing hopefully extend it and deal with his responsibilities. However, this is a difficult area. For patients to be autonomous, they must have the freedom to act upon information given and not feel adversely coerced into taking decisions with which they are unhappy – for whatever reason.

Legislation

In some instances, legislation has been introduced in an attempt to reduce deaths by careless driving, passive smoking and the transmission of AIDS and other potentially infectious diseases which may affect society at large.

Where does individual autonomy fit in with all of this? Recently in the UK a law has been passed that all taxi passengers should wear seat-belts in the passenger seats. Taxi companies had to have their cabs fitted with belts, and notices informing the public that this is now law are firmly fixed in front of them as they travel. In practice, very few people use them. There has been a lively correspondence on the issue in the national press and elsewhere. Many people feel that such an introduction increases rather than decreases risk. They also feel that such an imposition takes away their personal freedom. Such strong feelings were not the case a few years ago when seat-belts for private car use were introduced, or when crash-helmets were introduced for motorcycle riders.

Compliance for matters of safety and health is a complicated issue. It is well worth reading more detailed texts or studies related to this phenomenon, of which there are many.

CONFIDENTIALITY AND PRIVACY

Perhaps the most common scenario for the problems of keeping confidentiality in this context is research, although this is by no means the only one.

There have been and will continue to be consumer surveys on the values, attitudes and reactions of individuals to health promotion, and patient education. Frequently, those members of the well public, or indeed patients, want to know what will happen to the information they often so willingly give as part of those surveys.

The American Sociological Association has produced rules for ethical research and, as this falls mostly within the realms of the sociologist or at least, sociological research, it may be useful to quote some of these (ASA, 1968). The most significant one is,

> confidential information provided by a research subject must be treated as such by the sociologist (Rule 5).

In an extension of some of the other codes of conduct for protecting human subjects of research, every person is entitled to equal privacy and treatment as a private citizen.

However, most health professionals and anthropological and socio-logical researchers are able to make their own decisions about the confidentiality and privacy issues of researching these areas. In a way, many of the issues apply to ordinary social conduct or social convention rather than to just health care research. An exception would be the need for informed consent in areas of diagnosis or treatment.

For patients, the issues of informed consent are well documented (Faulder, 1985; Silverman, 1989; Gillett, 1989; McLean and Mckay, 1981) and it is not within the remit of this book to explore these in detail. Clearly, within the overall notion of autonomy, information-giving with a view to gaining consent for treatment is a real problem and is tied closely with privacy and confidentiality. People need time to absorb new information, the right venue to receive it where there is privacy, and a conversation can easily take place within the ground rules of confidentiality.

This all sounds ideal, but there are real problems with this in practice where facilities seldom give rise to this ideal scenario.

The business of confidentiality is currently being debated in the context of patient records (the Data Protection Act now being applicable to computerized records, but not yet to written ones). Also there has been lively debate about the idea of both patients and the public having access to their medical data. In many general practice surgeries now, decisions are keyed-in on the computer while patients are still in consultation with the doctor. Patients view the data on screen, agree it and only then is it stored as a correct and permanent record.

Individuals need to feel sure that medical data cannot be accessed by other bodies; that what has been disclosed as part of a confidential consultation will only be used by the two people who originally spoke and possibly the extended professional team at the practice or hospital.

Some of the ethical issues is this context related to HIV and AIDS, have been well debated but with no consensus as yet. In particular, there has been concern by some about the serosurvey begun in January 1990. Anonymous testing of blood serum to detect HIV and to predict the future pattern of HIV and AIDS is said by some to breach rules of privacy and confidentiality. Is this a case of sacrificing the needs of the individual for the greater good of the majority (that is, producing strategies to attempt to constrain HIV and AIDS from spreading further) (Government Paper, 1991)?

SUMMARY

It has not been possible within the confines of a book like this to give much detail to ethical issues. Much has been written about them in relation to health promotion and patient education; comprehensive references have been provided.

The three particular areas chosen for discussion in the context of this book – justice and fairness, autonomy and confidentiality/privacy – are considered to be those most frequently occurring in practice.

In the business of everyday practice, it is difficult to give time to those moral dilemmas, but it is our responsibility to think them through and reach decisions as individuals and as professionals. This often has to be at a time apart so that we are prepared for quick decisions when the real needs arise.

It is hoped that these arguments will stimulate further research and consideration that we may all be responsible in our dealings with those who consult us for help.

REFERENCES

Anderson, R. (1984) Health Promotion: an overview, *European Monographs in Health Education Research*. No. 6 (ed. Baric). Scottish Health Education Group, Edinburgh, pp. 4–126.

Apostolides, A.U., Hebel, J.R. and McDill, M.S. (1974) High blood-pressure: its care and consequences in urban centres. *International Journal of Epidemiology*, **3**, 105–18.

ASA (American Sociological Association) (1968) Towards a code of ethics for sociologists. *American Sociologists*, **3**, 316–18.

Ausburn, L. (1981) Patient Compliance with Medication regimes, in *Advances in Behavioural Medicine*, Vol. 1 (ed. J.L. Sheppard), Cumberland College, Sydney.

Baric, L. (1985) The meaning of words: health promotion. *Journal of the Institute of Health Education*, **23**, 10–15.

Birket, N.J., Evans, E., Taylor, D.W. *et al.* (1986) Hypertension control in two Canadian communities: evidence for better treatment and overlabelling. *Journal of Hypertension*, **4**, 369–74.

Blumberg, B.D., Kearns, P.R. and Lewis, M.J. (1983) Adult Cancer Patient Education: an overview. *Journal of Psychosocial Oncology*, **1**(2).

Boore, J. (1979) *Prescription for Recovery*, Royal College of Nursing, London.

Bowen, R.G., Rich, R. and Schlotfelde, R.M. (1961) Effects of organised instruction for patients with the diagnosis of diabetes mellitus. *Nursing Research*, **10**, 151–99.

Elms, R. and Leonard, R. (1966) Effects of nursing approaches during admission. *Nursing Research*, **15**, 39–48.

Ewles, L. and Simnett, I. (1992) *Promoting Health*, John Wiley & Sons Ltd, Chichester.

Faulder, C. (1985) *Whose Body is it? The Troubling Issue of Informed Consent*, Virago, London.

Gillett, G.R. (1989) Informed Consent and Moral Integrity. *Journal of Medical Ethics*, **15**, 117.

Government Consultative Document (1991) *The Health of the Nation*, HMSO, London.

Government Paper (1989a) *Working for Patients*, HMSO, London.

Government Paper (1989b) *Caring for People: Community care in the next decade and beyond*, HMSO, London.

Government Paper (1991) *The Health of the Nation*, HMSO, London.

Graham, H. (1984) *Women, Health and the Family*, Wheatsheaf Books, Sussex.

Hayward, J.C. (1975) *Information: A prescription against Pain*, Royal College of Nursing, London.

Johnson, J. *et al.* (1973) Psychological preparation for an endoscopic examination. *Gastrointestinal Endoscopy*, **19**(4), 180–2.

Levine, D.M., Green, L.W., Deeds, S.G. *et al.* (1979) Health Education for hypertensive patients. *Journal of the American Medical Association*, **241**, 1770–3.

Ley, P. (1988) *Communicating with Patients*, Croom Helm, London, pp. 53–71.

McLean, S.A.M. and McKay, A. (1981) Consent in Medical Practice, in *Legal Issues in Medicine* (ed. S.A.M. McLean).

Macleod-Clark, J. and Sims, S. (1988) Communication with Patients and Relatives, in *Oncology for Nurses and Health Care Professionals*, Vol 2: *Care & Support* (ed. P.A. Webb), Harper & Row/Beaconsfield, pp. 67–85.

Mitchell, J. (1984) *What is to be done about illness and health?* Penguin Books, Harmondsworth.

Morris, T. *et al.* (1977) Psychological and Social Adjustment to Mastectomy. *Cancer*, **40**, 2381–7.

Naidoo, J. (1983) GASP – a new anti-smoking initiative. *Journal of the Institute of Health Education*, **21**(1).

Nordberg, B. and King L. (1976) Third party payment for patient education. *American Journal of Nursing*, **76**, 1269–71.

Olsen, N.D.L., Roberts, J. and Castle, P. (1981) *Smoking Prevention: A Health Promotion Guide for the NHS*, ASH publication, 5 Mortimer Street, London Wl.

Pill, R. and Stott, N. (1982) Concepts of Illness Causation and Responsibility; some preliminary data from a sample of working class mothers. *Social Science & Medicine*, **16**, 13–51.

Powell, A.H. and Winslow, E.H. (1973) The cardiac clinical nurse specialist: teaching ideas that work. *Nursing Clinics*, **8**, 723–33.

Redman, B.K. (1971) Patient education as a function of nursing practice. *Nursing Clinics*, **6**, 573–80.

Schoenrich, E.H. (1976) The potential of health education in health services delivery. *Health Services Reports*, **89**, 3–7.

Silverman, W.A. (1989) The Myth of Informed Consent: In Daily Practice and Clinical Trials. *Journal of Medical Ethics*, **15**(6).

Somers, A.R. (1976) *Promoting Health: Consumer education and national policy*, Aspen Systems Corp., Germantown, Maryland.

SOPHE – Society for Public Health Education (1976) *Code of Ethics*, October, 15th, San Francisco, CA.

Stanley, B., Guido, J., Stanley, M. and Shortell, D. (1984) The elderly patient and informed consent. *Journal of the American Medical Association*, **252**, 1302–6.

Steele, D.J., Blackwell, B., Guttman, M.C. and Jackson, J.C. (1987) Beyond Advocacy: A review of the active patient concept. *Patient Education and Counselling*, **10**, 3–23.

Strehlow, M.S. (1983) *Education for Health*, Harper & Row, London.

Tones, B.K. (1985) Health Promotion – a new panacea? *Journal of the Institute of Health Education*, **23**, 16–21.

US Department of Health and Human Sciences (1980) *Promoting Health, Preventing Disease: Objectives for the Nation*, Washington, DC.

Vuori, H. (1980) The Medical Model and the Objectives of Health & Education. *International Journal of Health Education*, **XXIII**, 1–8.

Webb, C. (1983) Teaching for recovery from Surgery, in *Patient Teaching*. Recent Advances in Nursing 6 (ed. J. Wilson-Barnett), Churchill Livingstone, Edinburgh, pp. 34–55.

Webb, P.A. (1988a) Patient Teaching, in *Nursing the Patient with Cancer* (ed. A. Faulkner), Scutari Press, London.

Webb, P.A. (1988b) Teaching Patients and Relatives, in *Oncology for Nurses and Health Care Professionals, Vol. 2: Care & Support* (ed. P. Webb), Harper & Row/Beaconsfield, pp. 86–101.

WHO (1978) *Report on the International Conference on Primary Health Care*, Alma Ata, 6–12 September, 1978, WHO, Geneva.

WHO (1986) *Ottawa Charter for Health Promotion*, An International Conference on Health Promotion, 17–21 November, 1986, WHO Regional Office for Europe, Copenhagen.

Wilson, D. (1984) *Pressure: the A–Z of Campaigning in Britain*, Heinemann, London.

Wilson-Barnett, J. (1977) Patients' emotional reactions to hospitalisation. Unpublished PhD thesis, University of London.

Wilson-Barnett, J. (Ed) (1983) Keeping Patients Informed. *Nursing*, **31**, 1357–8.

Wiltshaw, E. (1985) Ovarian trials at the Royal Marsden. *Cancer Treatment Review*, **12** (Suppl. A), 67–71.

Wood, J. (1984) Patient Participation in General Practice, in *Public Participation in Health: towards a clearer view* (eds. R. Maxwell and N. Weaver). The Kings Fund Publishing Office, 126 Albert Street, London.

PART TWO

Health Promotion and Patient Education Across the Lifespan

CHAPTER 4

The mother and baby

Edith M. Hillan

INTRODUCTION

The process of childbirth has undergone radical change in most Western cultures over the last century. Prior to 1900 most deliveries took place at home with the woman attended by close female relatives or neighbours. The development of medicine, and in particular the sub-speciality of obstetrics, led to more and more deliveries taking place in hospital in an effort to reduce the maternal and perinatal mortality associated with childbirth. Although childbirth is now safer than ever before (DHSS, 1989; Rosen, 1981) many argue that this has been at the expense of women's dignity, sense of fulfilment and autonomy.

It should always be kept in mind that childbirth is a social and personal experience as well as a medical event, and, for most women a satisfactory pregnancy outcome involves delivery of a healthy baby and a good childbirth experience. Few women today view pregnancy and delivery as a series of biological events over which they have no control and, increasingly, they are demanding a more humanistic approach to obstetric care and a greater share of responsibility in decision making related to the care that they receive.

This increase in interest in the quality of childbirth can be seen in the amount of attention paid to pregnancy and delivery in the lay press and also in the realization by professionals of the importance of the delivery experience and early parent–infant bonding in establishing the family unit.

Maternity care is exceptional within the National Health Service because the vast majority of women who utilize it are healthy and merely come into hospital for assistance with a normal physiological process which, for most, also happens to be one of the most important events in their life.

Pregnancy, childbirth and parenthood require massive physiological and psychological adjustments on the part of the woman. Even under normal circumstances the transition to motherhood may be problematical especially if the woman's prior expectations of her delivery do not measure up to the reality. Oakley (1980) found that the most normal of births can involve elements of loss for the mother – loss of self-confidence, loss of body image, loss of previous employment and so on. She states that:

> Childbirth is a life event with considerable loss and uncertain gain. The response is liable to be hopelessness and the extent of this is determined in large part by the extent to which people feel able to take control over their own lives.

The issue of control in childbirth is complicated by confusions of terminology. Internal control relates to the woman's control over her behaviour during labour, for example in the way she copes with contractions or the amount of noise she makes. External control is concerned with women's influence over decisions that are made about them during labour, for example whether the membranes are ruptured or not, choices regarding analgesia, fetal monitoring or ambulation in labour. Probably the most important factor with regard to external control is the amount of information given. Women who feel they receive the right amount of accurate information are likely to feel more satisfied and in control.

Staff who work with women at this time need to remember that an understanding of the woman's feelings and social support may be as important as physical care in ensuring a safe and satisfactory birth experience. Pregnancy, childbirth and the puerperium should be seen as a continuum and care planned accordingly so that it is less fragmented and more individually tailored to the needs of women. This will help improve communication between all staff involved in care provision and help trusting relationships to be formed between the users and providers of the service.

Although most midwives and health care professionals would agree that women should have a free choice with regard to available options in maternity care, in practice this is often not the case. Choices may be restricted by either the amount of information that is made available or the way it is presented so that true choice is impossible.

This chapter will examine some of the issues related to the delivery of care throughout the antenatal, intrapartum and postnatal period to the mother and newborn. Particular attention will be paid to the information and support needs of child-bearing women and the opportunities for health education and health promotion by health care professionals throughout this time.

ANTENATAL CARE AND PREPARATION FOR PARENTHOOD

Antenatal care originally evolved as a medical service aimed at women who were ill during pregnancy. However, the service was rapidly extended to all women in an effort to reduce the maternal and perinatal mortality associated with childbirth and this was backed by successive government reports which urged women to attend for antenatal care during pregnancy. Over the years there has been considerable debate about the aims of antenatal care. Kerr (1981) stated that the goals should be:

- the detection of previously unrecognized maternal disease (e.g. heart disease);
- the prediction, prevention, early detection and management of complications of pregnancy;
- the amelioration of the discomforts and minor complaints of pregnancy (e.g. heartburn, constipation, leg cramps);
- preparation of the couple for child-bearing and child-rearing;
- preventive and promotive health education (for example, on smoking, diet, exercise, family planning).

Most women attend for regular check-ups in the antenatal period and professional and lay literature on the topic stresses that these visits should be used not only to monitor the clinical progress of the pregnancy but also to provide women with advice, information and reassurance. Many studies have shown that although women do attend antenatal visits (often at considerable expense and inconvenience), they are often dissatisfied with the quality of care that they receive. Lack of continuity, long waiting times, few opportunities to ask questions and inconvenient appointment times are usually cited as areas of general dissatisfaction.

In an effort to allay some of these criticisms, a number of innovative antenatal care systems have been introduced and evaluated over the past decade. In some, antenatal care has been provided by midwives and general practitioners in the community with only one or two visits to the hospital where the delivery will take place. In others, hospital based obstetricians and midwives have set up peripheral antenatal clinics within local health centres. Increasingly midwives are setting up their own antenatal clinics for low-risk women and referral to the general practitioner or obstetrician only occurs if problems develop during the course of the pregnancy.

Irrespective of where the antenatal care takes place, midwives and other health professionals involved must ensure that women are given the opportunity to ask questions, raise doubts and worries, discuss the progress of the pregnancy and the meaning of tests and procedures that might be carried out.

Antenatal education

A further important dimension of antenatal care is the provision of preparation classes which should play an important role in preparing women for pregnancy, delivery and parenthood. The goal of all antenatal education is to enhance the woman's confidence about childbirth, so encouraging her to make informed choices about the care she receives. Classes may be run by hospital or community based midwives, health visitors and physiotherapists or alternatively by organizations such as the National Childbirth Trust.

Recent research has criticized the content of antenatal classes and also questioned the teaching abilities of midwives and health visitors. Such criticism includes: poor preparation of sessions; conflicting advice being given; lack of realism about the burdens of parenthood (Murphy-Black and Faulkner, 1988).

A major problem of parentcraft teaching is the didactic style frequently adopted by the teachers. Inevitably antenatal classes will have participants of mixed needs and abilities and good antenatal teaching requires staff to be responsive to the needs of individual women and their partners. This involves allowing the participants to direct the choice of topics to be discussed – taking a **reactive** rather than a **proactive** approach. There is a tendency for health care professionals to overestimate knowledge and underestimate the desire for information by the women attending such classes.

Guidelines for effective antenatal teaching

The first starting point for all teaching, whether it is done on an individual or a group basis, is to try and find out what the audience already know about the topic you are going to teach. Start the session by asking some questions so that you can gauge what level to pitch your talk.

Outline the aims of your session and ask the women whether there are any other topics that they might like to have included. This helps to get people actively involved and will increase their motivation. Consider using a number of different strategies throughout the session – people get bored if they have to listen to one person for more than 15–20 minutes at a time. Some ways to prevent this are to:

- allow short question and answer sessions;
- use small discussion groups;
- get everyone in the group to make a brief statement about the topic under discussion.

Antenatal preparation classes may have different foci and forms. Some start in early pregnancy and are aimed at teaching self-care and basic hygiene, others are focused on physical preparation for labour and delivery, while others prepare women for parenthood and early child care. Sometimes the classes may be specifically geared to the needs of particular client groups, such as refresher classes for multigravidae, women undergoing caesarean section, women with multiple pregnancies or single parents.

As a general guide some of the topics which might usefully be considered for inclusion are outlined below.

Lifestyle during pregnancy

- Basic information about the anatomy and physiology of the reproductive tract and the changes which take place during pregnancy;
- pregnancy symptoms such as nausea, vomiting and backache, and ways of alleviating them;
- emotional changes in pregnancy;
- relationships with partners and other children;
- advice on diet, exercise, alcohol and smoking, sexual needs;
- welfare rights and maternity benefits.

Preparation for labour and delivery

- The mechanisms of labour and delivery as well as how to recognize when labour starts;
- medical and obstetric terminology;
- skills to cope with the stress of labour such as relaxation techniques, comfort measures, breathing exercises and diversion therapies;
- devising a birth plan;
- explanation of the different methods of pain relief available;
- deviations from the normal course of labour, including forceps delivery and caesarean section;
- information about fetal monitoring, augmentation and induction of labour, ambulation, etc.

Preparation for parenthood

- Caring for a new baby;
- feeding methods;
- clothing;
- hygiene;
- equipment needs;
- home safety and health education;
- the emotional needs of babies and how these can be met;
- where to seek advice and get help if problems or worries arise;
- discussion of the changes that occur within family relationships with the new arrival and coping strategies for times of stress;
- postnatal mood changes and postnatal depression.

Information should not come from the teacher alone; discussion with other participants allows experiences to be shared and reassurance to be gained. Many classes now encourage partners or friends to attend, so helping them to interpret the events which occur in labour and respond appropriately with emotional support and useful comfort measures.

Not all women are able to attend organized classes, and health care professionals must also develop and evaluate a variety of other teaching materials so that women can obtain information as they require. Such materials might include:

- printed information leaflets (preferably in a variety of languages);
- video materials which can be borrowed and taken home;
- computer-assisted learning programmes;
- posters and other display materials.

Some examples of these resources are given at the end of this chapter.

SOCIAL SUPPORT DURING PREGNANCY

Over the last few years there has been considerable interest in whether additional social support can favourably affect the outcome of pregnancy. Many women at risk of an adverse pregnancy outcome are known to be socially disadvantaged as well, and some researchers have hypothesized that the provision of additional support from family workers (for childcare, housework and generally providing a 'friendly ear') can improve pregnancy outcome for both the mother and child (Spencer *et al.*, 1989; Oakley, 1980). Although much of this research has been plagued by methodological difficulties, there is no doubt that social support improves the psychological health and satisfaction of women. Other beneficial effects have also been reported such as promoting breast-feeding and male domestic participation and reducing the occurrence of minor health problems in babies both in the short and long term (Oakley, 1989).

With current funding problems in the National Health Service it is unlikely that the provision of social support systems in pregnancy will be instituted in the near future. However, midwives and other health care professionals who care for women during this time should consider setting up more informal 'drop-in' and telephone advice centres that can be contacted at any time, day or night, by women who are experiencing problems or worries.

INTRAPARTUM CARE

As part of the antenatal preparation for delivery, women and their partners should be encouraged to visit the labour ward where they will give birth. This gives them the opportunity to meet some of the staff they may encounter and also to see the layout and equipment that are kept in the delivery rooms.

No matter how well prepared beforehand, many women will feel anxious, frightened or apprehensive when labour actually starts. Although labour wards are often busy places it is vitally important that when the woman presents in labour she is made to feel welcome by supportive and understanding staff. The woman's partner or a friend or relative should be encouraged to stay throughout the labour so that a familiar face is always at hand for moral support.

Ideally women should be looked after by one midwife for the duration of labour and delivery. Where staffing levels or shift patterns do not allow this, then it is important to explain the arrangements to the woman at the outset. The midwife allocated to the woman should ensure that the antenatal record of the pregnancy is complete and up to date and that any special wishes or preferences have been recorded.

Although the midwife is the key professional supporting the woman throughout labour, other staff such as obstetricians, anaesthetists and paediatricians may also be involved in intrapartum care. Teamwork between the different professional disciplines, in a calm unhurried atmosphere, is essential to ensure the well-being of the woman in labour. The woman should also be introduced to the doctor who is on duty in the labour ward, and if the unit is used for medical or midwifery student training then agreement should be obtained before they are allowed to participate in her care.

Birth plans

Every woman should have the opportunity to discuss and plan her care before labour and delivery. Many women may be happy to go along with normal unit policies if these are explained beforehand, although some will have particular preferences about aspects of the care they receive. Over the past few years there has been increased interest in the use of birth plans for the intrapartum period. These allow women to express their preferences on issues relating to labour and delivery, such as:

- pain relief;
- electronic fetal monitoring;
- ambulation during labour;
- position for delivery;
- the role of the father or other support person;
- interventions during labour;
- the use of episiotomy;
- contact with the baby at delivery;
- infant feeding.

Some hospitals may have designed their own birth plans for women to complete, although in other cases women may be encouraged to devise their own personal plan. No matter what kind of plan is used, in addition to verbal information about the various options available, supplementary written material should be available explaining both the risks and benefits of any procedures used in the hospital. Women can then make properly informed, considered choices about the options available to them. The midwife should ensure that the woman's preferences about the kind of delivery experience are recorded alongside any advice that is given.

Some hospitals introduce the birth plan at the booking visit and discuss it at each subsequent visit. Others would argue that this is too early and that the plan should only be introduced around the 34th week of pregnancy, when labour is more of a reality and some discussion of the options available has already taken place at the antenatal classes. For birth plans to be successful all staff need to be committed to the concept – they would be of little value if the couple's preferred wishes were not actually made available to them in the labour ward.

Birth plans, however, need to be flexible in case any unforeseen events, such as acute fetal distress or maternal bleeding, arise during labour. It is also important to stress that if the woman changes her mind at any time about the options she has chosen then this is perfectly acceptable.

Stress and support in labour

Over 99% of women in the UK will deliver their babies in a hospital setting. Although many labour wards have been upgraded and decorated to make them less clinical and more 'homely', there are still many features which make them potentially stressful for women in labour: unfamiliarity with both the people and the environment; the variable use of procedures such as routine electronic fetal monitoring, regular vaginal examinations, limitation of movement, restriction of food and fluids, perineal shaving, etc.

Some have suggested that fear, pain and anxiety are all exacerbated by these factors and that this in turn can affect the progress of labour and lead to increased obstetric intervention. Very few research studies have examined the effect of support on labour outcome; however, the available evidence suggests that support is very important to many women during this time (Green et al., 1988).

Support during labour has many dimensions and can be provided by both professionals and the woman's partner or friend. Physical contact is important and can involve rubbing her back, holding her hand or gently stroking her. Emotional support involves conversation and the provision of explanation, information and encouragement. A central feature should be that the woman is not left alone without either her partner/friend or the midwife present, at any time during the course of labour. A further important aspect is that of advocacy, which usually relates to the plans and expectations before labour, and helping women to participate in decision making during labour.

Pain in labour

Most women will experience pain during labour and many will request some form of analgesia during labour. The different options available along with the way that they are administered and their effects and side-effects should have been discussed with staff during the antenatal period. If this is not possible then provision should be made for discussion in the early stages of labour. No matter what the woman chooses, the midwife should be non-judgemental and supportive of her choice. Some of the commonly used methods of analgesia include:

- psychoprophylactic methods;
- Entonox;
- pethidine;
- epidural analgesia.

CONTACT WITH THE BABY AT DELIVERY

The promotion of bonding between the mother and her infant has become an increasingly important part of midwifery and obstetric care. The concept of bonding is characterized as being primarily undirectional, occurring rapidly and facilitated by physical contact (Reading, 1983). Several studies have shown that the hour after birth is a particularly sensitive time and that bonding between parents and their infants can be enhanced by allowing them the maximum opportunity to feed, feel and hold their baby (Klaus *et al.*, 1972; Kennel *et al.*, 1974; De Chateau, 1980). Klaus and Kennel (1982) have suggested that separation of the mother and infant after delivery may have adverse effects on maternal attachment which can persist for several months.

Restriction of early mother–infant contact can lead to less affectionate maternal behaviour and less confidence in caring for the baby. An association has also been found between restricted contact and the failure to establish breast-feeding.

For some women, early social contact with the baby might not be possible because they are too exhausted, in too much pain or the baby needs admission to the neonatal intensive care unit. Other women may not actually desire contact for less obvious reasons which are nevertheless important to them. However, contact should not be restricted by outdated hospital policies which still exist in some units. Staff need to be sensitive to the individual needs of women at this important time.

POSTNATAL CARE

The third report of the Maternity Services Advisory Committee (1984) recognized that postnatal care is as important a part of the child-bearing process as the actual delivery, yet noted that in many units it had the lowest priority. 'Inadequate and under-qualified care' resulted in communication failure, conflicting advice, confusion and lack of ma-ternal satisfaction. The report emphasized the importance of meeting both the physical and emotional needs of the woman during this vital time. This section will explore some of these needs and discuss strat-egies for ensuring that they are met by the health professionals in contact with women during this period.

Postpartum care should promote the following goals:

- comfort and relief of pain;
- physical rest from the stress of labour;
- emotional recovery of the woman;
- successful establishment of infant feeding;
- effective parent education;
- parent–infant attachment.

Comfort and relief of pain

Perineal pain, as a result of perineal trauma, is a common problem for women in the postnatal period and can interfere with the woman's enjoyment of her baby at this time. A wide range of measures and treatments are currently used in the management of perineal dis-comfort and include:

- local applications such as ice-packs, sprays, baths, local anaesthetic agents;
- physiotherapy treatments such as ultrasound, pulsed electromag-netic energy, exercises, relief of local pressure;
- oral analgesia such as paracetamol, aspirin, ibuprofen.

Recent research evidence suggests that the application of local cooling agents (such as ice-packs) is effective in reducing perineal pain al-though the relief is only temporary. The application of gels and sprays containing local anaesthesia (aqueous 5% lignocaine) is also effective and has a longer-lasting effect than cooling therapies.

Oral analgesics may be given in addition to local therapies but a number of factors should be considered when choosing the drug.

Drugs which are likely to cause constipation should be avoided, as should those which are carried in breast milk. The drug should also be relatively free of side-effects such as gastric irritation. Paracetamol or ibuprofen are the drugs of choice in treating perineal pain. There is little evidence to suggest that physiotherapy treatments are of any value, although the personal contact involved between the woman and the physiotherapist or midwife may enhance its therapeutic effect (Enkin *et al.*, 1989).

Physical rest from the stress of labour

One of the most important objectives of postnatal care is to promote the physical and emotional recovery of the mother from the stress of labour and yet hospital routines and practices remain extremely inflexible in many units, making this difficult to achieve. It is important for midwives working in postnatal wards to ensure that adequate time is set aside to allow mothers to rest. There should be a designated time each day when the ward is closed and women allowed to catch up on sleep. If possible a number of rooms should be specifically set aside for women who have experienced traumatic deliveries or who have fractious infants to allow extended rest periods.

When the woman returns home she should be encouraged to set aside time each day to catch up on sleep. Other family members should be encouraged to take over the care of the baby at this time to allow the woman to rest.

Emotional recovery of the woman

The birth of a baby results in role changes for the woman and in- creased responsibilities which make the immediate postnatal period a time of emotional stress. It is essential that midwives provide adequate support and encouragement during this time and allow women to build up their confidence in caring for their infants. The reality of caring for a newborn baby 24 hours a day is often very different from the expectation. Most women adapt gradually to the demands of motherhood and the speed at which this happens will be related to the woman's physical and emotional state. In many hospitals postnatal care is planned on a routinized basis with a chronological succession of increasing responsibility for the care of the infant by the mother irrespective of her age, condition after delivery or previous child- bearing experiences. Individual women will adapt at different rates and midwives must provide advice, help and encouragement to the women they care for. Professionals should be non-judgemental in their approach and women should be supported in decisions they make related to their care during this time.

SUCCESSFUL ESTABLISHMENT OF INFANT FEEDING

In the UK around 64% of women choose to breast-feed their babies, although many give up soon after delivery and in one study only 26% were still breast-feeding at 4 months, which is the minimum time recommended. These figures vary widely throughout the UK and between different social class groupings. There is some evidence to suggest that the majority of women who decide to breast-feed make this decision prior to or very early in pregnancy, whereas the decision to bottle-feed occurs later on in pregnancy (Royal College of Midwives, 1988). Some of the factors which may influence the choice of feeding method include:

- socio-cultural factors;
- perceived support from partner and friends.

Research evidence also suggests that once the woman has made up her mind about the way she is going to feed she is unlikely to subsequently change it.

The first breast-feed is extremely important and should be done at a time when the baby is receptive, in privacy and preferably with the father or another support person present. Skilled professional help can help build the woman's confidence and ensure that the baby is correctly positioned at the breast. The timing and duration of subsequent feeds should be determined by the baby's own individual patterns rather than institutional regimens or schedules. There is no research evidence to suggest that the gradual build-up of feeding times influences the incidence of cracked nipples or other breast problems. Similarly the widespread practice of supplementary feeds of water, glucose or infant formulas should be discouraged as they are more likely to result in women abandoning breast-feeding altogether. Accurate information and regular professional support throughout the postnatal period have been shown to positively influence the duration of breast-feeding. Professionals involved during this time need to base their advice on research evidence rather than preconceived ideas and historical wisdom (Enkin *et al.*, 1989).

EFFECTIVE PARENT EDUCATION

Although many aspects of baby care may have been taught in antenatal classes, it is important that education for parenthood continues throughout the postnatal period, both in hospital and the community. A planned programme of teaching should be prepared for each woman and should include topics such as:

- advice about feeding;
- sterilization of bottles and teats;
- infant hygiene, including how to deal with nappy and skin rashes;
- coping with wind, crying and sleeping problems;
- baby clinics and immunization schedules;
- the role of the health visitor;
- the postnatal visit;
- family planning and the resumption of sexual activity.

If possible the father and other family members should be included in these sessions. Parents should also be given the opportunity to express doubts and worries and ask any questions which they might have.

PARENT–INFANT ATTACHMENT

Klaus and Kennel (1982) maintain that certain influences which affect the formation of mother–child relationships are fixed, whilst others such as hospital practices and the attitudes of staff are alterable and may be changed to improve the establishment of such relationships. Ball (1987) found that the delivery of midwifery care had an effect on the transition to motherhood and could, by increasing or decreasing stress in mothers, make a notable difference to the way each adapted to the demands of mothering the child.

Some of the factors which have been shown to affect stress levels are:

- conflicting advice from midwives;
- lack of rest;
- poor continuity of care between midwives.

By providing the opportunity for adequate rest, alleviating pain and discomfort and offering advice and education to help build up confidence, midwives can help enhance the formation of strong relationships between the mother and her baby. Every effort should be made to ensure that the woman and her baby are not separated during the early postnatal period. The baby should be kept in a cot beside the mother's bed throughout the day and brought to her for feeding at night. A balance should be strived for which allows adequate rest and maximum contact.

CONTINUING CARE

The adjustment of the woman and her partner to the new arrival and change in structure of the family unit may take many months. The midwife has a statutory obligation to provide care for a period of not less than 10 days and not more than 28 days after delivery. After this time the responsibility for the woman and her baby is normally handed over to the health visitor and other members of the primary health care team.

Some women will need special care and support after delivery – those who have experienced a perinatal loss or given birth to a handicapped infant; women whose babies remain in a neonatal intensive care unit; mothers with handicaps or disabilities; women whose babies have been taken into care or put up for adoption, etc. One member of the team should assume responsibility for the co-ordination of care in these circumstances with referral to outside agencies as appropriate.

Although appropriate professional help and support are important in the postnatal period, women should also be made aware of community-based support groups in their area such as mother and baby groups, the local branch of the National Childbirth Trust and the Meet-a-Mum Association (addresses given in the Appendix).

POSTNATAL DEPRESSION

Estimates of the number of women who suffer from postnatal depression range from 7% to 30%. Some of the difficulties in determining exactly how many women suffer from this condition arise because of confusion over the definition of postnatal mood disorder. Cox (1986) defines **postnatal blues** as the transitory irritability, weepiness and depression that occurs in the first 2 weeks following delivery. Most women (as high as 80% in some studies) will experience some or all of these feelings after the birth of the baby. Postnatal blues are self-limiting, although the mood disturbance may merge into a more prolonged postnatal depressive illness. The diagnosis of **postnatal depression** is applied to women who experience a depressive illness without delusions or hallucinations and who do not require immediate in-patient treatment in a psychiatric hospital. It is distinguished from postnatal blues by its greater severity and longer duration. Kumar and Robson (1984) found that 16% of mothers were depressed 3 months after delivery and overall 22% were depressed at some time in the first year postpartum. On the other hand the woman suffering from **puerperal psychosis** is easier to recognize in that she is obviously disturbed and may have delusions as well as hallucinations. The incidence of puerperal psychosis is around 1 or 2 per 1000. Psychiatrists may be involved at an early stage with these women because of the severity of symptoms suffered.

Despite the fact that after discharge from hospital the woman is visited by a number of primary health care professionals – the midwife, health visitor and general practitioner – postnatal depression is rarely recognized. Professionals involved in the care of child-bearing women need to be alert to the possibility of postnatal mental illness in the mother, so that appropriate intervention can then be initiated. Several factors may indicate that a women might be suffering from postnatal depression:

- failure to keep appointments with health care professionals such as visits by the health visitor or attendance at the baby clinic;
- excessive preoccupation with the baby;
- need for constant reassurance and explanation.

The presence of some of these factors may alert the health visitor about the possibility of depression and if this is thought to be the case, then Cox (1986) recommends that a more detailed interview (including observation of the mother's non-verbal cues) should be undertaken to elicit further symptoms such as:

- depressed mood;
- sleep disturbance;
- ideas of not coping, self-blame and guilt;
- thoughts of self-harm or of harming the baby;
- rejection of the baby;
- impaired libido;
- anxiety.

If two or more of the symptoms are present in addition to a generally depressed mood then the woman is likely to be suffering from a mild depressive illness. If more than five symptoms are present, then the illness is more severe and speedy referral is needed so that appropriate treatment can be initiated. Useful literature and a telephone advice service are provided by the Association for Postnatal Illness.

CONCLUSIONS

Pregnancy and childbirth represent one of the most important times in a woman's life and one that is usually viewed with great clarity for years after the event. Midwives and other health care professionals have an important role to play throughout this time. Their attitudes and the quality of care they provide is central to women's memories of the experience (Green *et al.*, 1988). The main aim of care should be to ensure the safety of both the mother and the baby throughout the antenatal, intrapartum and postnatal periods. However, care providers can do much to ensure that the care is delivered in such a way that it takes account of the woman's wishes and promotes the formation of good parent–child relationships.

CASE STUDIES

Case study 1

Karen has come to the antenatal clinic for the first time. She is 22 years of age and is 11 weeks pregnant. When taking her history the clinic midwife discovers that Karen smokes 15 cigarettes per day and has done so for the past 7 years. Karen says that she has tried to cut down the number of cigarettes since she discovered she was pregnant but finds this very difficult. She asks if it is true that smoking means the baby will be lighter, and if so, will this mean an easier delivery with less likelihood of an episiotomy or a tear?

The evidence that smoking in pregnancy may have harmful effects on the baby is strong. Smoking reduces the average birthweight of the baby and increases the chance of preterm delivery. Women should be encouraged to give up smoking when they are pregnant, so reducing such hazards for the baby. Campaigns against smoking in pregnancy have tended to concentrate on the possible adverse outcomes for the baby and this can have unwanted side-effects for the mother. More than 50% of women who smoke during pregnancy are likely to worry about it and may spend the whole of the pregnancy in a state of guilt and inadequacy. The effects of such chronic stress and anxiety on the pregnancy and the mother's relationship with the baby after delivery have never been evaluated (Enkin *et al.*, 1989).

Although the midwife counselling Karen can give advice and information about the effects of smoking and pregnancy, she also needs to take into account Karen's social and personal circumstances. The midwife needs to help Karen make a choice about smoking and should focus on some of the following issues:

1. **the problem**
   why does she smoke? why does she smoke so much? encourage her to keep a diary to look at the factors which trigger her desire for a cigarette;
2. **identify the goal**
   in this case to stop smoking;
3. **identify strategies to help Karen reach her goal**
   coping strategies such as substituting chewing-gum for cigarettes, changing routines associated with smoking, keeping cigarettes in an inconvenient place, only travelling in non-smoking sections on buses and trains, encouraging a 'one day at a time' approach, etc.;
4. **help her learn to cope with stress**
   encourage her to learn relaxation techniques and other ways of coping with stress;
5. **set up self-help groups within the antenatal clinic**
   this encourages support from people who are in the 'same boat'.

Telephone numbers can be exchanged so that there is always a friendly voice at the end of the phone when the going gets tough. If it is not practical to start a group in the hospital, help her find out about groups in local health centres.

It is important that Karen is given help and not criticism from the midwife. Advice and information is important but encouraging strategies which focus more on self-help and behavioural change are likely to be more effective.

• Case study 2

Jane and Barbara are midwives working in a large inner city maternity hospital which serves a population where there are high levels of unemployment and marked social deprivation. They are concerned that women in social classes 4 and 5 don't seem to attend for antenatal care and education as regularly as those in social classes 1 and 2. They want to try and remedy this problem so they set about finding out which factors might discourage attendance so that they can then implement strategies to change this.

Some of the factors which might affect attendance include:

personal factors
- communication problems – language, literacy, medical jargon;
- lack of motivation;
- lack of awareness about the importance of antenatal care;
- lack of finance for bus-fares etc.;
- distance from home;
- difficult to get time off work if in part-time employment;
- problems with other children – no child minder, illness, no crèche facilities available within the clinic.

hospital factors
- waiting times at clinics;
- impersonal care from large numbers of staff;
- lack of opportunity to ask questions;
- clashes of appointment times between GP and hospital clinics;
- duplication of care.

Having identified some of the factors which might influence attendance Jane and Barbara then started to think about some of the aspects of hospital antenatal care which could be improved without major financial input. The provision of play areas and crèche facilities would allow mothers with young children to bring them along if it wasn't possible to find a babysitter. Such amenities could be provided by volunteers. It should also be possible to get refreshments supplied on the same basis.

The atmosphere in the clinics should be relaxed and stress-free. Long waiting times could be reduced by the implementation of a ticket system. It would also help if the actual number of antenatal visits was arranged on an individual basis as opposed to an institutional regime. The waiting areas should be comfortable and information leaflets, video materials and other health education materials readily available. Antenatal education classes should be run on the same days as the clinics so that women only have to make one journey to the hospital rather than two. If the clinic has large numbers of women from ethnic minorities, then link workers to help with translation should be recruited.

For low-risk women antenatal care should be undertaken by midwifery staff rather than medical staff. A relatively recent innovation in many areas has been the introduction of **team midwifery**, where a team of hospital and community midwives undertake the total antenatal, intrapartum and postnatal care for a group of women. This allows women to get to know the midwives that are looking after them, which encourages the formation of good relationships. Such schemes also encourage better continuity of care throughout the whole of the child-bearing period. A further advantage is that job satisfaction for midwives in the team is likely to be increased.

If staffing and finance allow then more radical changes might be implemented. Although many areas now have peripheral clinics attendance could probably be improved if opening times were extended to evenings and weekends. This might help women who find it difficult to attend because of child care difficulties.

Case study 3

Sarah, a 23-year-old married woman, has just given birth to her first son Ben. She decided fairly early on in pregnancy that she wished to breast-feed although she has not seen many women feeding by this method. Ben is just under an hour old and is in the phase of early responsiveness. Although Sarah is still in the delivery room and is keen to breast-feed her baby, Margaret, the midwife who delivered Ben, knows the importance of the first feed and wants to ensure that it is successful.

One of the most important factors in successful breast-feeding is to ensure that Sarah is in a comfortable position before starting. Margaret should offer her a bed pan and the opportunity for a quick freshen up before feeding. She should also reinforce the importance to Sarah of making herself comfortable for all subsequent feeds and that this should be done before the baby becomes hungry and distressed. Since the delivery bed is hard and uncomfortable, Sarah may require extra pillows to support her back and arms, or to raise the baby to a more comfortable level. Ben should be placed in a position which allows

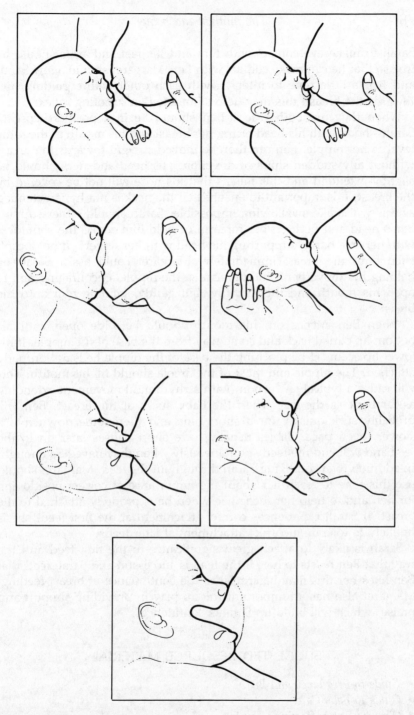

Figure 4.1 Successful breast-feeding.

Sarah to make eye contact with him and his feet and arms should be free so that he can make contact with her. Margaret should allow Sarah and Ben a little time to interact with each other before guiding him towards the breast; this may help stimulate Ben's rooting reflex.

When they are both ready, Ben should be in a position close to Sarah's body with his head facing her breast and his mouth at the same level as her nipple. Ben can then be moved straight towards the breast without any sudden shifts of direction. His head and neck should be slightly extended and this means that his nose will not be covered by the breast. It is important to ensure that the neck is not hyperextended as this will make swallowing impossible. Sarah should either support Ben's head and neck on her forearm or hold him across the shoulders with her free hand, supporting his head with her fingers. If he doesn't latch onto the breast immediately, Margaret could assist Sarah by helping her move Ben's mouth against the nipple, encouraging him to open his mouth and then swiftly, but gently, guiding him onto the breast.

When Ben latches on, his mouth should be wide open with his bottom lip curled back and some way from the base of the nipple. If his lower lip seems to be pinching the base of the nipple he is not properly attached. The nipple and most of the areola should fill his mouth. This will cause a typical jaw action, with a rhythmical movement extending as far back as the ear, when the baby sucks at the breast. Ben will probably suck quickly for a short time and then settle down into a slower, even pace. Babies usually have short pauses later on in the feed and will end the feed spontaneously when they have had enough. In addition to encouraging Sarah throughout the feed, Margaret should use this time to teach her about the importance of correct positioning for Ben and to help her recognize when he is properly attached to the breast. If Sarah experiences correct attachment at the first feed, she is unlikely to tolerate incorrect attachment at later feeds.

Sarah is likely to attach great significance to the first feed and the way that Ben reacts to her. If the feed is successful and Sarah feels that Ben likes her this may be crucial to the continuance of breast-feeding. Margaret also has an important role to play in providing support and praise, which will build up Sarah's confidence.

SUGGESTED RESOURCE MATERIAL

- *Guide to Pregnancy and Birth*
- *Guide to Baby Care*
- 'The parentcraft' video guide.

All available from Bounty Services Ltd., Owen Road, Diss, Norfolk IP22 3HH.

Other leaflets and information are available from the various agencies listed in the Appendix at the end of the book.

REFERENCES

Ball, J.A. (1987) *Reactions to Motherhood: The Role of Postnatal Care*, Cambridge University Press, Cambridge.

Cox, J.L. (1986) *Postnatal Depression: A Guide for Health Professionals*, Churchill Livingstone, Edinburgh.

De Chateau, P. (1980) The first hour after delivery – its impact on the synchrony of the parent–infant relationship. *Paediatrician*, **9**, 151–68.

Department of Health and Social Security (1989) *Report on confidential enquiries into maternal deaths in England and Wales 1982–84*, HMSO, London.

Enkin, M., Keirse, M.J.N.C. and Chalmers, I. (1989) *Effective Care in Pregnancy and Childbirth*, Oxford University Press, Oxford.

Green, J.M., Coupland, V.A. and Kitzinger, J.V. (1988) *Great Expectations: A Prospective Study of Women's Expectations and Experiences of Childbirth*, Child Care and Development Group, University of Cambridge, Cambridge.

Klaus, M.H., Jerauld, R., Kreger, B. *et al.* (1972) Maternal attachment. Importance of the first postpartum days. *New England Journal of Medicine*, **286**, 460–3.

Klaus, M.H. and Kennel, J.H. (1982) *Parent Infant Bonding*, Mosby, St Louis.

Kennel, J.H., Jerauld, R., Wolfe, L.C. *et al.* (1974) Maternal behaviour one year after early and extended postpartum contact. *Developmental Medicine and Child Neurology*, **16**, 172–9.

Kerr, M.G. (1981) Roles and Goals in Antenatal Care, *Providers and Alternative Patterns of Maternity Care Seminar*, Social Paediatric and Obstetric Research Unit, University of Glasgow, Glasgow.

Kumar, R. and Robson, K.M. (1984) A prospective study of emotional disorders in childbearing women. *British Journal of Psychiatry*, **144**, 35–47.

Murphy-Black, T. and Faulkner, A. (1988) *Antenatal group skills training*, John Wiley and Sons, Chichester.

Oakley, A. (1980) *Women confined*, Martin Robertson, Oxford.

Oakley, A. (1989) Can social support influence pregnancy outcome? *British Journal of Obstetrics and Gynaecology*, **96**, 260–2.

Reading, A.J. (1983) Bonding, in *Progress in Obstetrics and Gynaecology, Vol III* (ed. J. Studd), Churchill Livingstone, Edinburgh, 128–36.

Rosen, M.G. (1981) *Cesarean Childbirth: report of a consensus development conference*, NIH publication no 82–1067, NIH, Bethesda.

Royal College of Midwives. (1988) *Successful Breastfeeding: A Practical Guide for Midwives*. Royal College of Midwives, Oxford.

Spencer, B., Thomas, H. and Morris, J. (1989) A randomised controlled trial of the provision of a social support service dealing pregnancy. The South Manchester Family Women Project. *British Journal of Obstetrics and Gynaecology*, **96**, 281–8.

CHAPTER 5

The well and sick child

Steven Campbell

INTRODUCTION

The child's understanding of health and their acceptance of their own health conduct is an area of ongoing research. Substantial gaps in our understanding still remain. The reasons for some children employing healthy behaviours compared with others who do not are not clear. The child is influenced by his own developmental and psychological character as well as environmental factors, such as the family, school, peers and television. The child's health conduct may be associated with these influences, but the form in which they function to alter behaviour is not clearly understood (Hunsberger, 1990).

CONCEPTS RELATING TO HEALTH

There are two well-known and important paradigms in psychological theory which can be employed to analyse the child's beliefs about health. These are the cognitive developmental view, which is based on the work of Piaget and Inhelder (1969) and expectancy theory (Bandura, 1986).

The child's notion of health changes slowly with time in parallel with their cognitive development (Kalnins and Love, 1982). Younger children have problems in describing what they mean by health (Natapoff, 1978). These younger children seem to cluster events but these are not necessarily related. At this developmental stage, children can only concentrate on one incident at a time. They can catalogue healthy things to do, but do not grasp the reasons for these acts being healthy. However, by the time children start to think in a formal abstract manner, they can give physical examples of health, such as tooth brushing and the reasons for the action being important.

Children have differing abilities to understand healthy behaviours. The ability to understand will be related to their age, but children move through these stages at differing rates. The assessment of the stage in which a child thinks becomes a matter of clinical judgment. The child's understanding of health conduct is limited by his comprehension of cause and effect. The child will not understand the cause and effect until formal thought processes are gained, at about 11 years. The concept of prevention is not mastered until the child can relate a current cause to a future effect.

Expectancy theory is an essential paradigm in social learning theory (Rotter, 1954). It suggests that an action is performed when one expects that action to produce a required outcome. There is a mirroring of this expectancy theory within the health belief model (Pender, 1987). The health belief model suggests that the carrying out of preventative actions is set by the potential advantages of that preventative action being balanced against the potential difficulties of that action (Pender, 1987).

The discerned advantages of preventative action are altered by the susceptibility and threat of the disease as seen by that individual. Greater vulnerability and the more serious threat lead to a preventative action being more likely to be taken. Behaviours that can effect a constructive outcome are even more likely to be taken up. A child's view of health and illness and causality will have an influence upon healthy conduct. If a child anticipates that a desired health outcome will be achieved by specific conduct then the behaviour is more likely to happen.

The child's perception of vulnerability or feelings of susceptibility to illness have been studied by Gochman (1971, 1977) and Gochman and Saucier (1982). Children are not well motivated by health and do not see themselves as vulnerable to health problems. Whereas greater vulnerability has been shown to affect adult health conduct in a positive manner, the same is not true of children. In contrast, when a sense of vulnerability increases in children, healthy behaviours decrease (Gochman and Saucier, 1982). The discerned vulnerability of children was shown to be negatively correlated with self-concept and positively correlated with anxiety. One explanation of children's behaviour is that perceived vulnerability could be viewed as an anxiety state that leads to an individual being incapable of coping and perceiving himself in a negative manner. It was concluded that vulnerability of an individual is a personality characteristic and an aspect of the child's cognition. The receptivity of children to education may be affected by their individual differing levels of perceived vulnerability or anxiety state.

Green and Bird (1986) have studied children's ideas about how people become ill or remain healthy. Children mentioned health behaviours over which they had some control as reasons for health or illness, such as eating. When children become older they view germs and bad weather as major reasons for illness, although the young child pictures germs and weather in a similar manner to the conduct that they have control over. Green and Bird (1986) suggest that during the child's maturation there is acceptance of culpability for health but not the blame for illness.

Gochman (1971) suggests that locus of control is important in the health behaviour of children. The child who sees a reward as the result of destiny, fortune, or coming from other than themselves is externally controlled. Children who see a reward as a result of their own conduct are internally controlled and are more likely to be able to change life conditions. Adults, internal individuals, when confronted by difficulties, adapt more appropriately than do external individuals. Gochman (1971) demonstrated that the degree of internal control is important in influencing perceived vulnerability to health problems and appropriate adaptation. The phenomenon of the child's manner of control affecting vulnerability is intricate and is influenced by the extent to which health is of relevance to the child. Internally controlled children feel less susceptible to health problems than the externally controlled, but if health is irrelevant to the child the association is not present.

Cognitive development and the child's style of control are factors in children's understanding about healing (Neuhauser *et al.*, 1978). The style of control influences the awareness of the body; internal children have more access to internal signs. However, this was only present when the task demanded the child's abstract cognitive skills. If the task is made too difficult or too easy for the child's cognitive ability, the child's style of control did not alter their understanding. Internality has been shown to increase with age, socio-economic status, and be higher in females (Perrin and Shapiro, 1985).

EXTERNAL FACTORS

Children learn actions from individuals who are important in their lives and from other factors that they hear and see. Children respond in an individual manner to the environment, but all children learn from their family, friends, school and the media. Dielman *et al.* (1982) have studied the relationship of the child with their parents' health behaviours and beliefs. The conduct of the parents appears to have an effect upon children, but their beliefs concerning health are rarely communicated verbally (Dielman, 1982). The greatest influence of the family is during early childhood, but by early adolescence peers have assumed this role (Mullen, 1983). The influence of parents on young children may be diminishing as patterns of child care change. The time parents spend with their younger children may be reducing and so it is more significant that the family's influence is positive. These behaviours might be those that are modelled. These might be the way family members relate to each other, the reinforcement of certain behaviours by encouragement, as well as the occasions children have to be involved in health behaviours (Bruhn and Parcel, 1982). This conduct models both the bodily and psychological behaviour for children. Children learn principles underlying hygiene, diet and sleep as well as the parents' coping methods and the manner they relate to others.

The maturing child is progressively influenced by the school and his peers which affect his health conduct. Schools have an influence in a variety of ways, whether in the classroom, in providing support and discipline, physical education or school health services. Schools can also provide humanistic education where values are examined with its implications for improved insight into mental health and self-concept (Black and Newton, 1981). Other schools have designed courses to understand the provision of health care and how children can get access (Grasser and Craft, 1984).

Peers become most important for the child nearing teenage. It is paramount for these children to be part of a group, and so the adolescent imitates the conduct of peers to guarantee social support. Mullen (1983) suggests that productive approaches to prevent difficult behaviour improve an adolescent's sense of worth and produce improved academic performance.

Adults have shown concern about children watching television in social isolation, with little physical activity or two-way communication. This has the potential to disrupt the healthy development of the child, but can bring informative and imaginative experiences to children. In contrast, advertisements have specific effects through the representation of certain foods and drinks and products like non-prescription drugs. In the USA a child can see the equivalent of three hours a week of continuous advertisements (Comstock, 1981). This may not be the case at present in the UK, but with the advent of satellite television this may become so. Television has the capacity to affect health conduct. There are attempts by responsible television producers to address health topics and these are to be praised. Other countries have introduced whole stations devoted to issues of health, such as Canal Santé from France.

SELF-CARE

The consideration of what is health or what is required to preserve health is established by the individual's perceived need. Health conduct which children or their primary care givers see as appropriate or beneficial affects their engagement in health-promoting activities. The perceived health needs of the child or the family may vary with age, sex, or cultural orientation, as well as financial and social class considerations. The child who is highly prone to a health problem, which has serious consequences, is most likely to have parents who will assist the child to adopt a preventative strategy. Children do not appear to react in a similar manner. The approach of the health care professional will differ from parent to child. For the parents, the task of the health care professional is to aid in the recognition of the child's vulnerability to the health problem and the consequences to health if a preventative strategem is not adopted. In the case of the child, the health care professional assesses the child's developmental level in relation to their understanding of health and gives explanations in an appropriate manner.

It is important to gather an understanding of the child's perception of the health problem along with any other relevant experience. A major part of this is the child's comprehension of cause and effect, which must be appraised before relating consequences.

The family must take the final responsibility about whether a health problem requires action. The health care professional must be led by the values and beliefs of the family if the family is to see health as critical or essential. These efforts will be more productive if the effort required to preserve health is practicable for the family's lifestyle and finances.

The recognition of a health need does not mean that the child or parents will take any action. There is a requirement to know the potential actions that could be taken to deal with the need. The family obtains its problem-solving choices from many roots, a comprehension of which allows the health care professional to understand and advance the conclusion of the child or family.

There are many potential sources. These might be the family or cultural tradition: when the choice a family has made in the past to deal with a health problem will be taken until it does not work. There are also social or peer incentives, where the more a child or parent requires the group's approval, the more likely the option is to be selected. Information from the mass media is also important, but this depends upon how much personal meaning the message has to the child or parent. There have been studies which show that mass media which stress personal and social results are more productive in altering behaviour than those that stress corporeal harm (Wu, 1973).

An interpretation of the role of the health professional would be to assist the family or child in the evaluation of the various options available. There might be a consideration of the consequences of an action, followed by impartial support of the efforts made by the family to attain the goal. An example might be when a family decides to eat vitamin tablets rather than fruit and vegetables in their diet. The professional would prefer the latter on many grounds but does not state this; the family is supported in their decision, in recognition of the improvement in health behaviour. The child and family could be encouraged to evaluate the consequences of an action if it is adopted by listing the things they will enjoy as a result of it. These could be compared with the things they enjoy which could not be expected to be continued if an action is not adopted. This approach adheres to the social consequences of the action rather than the corporeal or physiological result.

The impartial support of the child and family is essential, even when the professional considers that the choice may not have been the judicious one. The feelings such situations engender are not uncommon, but need to be controlled in order to protect the quality of the relationship. Normally, there is no single correct manner to preserve or promote health. It is possible that the favoured option is not feasible for the child or family. Success in the family's choice, even though the outcome may be restricted by that choice, prepares the family for an option with greater potential for health.

The direct involvement of the professional in the family's decision-making process may well be appropriate at the beginning of their health career. However, continued active involvement restricts the family's opportunities to develop their own problem-solving abilities. The availability of the health care professional when the family are learning greater skill in problem solving is critical to the family's health education and care.

The proportion of responsibility that care givers and professionals give to growing children is important. There seems to be a need to allow children to be given progressively more opportunity to be involved in their own health care. This progression would allow children to gradually assume responsibility for their own healthy and unhealthy habits and their consequences, and assume responsibility for relating to professionals. The needs of children, such as those with cystic fibrosis, are often not recognized in relation to cognitive development. Explanations, which have sufficed in the past, are maintained until a crisis. There is then a belated necessity to update the child's knowledge. The child may feel aggrieved that his right to the information has been overlooked.

HEALTH PROMOTION

Strategies used to promote health are the same in all arenas. These might include initiating rapport, giving support, teaching, counselling and making referrals where necessary. A relationship is rarely established straight away, and it is common for the child to test the professional about the stability of the relationship. Shared play can provide good opportunities to consolidate the relationship, but needs to be done with permission of the parents and most importantly the co-operation of the child. Parents are most receptive to the professional whose method regards the needs of the family first. This is especially important in large institutions where the apparent needs of the organization can overwhelm the family at the expense of the child.

The extended family has led to the resource of some families being stretched, with relatives living at some distance. There is a resultant loss of the health-promoting role of grandparents and other more experienced members of the family. It also represents an opportunity for the professional to break patterns of poor health practice without the repercussions within the family. This has been recognized by professionals who offer information and support that was previously available within the family (Hansen and Aradine, 1974). Parents expect the professional to understand and augment their strategies of parenthood. Acquaintance with the characteristics of the family is a good use of both the professional's time and resources. Primary care givers need to meet their own dependent needs, otherwise we cannot expect that they will be able to meet their children's developmental needs.

The professional uses every opportunity to develop the awareness of the parents to their child's resources and deficiencies. The establishment of the child's assets assists in the characterization of the child in a positive manner to both the parents and the professional. This is especially important for the family with a chronically ill child where emphasis on the child's normal development and those behaviours that communicate the child's personality reassures the parents that their child is advancing, whereas developmentally negative behaviour is temporary and not a result of inappropriate parenting techniques.

The professional is required to encourage families with respect for their cultural beliefs, style of parenting and lifestyle. There is a duty to introduce, subtly, those scientific principles which are integral to health with deference to their beliefs and parenting styles. The professional must give recognition to the family or child's purpose as well as their abilities. This might be that the family have noticed a health problem, but have adopted an outmoded strategy to deal with it. The intention is certainly correct and to be applauded, but it requires a great deal of tact to correct the intervention.

A large proportion of professional care is teaching. Through the medium of teaching the professional engenders an aura of caring and helps the family to gather information to introduce problem solving to master the impediments to healthy modification of their lives. There is an abundance of advantageous information for parents and children, and the professional feels obliged to relate it all in the fleeting contacts with the family. Therefore, the times when a family waits are valuable teaching opportunities, and each procedure or treatment offered lends itself to simultaneous teaching. Some children's out-patients departments have built these ideas into their philosophy of care. Whereas in the past families might have complained about the wait for an appointment, this time is now being used productively by dynamic professionals and the families.

Children undergoing day surgery have become major consumers of the care provided by children's units throughout the UK. Out-patient clinics are useful arenas in which to start the preparation for the anticipated procedure and its consequences for the child and family. Southampton General Hospital has produced a series of booklets about specific surgery such as inguinal hernia and undescended testes. These augment the booklet which deals with the general problems for the child and family having day surgery. Sub-headings include, 'After the operation', 'When can my child return to his normal activities?' and 'Looking after your child at home'. The text and illustrations in these booklets are well suited to the needs of families and have been well received.

Teaching may be in a planned or formal situation, such as parent classes or personal health classes in school. The majority of teaching is either casual or by chance, occurring when prompted by recognized need. Hunsberger (1990) suggests that there are three forms of incidental learning: imitation or role models; task repetition; and positive environmental feedback.

Role modelling is productive at any stage of development, when children or adults learn more from the educator's deeds than words. Children and those adults who feel insecure in the parent role respond well to this form of teaching, by imitating to learn skills. A demonstration clarifies verbal instruction. Role play, puppet play, games which use role reversal, and psychodrama also have their place. These techniques make children and families more aware of the roles and feelings of others. Learner participation with clear and concrete rewards for effort and achievement gives good reinforcement and practising of skills. Hunsberger (1990) suggests that 'the more educated the learner, the more likely learning can take place through verbal or written instruction and logical explanation, with or without the use of active teaching techniques'.

The approach of the teaching should be family centred. Children who have no opportunity to see healthy behaviours in people important to them are unlikely to adopt such behaviours. Promoting children's health cannot stop at the child: it is obviously necessary to help parents to become better role models. These matters are addressed in further detail in Chapter 2.

Professionals have a clear role in helping parents to be aware of the potential outcomes, whether good or bad, of their intended actions. Such teaching circumstances have been referred to as anticipatory guidance (Hunsberger, 1990; Pridham, 1977). In child care this might relate to developmental issues so that families have ideas about the future and its management. In acute health care it might be as simple as warning the parent that a child's urine might be coloured red by the excretion of a drug. The Public Health Association defined anticipatory guidance as 'teaching the mother what to expect before she begins to worry or make mistakes' (Committee on Child Health of the American Health Association, 1955). Such anticipatory guidance is time consuming, but it may be possible to group together families with similar health problems or at the same developmental level to maximize the use of the time (Osborn, 1982).

Parents have a fundamental desire to succeed in the care of their child. They need to receive reassurance from their family and friends as well as from professionals that their approach to parenting can prosper. Health-related subjects are often in the view of the media and cause the level of debate among parents to rise. Professionals need to be aware of this. They need to answer questions about this information, substantiate accurate information, and redress the balance when the information is misleading.

TEACHING CHILDREN

Hunsberger (1990) suggests that 'too often health teaching about children is directed mostly toward their parents'. This is a temptation which is difficult to avoid when the professional is busy, short of time and can relate to a fellow adult whose cognitive developmental level is known. Pidgeon (1977) notes, 'Like sponges they (children) silently absorb and ruminate over what they hear . . . health teachings should be aimed at children as well as their parents.' Stress is a universal problem, which causes severe long-term health problems. Children suffer stress and without their parents and being immature have few abilities to cope with it. They need to learn ways to alleviate stress, acquire competent coping abilities, as well as attitudes that err toward health rather than illness. A clear example of such a situation might be a visit to the hospital for a child to have an unpleasant procedure. Children need information about what to expect during such health care experiences (Rodin, 1983).

Hunsberger (1990) suggests that acquisition of healthy behaviour by children involves four processes. They must develop an awareness of health from role models. They must be exposed to developmentally appropriate information about health and care practices. Children who are to learn about responsibility must be included as active participants as early as possible. They must be supported in their attempts and during their accomplishments in practising healthy behaviour.

Teaching children has regard for the child's reasoning ability at differing ages, the notion of health that is appropriate for the age, and the amount of autonomous action that a child is capable of at that age. These teaching opportunities are best aimed at helping the child to develop problem solving and coping abilities in health promotion.

COUNSELLING ROLE

The successful counsellor cultivates skills of observation, judicious questioning, impartial listening and letting the client decide upon the answers. Those family members who will be affected by the situation should be included in such counselling. This allows all appropriate members of the family to achieve an understanding of the problem and their role including that of the counsellor. The professional's role as a counsellor is aimed to elicit a feeling of confidence in dealing with problems, and by leading through the decision-making process.

REFERRALS

Health promotion is a multidisciplinary role that dictates an imaginative approach to the use of skills and the share of work. An appropriate referral will be based on a thorough knowledge of the multitude of potential health team members whether local, regional, statutory or voluntary (Mesters *et al.*, 1991). This knowledge might be of the potential of the resource, its ability to succeed and the method by which the family can obtain these services (Hunsberger, 1990). When considerable resources are required by the family, the professional may act as co-ordinator in order to maximize their efficient use.

CONCLUSIONS

The child's conception and the consequences of his behaviour are fundamental to appropriate delivery of educational and promotional ideas. In a great many ways the current theory only leads the professional to guess at the comprehension of the child at difficult stages of development. There would appear to be a central and crucial need for further psychological research to develop theory and so increase our understanding and improve our interventions.

Health promotion for the child and his family is an area of great creativity. The potential is never ending and, although the activity needs the co-operation of all health care disciplines involved, such team-work is not always achieved. An integrated approach must be the aim, to prevent fragmentation and confusion.

CASE STUDIES

Major study – the ill child – the child with asthma

Asthma currently affects 5% of the adult population and 15% of children (Horsley, 1987). It is a particular problem for carers and professionals involved with children. Ellis (1990) reports that asthma is responsible for around 2000 deaths per calendar year in the UK, although he does not suggest the proportion of these deaths which might be children. These mortality figures might be reason in themselves for the use of the child with asthma as a case study in a book about health promotion. However, there are also pertinent effects of the altered physiology upon morbidity and the quality of life of both the individual sufferer and the family (Nocon and Booth, 1989; Usherwood *et al.*, 1990). The cause of asthma is not clear, but there appears to be both an allergic and a nervous component.

A child with asthma may initially visit the general practitioner suffering from a chest infection, which disguises the underlying biological problem. In unfortunate circumstances this may be followed by an emergency call out to visit the child at home because the child is having great difficulty in breathing. It is possible that an emergency admission to the local paediatric unit may be required. The child may not have been prepared for an admission to hospital, which may become a potential source of exacerbation of the nervous source of the problem. The parents may be concerned for the loss of their child and are likely to pass this stress on to the child. Such a situation is traumatic for both the child and the parent and requires sensitive handling by appropriately trained staff.

This acute admission might be considered to have an effect on the feelings of vulnerability of the child, but this will depend on how close the child is to maturity. Older children, more than 12 years, are nearing maturity and have further motivation to learn how to avoid such situations again; whereas the younger child does not have a clear idea about cause and effect and would be less motivated by feelings of vulnerability. The older child would be expected to be more susceptible to health promotion strategies aimed at preventing the situation from occurring again. The younger child might even regard the illness as some form of punishment (Eiser, 1991).

A measure of the efficiency of the respiratory system, which is used in the assessment of the effectiveness of treatment, is that of Peak Expiratory Flow measurement (PEF). It is important that this measurement is carried out in a correct and consistent manner. The professional must work closely with the parent and the young child, if this method is to be employed. Each test produces a score and it is possible to use this score as competitive motivation for the young child. Attractively presented graphs filled out with the parent and child will involve the child in the care. Some ingenious methods have been employed, such as blowing bubbles under water or blowing candles out to get the younger child to co-operate.

There are various systemic medications which are beneficial in the treatment of asthma, such as salbutamol elixir and soluble prednisolone. However, these are not the preferred route, because they have an overall effect upon the individual including the side-effects. The preferred route is via the lungs where the medication has its effect directly upon the smooth muscle. However, these medicines are highly unacceptable to the younger child, who perhaps sees the inhalers as being difficult to use and frightening. It would be impracticable to teach the child about the avoidance of the systemic side-effects, and so the professional directs such education towards the parent. This must be balanced against the potential clinical necessity to use systemic drugs at times of exacerbations of the disease. These two drugs have well-documented side-effects, such as increased appetite which is associated with oral steroids or the changes in behaviour which have been noted with systemic salbutamol. Such information given to the parents would constitute anticipatory guidance.

Inhalers are very useful, but difficult to teach to the young child. Their comprehension of their own bodies is poor (Bibace and Walsh, 1981). Initially they may have problems in co-ordinating inhalation with the dose of drug. However, there are some useful parallels: the use of straws to suck drinks means that the skill is known to the child, but needs to be adapted. By the use of placebo doses, the professional, parent or even sibling has an opportunity to role model the technique. Some children complain that there is nothing to suck, such as with the sucking of Rotahalers. The powder also can be irritant and cause coughing, which can be a further disincentive to the child to completing the treatment. Innovations, such as the Spinhaler, give the child a feeling of accomplishment by having a discernible effect (Figure 5.1).

The causes of asthma are many and various, but a major component is allergy. Some of these causes are preventable, such as that of smoking. Parents whose child is admitted in status athmaticus are highly vulnerable and it could be considered unethical to take advantage of this vulnerability at an early stage to alter their behaviour. The motivation caused by the parents' perceived vulnerability to the ultimate failure as parents, the death of their child, would be countered by the potential destruction of the therapeutic relationship. However, smoking might well predispose the child to an asthmatic attack and there is a need to alter this behaviour. Physiological dependence upon cigarettes will mean that it will be difficult if not impossible for the parents, even if highly motivated, to stop immediately. It may be that subtle changes to their lifestyle can be made, such as not smoking in

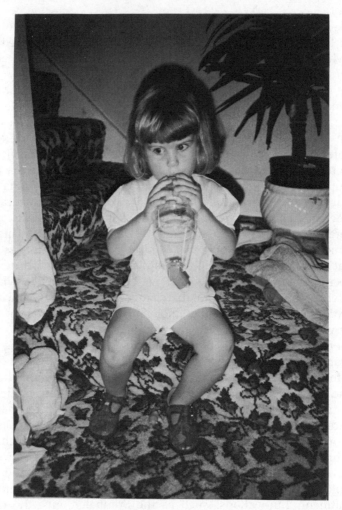

Figure 5.1   Child with nebulizer.

the same room as the susceptible child. If it is possible for the parents
to do this they may well be rewarded by an improvement in their
child's condition. The health professional also has a valuable role to
play in positively reinforcing this change in health behaviour which
reflects well on their abilities as parents.

Young children who are not yet able to think in an abstract manner
will not be able to cope with the concept of causality. They will therefore not be able to see that being in a room with their grandfather who
is a heavy pipe smoker might well lead to an asthmatic attack. Indeed,
the emotional stress of denying the child access to the much beloved
grandfather might cause an asthmatic attack itself. This demonstrates

the complex nature of health promotion in most situations but especially that of the child with asthma. The child's lack of comprehension of cause and effect may mean that drugs which prevent asthma may be poorly accepted. It is difficult enough to get some children to take medication when it is to make them better, but it is even more difficult when it is to keep them well.

There is a great pressure upon children's wards to get children home as soon as possible. This is part of their philosophy to reduce the trauma caused to the child by hospitalization. However, it is also because beds are constantly required by others. The result is that teaching is done at great speed and requires further reinforcement and support by the primary health care team, teachers and out-patient staff (Mesters *et al.*, 1991). The use of specific clinics (Charlton, 1989) may have a role to play.

Major study – the well child – childhood accidents

Accidents cause more mortality and morbidity from 1–14 years than any other cause. The Department of Health (1991) suggest that 21% of deaths in the age group 1–4 years are caused by accidents and 36% in the age group 5–14 years. The Department of Health (1991) present the changes in the distribution of death by cause between 1931 and 1988. The analysis of these changes is notable for the absence of comment about the increase in the percentage of deaths in childhood caused by accidents to its current level of three times that in the past.

Childhood accidents represent the largest challenge to health promotion and health education (Jackson, 1977). Even the term 'accident' denotes an unexpected, unavoidable, or unintentional event which implies that nothing can be done to prevent such an occurrence. This is not the case: there are things that can be done to prevent such occurrences. *The Health of the Nation* outlines the goal in child health care as being 'To reduce preventable death and ill health in . . . children' (Department of Health, 1991). Accidents are preventable, and so should fall within these Department of Health guidelines.

The retrospective analysis of childhood accidents may give information about the underlying patterns leading to a possible strategy for intervention. Walsh and Jarvis (1992) suggest that there are more accidents after school than those before school. A strategy based on this information is rather more difficult to contrive. Each child's accident has its individual circumstances, unless there is a problem with the design of particular equipment, such as that of a bicycle, or of the environment, such as the need for a pelican crossing. It is difficult to perceive a natural responsibility within the current system of care to collate the information on childhood accidents. The Department of Health (1991) state that accidents cause one child in five to attend a hospital. Therefore, there might be a role for the Accident and Emergency Department to keep a full register of accidents by cause. The Walsh and Jarvis study has included the grid reference of the actual accident site (supplied by the police), which gives more useful information than merely the address of the family. Unfortunately this would not be full information, because it will exclude those children who receive treatment from the general practitioner, practice nurse or skilled neighbour or relative. The collation of this information might provide information which could inform policy makers about the required changes to the environment, such as fences etc.

The relationship to health concepts

Young children with immature cognitive development cannot assess cause and effect relationships and so present a particular challenge. They will not be able to predict the potential danger of a situation, nor produce an appropriate strategem. Parents and the state have attempted to deal with the problem by rote learning, so that the child has a set procedure to deal with, for instance, crossing the road. Such an approach is innately inflexible.

The ability of children to react to potential dangers within their environment will depend upon their cognitive development. However, those children who are internally controlled are more likely to be able to produce strategies to prevent potential accidents. A current major study in Newcastle is attempting to address some of these issues (Walsh and Jarvis, 1991). One child in answering a question about the potential dangers between school and home was not only able to identify one particularly dangerous junction, but also to draw a diagram of how this junction could be improved and made safer. This child would appear to be an internally controlled individual. Other children, whose parents have life happen to them (are externally controlled) would be less likely to be able to produce such a strategy. They may also be in more danger, they may walk to school more often than internally controlled children or have to cross busier roads. While the external control, or fatalism, may not be linked conclusively to social deprivation, the lack of resources, gardens or other safe play areas certainly are. The potential link of a child who is less likely to be able to develop strategies to deal with a more dangerous environment or lifestyle would seem to be a recipe for childhood accidents with resultant morbidity or death.

The Newcastle study (Walsh and Jarvis, 1991) seems to present a useful strategy. Education and awareness of potential dangers for the child has been an essential tool targeted at children in school (Figure 5.2). These children are also used as a resource to assess the potential

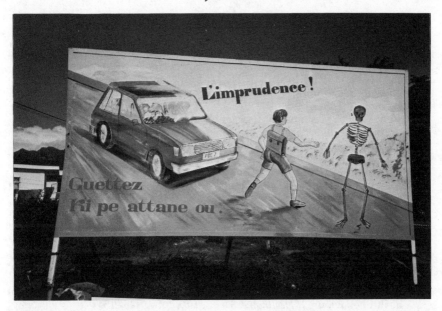

Figure 5.2 A safety sign at the road side of one of the few dual carriageways in Mauritius.

dangers of their environment. Such information could then be used in a preventative manner.

Multidisciplinary approach

The problem of childhood accidents is so large that it would not be appropriate for one profession to take responsibility for it. Schools and related professions seem to have a clear role to play. Similarly, the members of the primary health care team would seem to have a role in identifying and dealing with local need. However, co-ordination of an accident register with a geographical database would serve all of these professions well.

> The range of those with the opportunity to contribute is equally wide – accident prevention is par excellence an example of an area where the best results are achieved by cooperation and collaboration. (Department of Health, 1991, p. 73)

REFERENCES

Bandura, A. (1986) *Social foundation of thought and action*, Prentice Hall, Englewood Cliffs, NJ.

Bibace, R. and Walsh, M.E. (1981) *Children's conceptions of health and illness and bodily functions*, Jossey-Bass, San Francisco.

Black, J.L. and Newton, J. (1981) Should health behaviour change be an object of school health personnel? *Journal of School Health*, **51**(3), 189–91.

Bruhn, J.G. and Parcel, G.S. (1982) Current knowledge about the health behaviour of young children: a conference summary. *Health Education*, **9**(2 and 3), 238–61.

Charlton, I. (1989) Asthma clinics: setting up. *Practitioner*, **233**, 1359–62.

Committee on Child Health of the American Health Association (1955) *Health supervision of young children*, American Public Health Association, NY.

Comstock, G. (1981) Influences of mass media on child health beliefs and behaviour. *Health Education Quarterly*, **8**(1), 32–8.

Department of Health (1991) *The health of the nation. A consultative document for health in England*, HMSO, London.

Dielman, T.E. *et al.* (1982) Parental and child health beliefs and behaviour. *Health Education Quarterly*, **9**(2 and 3), 156.

Eiser, C. (1991) It's OK having asthma . . . Young children's beliefs about illness. *Professional Nurse*, **3**, 342–5.

Ellis, P. (1990) Asthma: meeting the demand for pain relief. Drugs and inhalation devices. *Professional Nurse*, **2**, 76–81.

Gochman, D.S. (1971) Some correlates of children's health beliefs and potential health behaviour. *J. Health and Soc. Behav.*, June, 148–154.

Gochman, D.S. (1977) Perceived vulnerability and its psychosocial context. *Soc. Sci. Med.*, **11**, 115–20.

Gochman, D.S. and Saucier, J.F. (1982) Perceived vulnerability in children and adolescents. *Health Education Quarterly*, **9**(2 and 3), 142–54.

Grasser, S.C. and Craft, B.J. (1984) The patient's approach to wellness. *Nurs. Clin. North Am.* **19**(2), 207–18.

Green, K.E. and Bird, E. (1986) The structure of children's beliefs about health and illness. *J. Sch. Health*, **56**(8), 325–8.

Hansen, M. and Aradine, C. (1974) The changing face of primary pediatrics. *Pediatric Clin. North Am.*, Feb, 245.

Horsley, M. (1987) Diseases and their treatment: Asthma. *Pharmaceutical Journal*, **239**, 552–4.

Hunsberger, M. (1990) Health concepts: children's perceptions and behaviours, in *Family-centred nursing care of children* (eds. R.L. Foster, M.B. Hunsberger and J.J.T. Anderson), W.B. Saunders Co., London.

Jackson, R.H. (1977) *Children, the environment and accidents*, Pitman Medical, London.

Kalnins, I. and Love, R. (1982) Children's concepts of health and illness and implications for health education. An overview. *Health Education Quarterly*, **9**(2 and 3), 104–15.

Mesters, I., Meertens, R. and Mosterd, N. (1991) Multidisciplinary co-operation in primary care for asthmatic children. *Soc. Sci. Med.*, **32**(1), 65–70.

Mullen, P.D. (1983) Promoting child health: channels of specialisation. *Fam. Community Health*, **5**(4), 52–68.

Natapoff, J. (1978) Children's views of health: a developmental study. *Am. J. Public Health*, Oct, 995–9.

Neuhauser, C. *et al.* (1978) Children's concepts of healing. Cognitive development and locus of control factors. *Am. J. Orthopsychiatr.*, April, 335–41.

Nocon, A. and Booth, T. (1989) The social impact of asthma: a review of the literature. *Social Work and Social Sciences Review*, **1**(3), 177–200.

Osborn, L. (1982) Group well-child care: an option for today's children. *Pediatr. Nurs.*, Sep/Oct, 306–8.

Pender, N.J. (1987) *Health promotion in nursing practice*, Appleton Century Crofts, East Norwalk.

Perrin, E.C. and Shapiro, E. (1985) Health locus of control beliefs of healthy children, children with a chronic physical illness, and their mothers. *J. Pediatr.*, **107**(4), 627–33.

Piaget, J. and Inhelder, B. (1969) *The psychology of the child*, Basic Books, NY.

Pidgeon, V. (1977) Characteristics of children's thinking and implications for health teaching. *Matern. Child Nurs.*, Spring, 1.

Pridham, F. *et al.* (1977) Anticipatory care as problem solving in family medicine and nursing. *J. Fam. Pract.*, **4**(6), 1077–81.

Rodin, J. (1983) *Will this hurt? Preparing children for hospital and medical procedures*, Royal College of Nursing, London.

Rotter, J.B. (1954) *Social learning and clinical psychology*, Prentice Hall, Englewood Cliffs, NJ.

Usherwood, T.P., Scrimgeour, A. and Barber, J.H. (1990) Questionnaire to measure perceived symptoms and disability in asthma. *Archives of Disease in Childhood*, **65**, 779–81.

Walsh, S.S. and Jarvis, S.N. (1992) Measuring the frequency of severe accidental injury in childhood. *Epidemiology and Community Health*, **46**(1), 26–32.

Wu, R. (1973) *Behaviour and illness*, Prentice Hall, Englewood Cliffs, NJ.

CHAPTER 6

The well and sick adolescent

Jayne Taylor

Adolescence is a period of the lifespan that is characterized by distinct physiological, psychological and social change. The change is often rapid, occurs at different rates in individuals of the same chronological age and brings with it shifting needs. It is a period which involves making adjustments, as the adolescent and the family focus on issues such as independence, trust, norms and values. Sometimes, it is a period of conflict and occasionally a time of extreme sorrow and torment.

The majority of adolescents survive relatively unscathed, having acquired the social, cultural, academic and vocational skills required to take them into adulthood. Health promotion during this period can provide the adolescent and the family with the relevant information necessary to help them make healthy choices in relation to both their physical and psychological well-being. It can also help them to develop a positive self-image and feel comfortable with their changing bodies. However, the environment, the nature of the information and the way it is given must all reflect the adolescent's special needs.

For a few, adolescence marks the beginning of an acute or chronic health problem, whilst for others, chronic childhood illness is further complicated by the normal physiological and psychological changes experienced during this period. Many health care professionals are acutely aware of the complex needs of the sick adolescent and of the difficulty of ensuring that health education is effective. Health educators working with acutely or chronically ill adolescents and their families must be both knowledgeable and skilled about the many factors that influence their needs, as well as being able to constantly adapt as needs change.

In order to begin to look at health promotion and patient education, it is important to consider some aspects of normal physical and psychological development during adolescence. These developmental features help to put many of the problems encountered by adolescents into context and can assist health educators in their task of ensuring that education is effective and appropriate.

PHYSIOLOGICAL DEVELOPMENT

Physiologically, adolescence is characterized by an increase in the secretion of gonadotrophins from the pituitary gland resulting in the stimulation of the testes to produce testosterone in boys, and the stimulation of the ovaries to produce oestrogen in girls. Oestrogen production starts to undergo cyclical changes at around the time of menarche (the first menstrual period). Graham and Rutter (1985) suggest that menarche usually occurs at some point between 10 and 16 years in girls. Testicular growth is usually complete at some point between 13 and 17 years in boys.

Whilst these primary characteristics are important events in the lives of young people, it is the development of the secondary sexual characteristics that is seen by the adolescent to be most significant in terms of their physical appearance. The development of breasts in girls is the first outward sign of puberty. Both sexes grow pubic hair, experience apocrine secretions (body odour) and an increase in the size and secretions of the sebaceous follicle, which leads to the development of the dreaded 'spots' (Vaughan and Litt, 1990).

Adams (1983) also points to the early adolescent growth spurt as being significant. In girls the growth spurt is an early sign of puberty whereas in boys it is a later manifestation. Apart from an increase in height, girls show an increase in hip width and boys in shoulder width. Fat distribution also changes with boys tending to lose fat whilst girls remain relatively stable, followed by a rapid rise in body fat as height velocity slows down.

It is not surprising that adolescence is the period of greatest risk for developing eating disorders such as anorexia nervosa (Agras and Kirkley, 1986) as the young person attempts to control a body that appears to be out of control. Those particularly at risk appear to be individuals who perceive body shape as being important to their lifestyle. Russell (1985) in his discussion of anorexia nervosa cites research which shows that the incidence of anorexia nervosa is exceptionally high in fashion and ballet students.

The development of anorexia nervosa is, however, much rarer than what Burkitt (1973) has described as the commonest form of malnutrition in the Western world – obesity. Over the past decade obesity has increased rapidly (Mansfield and Emans, 1989) and by late adolescence Graham and Rutter (1985) found that nearly 50% of girls feel fat. These findings were confirmed by one innovative adolescent screening clinic where it was found that the most common medical complaints among 16 and 17-year-olds were 'obesity, depression and acne' (Donovan, 1988).

Other changes in appearance can also be very distressing for the adolescent. For example, they may be disturbed about their height, their teeth, their skin and nose shape. In addition, boys may worry about early hair recession and their genital development, just as girls experience anxiety over their breast size.

Late or early development

Adams (1983) suggests that adolescents tend to compare their own growth and development with that of their peers and very early or very late development can be very threatening. Bee (1989), however, suggests that the age of onset of puberty is not important, but whether the onset coincides with what the adolescent perceives to be 'right' or 'normal'. In other words, it is the perception of what constitutes lateness or earliness by the individual that is crucial, rather than the actual timing.

Late or early physical development does have implications for anyone involved in health promotion, as it may be difficult to remember that a 12-year-old, who has the physical appearance of a 16-year-old, will not have the life experience or cognitive ability of someone who is actually 16 years old. Alternatively, Mussen *et al.* (1990) suggest that late maturation can lead to the adolescent being 'treated like a child'.

PSYCHOLOGICAL DEVELOPMENT

The psychological processes that occur during adolescence are more difficult to define. Adams (1983) suggests that adolescence should be seen as a transitional period which involves several psychosocial 'tasks' and this provides a useful framework for considering psychological development. The 'tasks' are:

- becoming comfortable with their own bodies;
- striving for independence;
- building relationships with the same and opposite sexes;
- seeking economic and social stability;
- developing a value system; and
- learning to verbalize conceptually.

Clearly these tasks are not completed overnight nor is it certain that all individuals complete all tasks. A successful outcome is dependent on many internal and external factors. In addition there are many theories about cognitive development, the development of personality, and about how individuals become socialized to their changing roles which are important when considering psychological adjustment to adulthood. It is not feasible to outline more than two of the most influential theories here, which are Piaget's theory of cognitive development (Mussen *et al.*, 1990) and Erikson's theory of identity formation (Erikson, 1963).

According to Piagetian theory, the final stage of cognitive development begins in adolescence with the development of formal operational thought. In practice, a knowledge of Piaget's theory is very useful to anyone involved in adolescent education. If adolescents have not reached formal operations, and are still in the previous stage (the concrete operational stage), they will not be able to consistently reason about things which they have no experience about. In'other words, until adolescents are capable of formal operational thought they can reason about real problems but not hypothetical ones. Some of the changes that occur with this final stage are summarized below.

Concrete operations	Formal operations
Grasps concept of conservation	Able to think conceptually
Able to use inductive logic	Able to use deductive logic
Understands rule of reversibility	Can think hypothetically
Grasps rule of class inclusion	Can systematically problem-solve

Figure 6.1 Piagetian theory.

The formal operations stage can bring with it doubt in relation to previous knowledge, as adolescents identify inconsistencies in what they have previously been taught. For example, they may start to question why parents forbid smoking and yet smoke themselves, as well as recognizing that there are exceptions to established rules (Botvin, 1984) such as, for example, that not all smokers get lung cancer. This questioning results in the adolescent considering available evidence about smoking and a decision will be made about personal behaviour. Botvin suggests that many factors will ultimately influence the decision-making process during adolescence. Social influence from peers, parents or media personalities can affect decisions in both positive and negative ways so that if close friends are smokers it could be a negative influence. However, peer pressure to conform to negative health behaviours is not always successful. Botvin (1984) discusses that self-esteem, self-confidence and personal autonomy are important factors in predicting conformity to peer pressure. An individual who has a strong internal locus of control would be unlikely to adopt negative health behaviours just because their friends have.

Mussen *et al.* (1990) suggest that the tendency for some adolescents to become pre-occupied with societal, religious and political issues is also dependent on the capacity for formal operational thinking. This pre-occupation is sometimes linked to what Erikson describes as 'identity formation' (Erikson, 1963). In some societies identity formation is not difficult because there is little social change, limited extraneous influence and the adolescent has a clear view about their adult role. The adolescent may comply with cultural, vocational and societal expectations and indeed be quite content to do so. However, in complex societies there are many external influences which can potentially cause problems in the search for identity. Erikson suggests that the adolescent's inability to decide about future roles can be particularly disturbing and can result in 'identity confusion' as adolescents

> temporarily overidentify, to the point of apparent complete loss of identity, with the heroes of cliques and crowds. (Erikson, 1963, p. 253)

Further conflict may also arise if parents and adolescents disagree about educational options, career choice and other future plans. This conflict is particularly traumatic if the adolescent's choices challenge the beliefs and traditions of the parental culture.

Whilst many adolescents undergo a period of active searching for an identity, the process and the outcome are usually both positive and constructive. Unfortunately, a minority seem to be transiently or permanently in role confusion. Parry-Jones (1985) discusses some of the many manifestations of adolescent disturbance which include anxiety, depression, eating disorders, parental–adolescent estrangement, social alienation, anti-social behaviour, sexual problems and problems at school. Whilst some of these young people can be helped to cope with their distress, a few will become homeless, jobless and friendless. The prospects for these young people are dreadful.

The implications of the theories of Piaget and Erikson for health educators are vast and raise several questions about how educators can ensure that their teaching is appropriate. How, for example, do health educators know if an individual has reached the formal operational stage? Once reached, do individuals remain there constantly? Can adolescents be helped with their identity formation? What changes should be made in terms of the educative approach? Do all individuals reach formal operations and is identity formation permanent? The answer to the last question is probably that not everyone does progress beyond the concrete operational stage or at least that not everyone consistently remains there (Keating, 1980; Overton et al., 1987). Graham and Rutter (1985) also express doubts about the permanence of identity formation. Social situations frequently change and it is probable that individuals undergo periods of identity diffusion throughout life.

It should be said that the theories of Piaget and others have been questioned by some psychologists and will, no doubt, continue to be the source of some speculation. Within the context of health promotion with adolescents, the accuracy and precision of theory are not the issue. What is important is that by having some knowledge of psychological theory, the health educator can appreciate that adolescents do not all possess the same abilities when it comes to cognitive thought. Therefore, those who possess knowledge about cognitive domains will undoubtedly be in a better position to offer appropriate education (Tauer, 1983).

HEALTH PROMOTION

Health promotion during adolescence involves facilitating young people to explore their feelings and attitudes about health issues, influencing behaviour, raising awareness of the function of the health services and assisting with the development of skills required to achieve and maintain good health. Health promotion activities should be appropriate to the physiological and psychological developmental stage of the adolescent. However, this is sometimes very difficult as the first sections of this chapter have highlighted. Chronological age and physical appearance are not accurate guides as to an individual's level of cognitive development, and in practice this can mean that in a group of 14-year-old adolescents there will be a vast variation in the ability of individuals to comprehend information. Unfortunately, if the level of information is aimed too high some students will switch off, and equally, if the pitch is too low, others will become bored and will also switch off.

The Health Education 13–18 Project (Schools Council/Health Education Council, 1982) suggests principles for ensuring that health promotion is effective in meeting the educational needs of adolescents. These principles are to:

- encourage individuals to identify with real situations and experiences;
- give individuals opportunities to clarify their own attitudes and values;
- give individuals the chance to explore and discuss their personal perspective;
- ensure that information is given in a non-didactic way.

By adopting an adolescent-centred approach to health education, each individual is encouraged to look at their own practices and situation in a way that is appropriate to their age, cognitive development, family situation and cultural group. It is also important that consideration should be given to the previous knowledge and experience of each individual. French writes,

the power of these internal systems, alongside those of beliefs and attitudes, to provide a very effective filter through which perceptions of the outside world are selected and interpreted, often seem forgotten . . . (French, 1984, p. 262)

It is important, therefore, that those involved in health promotion are aware of the external influences that colour both the perception and perspective of adolescents. Acknowledgement of the power of these external influences gives support to the view that health education in schools, for example, should be integrated into the curriculum, facilitated by people with knowledge of individual adolescents, should emphasize parental links and should be entirely flexible. In addition, Gibson (1987) suggests that it should be affective and action orientated, group/activity based, should assume a process rather than a product approach and should use an educational rather than a medical model. The power of what Gibson describes as the 'hidden curriculum' should also be recognized. Just as adolescents will question the wisdom and authority of parents who demonstrate contradictory behaviour so they will question the behaviour of teachers who, for example, smoke on school premises.

Kolbe (1984) emphasizes the need not only to influence individual behaviour, but to ensure that community organization enables behaviour to change and that positive behaviour is reinforced. If health promotion strategies are not widely supported, research shows that the effectiveness of, for example, an anti-smoking programme will be limited. Reid writes that

> effective health promotion for the young must begin by considering all factors involved in a particular health related behaviour. This will usually require a whole community approach, involving parents, shopkeepers, clinics, and the support of the local media. (Reid, 1984, p. 75)

The organization of such a wide approach is far from easy and involves a sophisticated level of communication and co-operation between many individuals and groups.

Methods of achieving effective education

Much emphasis has been placed on ensuring that education is appropriate to individual adolescents and of being aware of the power of external influences. There is a great deal of literature and other resources available to help those involved in health promotion programmes and lists of material can usually be obtained through Health Promotion Units. It is however very important that material is carefully assessed for its appropriateness before it is used. Whilst it is not the intention to be prescriptive here, Figure 6.2 gives some additional hints about working with adolescents.

PRACTICAL APPLICATION

The scope of health promotion during adolescence is extremely wide and it is not possible to cover all the issues that are relevant during this part of the lifespan. However, the emphasis of this book is on practical

Do	Don't
Involve adolescents	Embarrass anyone
Use group work/discussion	Isolate anyone
Use peer teaching	Force participation
Use case studies/role play	Use shock-horror tactics
Use appropriate videos	Over-use teaching methods
Lay down clear ground rules	Break your own ground rules
Refer to media figures	Let yourself get out of date
Involve parents	Be afraid to make mistakes
Facilitate sharing of views	Break the law*

* refers specifically to the 1986 Education Act and the circular *Sex education in schools* Department of Education and Science circular 11/87 Welsh Office circular 45/87.

Figure 6.2 Do's and Don't's of working with adolescents.

application and the next section, therefore, takes one area of need in order to illustrate how an effective programme can be developed.

Building relationships with the same and opposite sexes

The role of peers in adolescence is crucial. Relationships between individuals of the same and opposite sexes serve as 'prototypes' for relationships in adulthood (Bee, 1989) and it is important that individuals learn to communicate and interact proficiently. In the search for independence, family ties become looser and peers become influential. This peer influence can be beneficial and a supportive peer group can help adolescents through some of the commonly experienced conflicts that arise. There is also considerable pressure to conform to the norms and values of the peer group, which can have positive or negative consequences, although Parry-Jones (1985) suggests that parental influence remains strong in the majority of adolescents.

Having close friends with whom the adolescent can share their experiences, successes, failures and hopes is particularly important. Friends will criticize but the criticism will usually be readily accepted, whereas criticism from parents is seen to be authoritative and autocratic. Friendship can limit extremes of behaviour and be a constructive part of identity formation (see p. 100). However, variations in development between peers of the same chronological age can result in adolescents sometimes feeling distanced from their friends and peers. Parry-Jones suggests that is an not unusual experience and

> feelings of sadness, apathy, emptiness, loneliness, boredom and isolation from peer groups may occur in normally adjusted young people (Parry-Jones, 1985, p. 586).

However, for some adolescents the feeling of 'isolation' can lead to despondency and depression. This depression can manifest itself in a number of ways, including drug, solvent and alcohol abuse, aggression, somatic complaints and sexual promiscuity. Rejection by peers has also been implicated in studies of suicide in adolescence (McClure, 1988). The following example illustrates the power of friendship.

Two 13-year-old girls were admitted to the Accident and Emergency department after taking an overdose of Temazepam, which had been prescribed for the mother of one of the girls. The reason given for taking the overdose was an argument between one of the girls and a close school friend the day before. One girl had brought the tablets to school and both had taken them during first break. The girl who took the tablets from her mother had many social problems and the loss of a friend seemed to be the last straw. The other girl took them so that she could 'die' with her friend.

Without doubt, adolescents have a need to feel that they belong and not belonging can influence behaviour. The lonely adolescent who desperately wants to belong to a group may well conform to their practices just to feel a sense of belonging. Parry-Jones (1985) describes the typical solvent abuser as feeling 'lonely and friendless' and Pallik-kathayil and Tweed (1983) suggest that adolescent drug users often begin taking drugs because they want to associate with a peer group. The following extract illustrates how taking drugs gave one 13-year-old adolescent a sense of belonging.

The first tab was a profound experience . . . sitting in a darkened room with hippie music playing and blissing out . . . that feeling of belonging, not feeling isolated from people any more, a sense of wonder . . . It was spiritual, it was colourful, it held out a promise of something better to come (Masterson and Mordaunt, 1989, p. 15)

This need to feel a sense of belonging to a group and to have friends with whom to share innermost thoughts and feelings has many implications for those involved in health promotion. Exploring the power of friendship with adolescents is useful in helping them to identify their own needs as well as looking at how decisions are made. It is also helpful to look at the influence of the media in the personal decision-making process. Dixon and Mullinar (1983) suggest the use of group collages for exploring media influence. The collage is collated from various magazine and newspaper cuttings and each group is responsible for explaining what they feel the media message is.

Another useful method for exploring the issue of peer group pressure is the use of peer teaching, which can be very effective (Gray *et al.*, 1987), especially as all individuals will have experience (either positive or negative) of peer groups. Keeping personal diaries of interactions can also be used to initiate discussion and act as *aides-mémoire* and role play can be a powerful method of facilitating identification with issues. Some suggested discussion points are outlined below:

- how behaviour changes in groups;
- how personal behaviour can be controlled in a group;
- factors relating to personality (shy, extrovert, etc.);
- characteristics of groups;
- characteristics of 'a friend';
- influences on friendship.

Relationships with the opposite sex

As adolescents develop physically and psychologically, the structure of peer groups change. Research by Dunphy (1963) showed that initially same-sex peer groups are the norm, but eventually small peer groups combine to form small heterosexual 'crowds'. These crowds allow adolescents to mix socially with members of the opposite sex and eventually couples will pair off although it should not, however, be assumed that all pairing off will be heterosexual. Patrick suggests that '10 per cent of pupils . . . are estimated to be lesbian or gay' (Patrick, 1988, p. 201).

Adolescent sexuality involves looking at the search for identity, feelings and relationships, learning to care, sexual attitudes, developing gender roles, touching and being accepted as sexual beings (Tauer, 1983). There is a very definite role for the health promoter to help the adolescent explore personal feelings and attitudes, as well as encouraging them to listen to the perspectives of peers.

Another role of health promotion is the facilitation of effective decision making in potentially sexually active young people. A recent English survey by Curtis *et al.* (1989) of 761 teenagers aged 15–17 years showed that 56% of both sexes had already had a steady relationship and 40% of these relationships had involved sexual intercourse. Another study by Bowie and Ford (1989) showed that 47% of 16-year-olds had engaged in heterosexual intercourse. The implications of these findings are significant on several counts. First, many studies have shown a correlation between early sexual intercourse and cervical cancer in young women (Broadley, 1986). Secondly, Hersov (1985) discusses studies from the UK and the USA which indicate that many teenage girls become pregnant, of whom many will have terminations of pregnancy. Davis (1989), in her review of research, suggests that adolescent pregnancy and child-bearing carry increased physiological risks for both mother and baby as well as longer term psychosocial disadvantages for the family. The third implication for homosexually and heterosexually active adolescents is the risk of contracting sexually transmitted infections, particularly human immunodeficiency virus

(HIV). HIV infection is spreading rapidly among the heterosexual population, and adolescents who engage in sexual intercourse are putting themselves at risk. Moriasy and Thomas, in their excellent book about women and HIV, write

> whatever the prevailing social norm, many young people do engage in sexual activity, some at very young ages and many with a high degree of ignorance about how to avoid unwanted pregnancy or sexually transmitted diseases, including HIV infection (Moriasy and Thomas, 1990, p. 21)

Clearly if health promotion is to be effective in reducing the number of adolescent pregnancies and terminations, and preventing the spread of HIV infection, it must reach young people before they become sexually active. Strategies should also include educating those who are already sexually active, and therefore at risk, about safer sex. Great care should be taken, however, not to make assumptions about which adolescents are sexually active and which are not. Information must be given in a general, value-free way and should not embarrass individuals.

Health educators must also take care to ensure that they are not in breach of the law. The whole spectrum of sex education in schools is complex because of legal and cultural factors. The 1986 Education Act

> amounts to an enhancement of the power of parents and the local community to decide and influence whether sex education is taught at all, and if so, how (Scowen, 1988, p. 143)

In addition, there are restrictions upon teaching about contraceptive advice and Clause 28 of the 1988 Local Government Bill makes it illegal for any maintained school to teach about the acceptability of homosexuality (Patrick, 1988). Thus there is the danger that a school may not include comprehensive sex education in their curriculum and that adolescents will not get the advice they need about practising safe sex.

Where sex education programmes are included in the school curriculum, those involved should ensure that programmes include clear statements that early intercourse and multiple sexual partners are correlated with several important medical risks, including HIV infection (Curtis *et al.*, 1989). Programmes should be appropriate to the level of cognitive development of the adolescent as well as being language and culture sensitive. Several points are suggested below, for initiating discussion with individuals and groups:

- development of sexuality; building relationships;
- physical and psychological development;
- who owns your body?
- developing a value system;
- sexuality and health myths;

- AIDS: the facts; spread; myths; prevention; the future;
- pregnancy and its implications: preventing pregnancy;
- making decisions – what influences decision making.

Parental education

It is also useful to help parents through some of the conflicts of adolescence. Parents have usually had no first hand experience of what it is like to live with an adolescent and it can be a very confusing and conflict-ridden time for them. Gunn (1987) described a scheme where parents were invited to a boys' school for a health education evening to help prepare them for some of the pitfalls of adolescence. Gunn writes of the evenings,

> Various topics have been discussed: pocket money, parties, homework, girls, evenings out and time of return, drink, drugs, smoking and sex – with its associated problems including . . . AIDS. In some cases there was merely an exchange of ideas . . . In others there was an attempt to agree on 'collective guidelines' so that boys would find it hard to refer to the supposed practice of 'other parents' in their own quest for concessions (Gunn, 1987, p. 76)

This strategy of including parents is useful and this idea could be expanded to include other topic areas. For example, 'second generation' adolescents from some cultural groups find that they are torn between their family culture, with its associated rituals and traditions, and the culture of their school life, their peer group and their close friends. It may well help parents to openly discuss their fears regarding their sons or daughters, and would go some way towards breaking down the ethnocentric barriers of some health promotion strategies.

EVALUATION

Measuring what kinds of health promotion strategies are effective among specific groups of the population is an important part of health promotion. When strategies are designed and goals set, evaluation criteria should be identified along with the proposed methods for collecting information about the effectiveness of a particular programme. Figure 6.3 gives a diagrammatic representation of the evaluation process.

When evaluating health promotion programmes with adolescents it is useful to look at effectiveness from a variety of perspectives, because many problems of adolescence involve families and the wider community. This point is taken up by Tones *et al.* (1990) who suggest that evaluation of school health promotion programmes should look at the individual pupil, the school, the family and the community. In

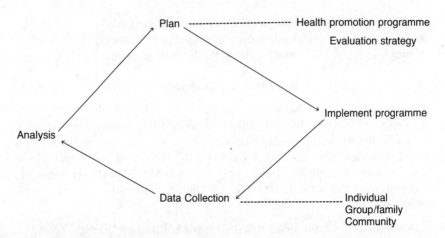

Figure 6.3 The health promotion process.

addition, any evaluation should include short-term measurements and longitudinal measurements in order to look at the most effective ways of promoting permanent changes in behaviour (Williams, 1986).

THE SICK ADOLESCENT

Adolescence is usually a time of life that is associated with good physical health and the first part of this chapter has looked at the needs of healthy adolescents and at how those involved in health promotion can ensure that their teaching strategies are effective. However, considerable morbidity is evident among adolescents, with injuries following road traffic and sporting accidents occurring with relative frequency, as do problems such as appendicitis and glandular fever. Accidents account for more deaths among adolescents than any other cause (OPCS, 1990).

For other young people, adolescence marks the beginning of a chronic or even life-threatening health problem. For example, cancers such as leukaemia, lymphomas, central nervous system tumours and bone tumours, whilst rare, do account for significant morbidity and mortality during adolescence (Thompson, 1990). Other problems which potentially affect the appearance such as scoliosis can also develop during adolescence as well as chronic skin conditions, such as acne. Adolescence may also be the period when chronic psychological disturbances become apparent, with schizophrenia being by far the most frequently occurring chronic psychological disorder among adolescents (Mussen *et al.*, 1990).

For other young people, existing childhood problems continue into adolescence, and some problems may be further complicated by the physiological and psychological changes that occur normally during this time. For example, as cognitive abilities develop, adolescents with cystic fibrosis face the realities of the future in terms of their potential roles as adults, as well coming to fully understand the implications of their illness in relation to their mortality. Some young people find that their health deteriorates rapidly and they find it difficult to keep pace with their healthy peers. Some adolescents find that differences between themselves and their peers which were not seemingly apparent, or indeed important, during childhood, are so marked that they no longer feel comfortable with their friends. These times are emotionally painful for the individual and leave friends with feelings of guilt and sadness.

Patient education

Patient education during adolescence usually involves helping young people to recover from acute illness, helping those with chronic illness to seek independence and come to accept their health problems, and helping those with terminal illness cope with their impending death. Arguably, the skills required by health care professionals involved with adolescents, regardless of the extent or prognosis of their illness, are similar, although the content and timing of education will vary. The importance of possessing good communication skills, patience and an understanding of normal adolescent development cannot be overemphasized. Outlined below are several principles for communicating effectively with adolescents which can be applied to all situations.

- Break initial silence by discussing something familiar, e.g. school, the environment, a recent event.
- Address obvious anger or aggression directly – it will be a barrier to communication if you do not.
- Assess previous knowledge and understanding before giving information – this tells you where you need to start from.
- Ensure information is language, culture and age appropriate – back up verbal information with written information.
- Keep interviews fairly short and be flexible about timings and venue of future meetings if you can.
- Help the adolescent to explore possible choices and make their own decisions – be accepting of those decisions in a value-free way.
- Don't overidentify with the adolescent – it will not help you to help them.
- Utilize informal opportunities to educate as well as formal ones.

In addition to these general principles relating to communicating with the adolescent, it is important to consider the role of parents. They will usually be involved to some extent in the ongoing care of the adolescent and should therefore usually be included in discussions. It should also be remembered that until the age of 18 years, adolescents are considered to be minors in law and parents have the right to give or withhold consent to treatment, although the 1989 Children Act rules that

> parental responsibility itself diminishes as the child acquires sufficient understanding to make his own decisions. (Department of Health, 1989, p. 9)

It may also be appropriate to include other members of the family, particularly siblings, in discussions about diagnosis, treatment and future care. If adolescents are sent home from hospital following acute illness or if they are to receive ongoing care because of chronic illness, the lives of siblings will inevitably be affected. Involving them can help to develop trust and avoid family problems which arise because family members do not share information honestly, particularly when the adolescent's illness is serious.

It is, however, important to see the adolescent on their own so that they have the opportunity to discuss issues that they don't wish to discuss in front of their parents. For example, a male adolescent about to start radiotherapy for testicular cancer may not wish to discuss sperm banking in the presence of his parents and siblings. Privacy should always be afforded when discussing issues that may embarrass the young person.

The ill adolescent and body image

Adolescents with acute and chronic illness have to cope not only with the normal physiological and psychological changes of adolescence but also with additional demands of their illness. Adolescents who are first diagnosed as having chronic health problems such as cancer, for example, have to cope with a normally changing body as well as the potential prospect of mutilating surgery, aggressive treatment and death. Wilburn (cited in Thompson, 1990) discusses the reaction of some adolescents to the prospect of alopecia after cancer treatment. Wilburn found that in some instances hair loss was considered to be so repulsive that treatment was refused. When talking with these young people about their treatment, Thompson warns that it is important that efforts are made to 'reduce the prevalent over-emphasis on physical appearance in our culture' (Thompson, 1990, p. 138). Information about treatments, their benefits and their short and long-term effects should be given accurately and honestly. Young people should be given time to think about their options and every opportunity given for them to ask for clarification. It may be appropriate for the adolescent to meet others who have had similar treatments.

Other adolescents also face permanent disfigurement due to skeletal problems such as idiopathic late onset scoliosis, which occurs during adolescence. Whilst advances in surgical techniques have been made, many young people are treated with a brace worn for 23 hours per day. Jackson (1988) has found that some adolescents find it difficult to cope psychologically with the brace regime. Sensitive education can help adolescents through the initial trauma of coping with both the knowledge of the deformity and the inconvenience of the treatment. For example, simple advice about clothing, available from the Disabled Living Foundation, can help in a very practical way.

Independence

It is not only illness that results in outward body change that causes problems with body image. Simmons *et al.* (1985) highlight the problems experienced by some adolescents with cystic fibrosis of coping with a body that they do not perceive to be normal. Being dependent on parents for physiotherapy can enhance these feelings of being abnormal and it may be possible to look at the young person's lifestyle to see if adjustments can be made. It is important where parents have been very involved in care to be aware of the parental perspective as well as that of the adolescent. Dragone (1990), in her research, found variations between chronically sick adolescents and their parents about the difficulties and needs of the adolescent.

Those involved in patient education should be prepared to negotiate and compromise with adolescents so that they can be as independent as they wish to be. Kelly (1991) suggests that adolescents should be allowed as much freedom as possible, and can successfully be involved in planning their own care. Dryden (1989) discusses teaching adolescents practical skills such as passing nasogastric tubes so that they can be less dependent on parents.

Litt and Cuskey (1980), in their discussion of adolescent compliance, suggest that giving adolescents insight into their own situations may help in securing their co-operation. Putting trust in their abilities to comply with advice is important to the adolescent, and setting mutually acceptable goals, monitoring progress and praising goal achievement may well motivate young people and raise their self-esteem.

Coping with sexuality

Some adolescents face great emotional trauma during adolescence because of their developing sexuality. During the first part of this chapter, issues relating to forming relationships with members of the same and opposite sex were explored, and many young people will eventually become involved in a heterosexual relationship. Of these, a proportion will eventually have children of their own. For some young people with chronic illness, that could be either vertically or genetically transmitted to their children, this path cannot be taken without considering the wider implications. For example, adolescents with sickle cell anaemia, thalassaemia, haemophilia and cystic fibrosis have to live with the knowledge that their children may inherit the same illness that has possibly caused them great personal pain and distress. In addition, they have to acknowledge their own mortality and recognize that they themselves may die, leaving a child to be brought up by a partner, or in the absence of a partner, by extended family or even social services.

Another group of adolescents who face similar problems are those who are infected with the human immunodeficiency virus (HIV). They may infect sexual partners and HIV-infected women may transmit the virus to their child *in utero* or during birth. Studies in Europe and the USA have shown that the transmission rates from HIV-infected mothers to their babies are between 24 and 35% (Husson *et al.*, 1990). It is thought that the number of HIV-infected adolescents is small at present and making accurate projections about the future is difficult. However, as HIV spreads through the heterosexual population, more adolescents will become infected by sexual contact or by sharing infected needles when injecting drugs.

Patient education with adolescents who have to make decisions about their future roles as sexual partners and parents is a particularly sensitive issue and there are skilled counsellors who are specially trained in this field. For example, genetic counsellors are expert at helping young people work through their options and other health care workers can best help the adolescent by liaising with the counsellor, reinforcing their work and not being contradictory. Whilst it may be difficult to involve outside agencies, especially if a good relationship has developed with an adolescent patient, one of the skills of being an effective health educator is recognizing situations that require special skills.

Denial

Adolescents who develop chronic ill health problems or who, because of their increased cognitive abilities, have a different perspective of a longstanding chronic problem may go through stages of denying the severity of their ill health (Mackenzie, 1988). Mackenzie writes,

> the patient may be extremely hostile or unwilling to discuss the illness and treatment and it may take time to break down this hostility and establish a bond of trust. (Mackenzie, 1988, p. 61)

A great deal of patience and time are needed to help the adolescent through the denial stage and in some instances the help of psychologists will be needed in order to help the young person. However, it should be remembered that denial is a coping mechanism and the individual will give clues as to when it is appropriate to discuss a particular issue. The professional should be guided by them rather than picking their own time. Denial can be a feature of both physical and psychological illness, and until it is resolved progress is difficult. Compliance with health education advice is likely to be poor.

Holistic care

Patient education should be concerned with the whole individual, regardless of their health status, and health care professionals should take advantage of opportunities to look beyond the health care problem that has brought the adolescent into contact with the health services: for example, teaching an overweight adolescent admitted to hospital with a fractured femur about healthy eating or an adolescent who has diabetes mellitus about foot care. There are also obvious times when it would not be appropriate, for example, when an adolescent has just been informed of a distressing diagnosis, or when the young person is feeling unwell.

The future

There is currently much debate about the care of adolescents in hospital. Ideally, they should be cared for on units designed and organized for their special needs (Kelly, 1991) with staff who have undergone further education in adolescent care. The education of ill adolescents both in hospital and the community is dependent upon the skill of the educator to communicate effectively and to have knowledge about available resources suited to adolescents.

Unfortunately the reality is that they often end up on adult wards with nurses who have no experience of their special needs and whose knowledge is generally based on personal experience. Adolescents who are admitted to children's wards may also experience problems because of the lack of recreational facilities and privacy.

It is unrealistic to expect that adolescent care will improve overnight but there are measures that will make patient education more effective. For example, developing clinical specialists in adolescent care to liaise with staff, parents and adolescents and act as a resource person for community and hospital staff would avoid some of the potential problems commonly experienced. In addition, the Action for Sick Children (formerly the National Association for the Welfare of Children in Hospital (NAWCH)) have published a report *Setting Standards for Adolescents in Hospital* (NAWCH, 1990) which contains checklists so that hospitals can look at their adolescent services and identify areas where change is needed. Finally, to conclude this section on education and the sick adolescent it seems appropriate to quote Thompson, who sums up the essence of the issues that have been explored.

Adolescent patients must be cared for not as children or adults but as an age group with specific needs. It is important to understand their development and how medical problems affect their mood, behaviour and coping. It is a special time in their lives, both psychologically and biologically. They need and deserve a special kind of understanding. (Thompson, 1990, p. 138)

SUGGESTED RESOURCE MATERIAL

Peer relationships

'Talking with Young People' (Video/Resource Pack) Open University Youth Services Project (1988).

'Health Education 13–18 Project' (Resource Pack) Schools Council/ Health Education Authority (1982).

'Double Take' (Drug Abuse – Video) DHSS (1985).

'TACADE' (Teachers Advisory Council on Alcohol and Drug Education) provides a great deal of information and teaching material relating to drug and alcohol abuse, including:

  Dealing with Solvent Misuse (1982)

  'Free to Choose' (Resource Pack)

  'Drugwise' (Resource Pack) – TACADE/HEA/SHEG.

Sexuality

Elliott, M. (1990) *Teenscape: A Personal Safety Programme for Teenagers*, Health Education Authority, London.

AIDS Facts (Folder and loose leaf sections) (1987) Cambridge Science Books.

'Choices' (Teachers pack and video), Bloomsbury Health Authority.

'Your choice for life: AIDS education for 14–16 year olds'. (Video) DES/Welsh Office (1987).

'Nursing and AIDS: Issues relating to young people' (Video) Department of Health (1990).

'Chances and Choices Ministry of Education', Western Australia (1991) (Video containing 5 trigger programmes about sexuality for 14–17-year-olds).

REFERENCES

Adams, B. (1983) Adolescent health care: needs, priorities and services. *The Nursing Clinics of North America*, **18**(2), 237–48.

Agras, W.S. and Kirkley, B.G. (1986) Bulimia: theories of etiology, in *Handbook of Eating Disorders* (eds. K.D. Brownell and J.P. Foreyt), Basic Books, New York.

Bee, H. (1989) *The Developing Child*, 5th edn, Harper and Row, New York.

Botvin, G. (1984) The Life Skills Training Model: A Broad Spectrum Approach to the Prevention of Cigarette Smoking, in *Health Education and Youth* (ed. G. Campbell), The Falmer Press, London.

Bowie, C. and Ford, N. (1989) Sexual behaviour of young people and the risk of HIV infection. *Journal of Epidemiology and Community Health*, **43**(1), 61–5.

Broadley, K. (1986) Falling Through the Net. *Nursing Times*, **82**(24), 29–30.

Burkitt, D.P. (1973) Some diseases characteristic of modern Western Civilisation. *British Medical Journal*, **1**, 274–8.

Curtis, H., Lawrence, C. and Tripp, J. (1989) Teenage Sexuality: implications for controlling AIDS. *Archives of Disease in Childhood*, **64**, 1240–5.

Davis, S. (1989) Pregnancy in Adolescents. *The Pediatric Clinics of North America*, **36**(3), 665–80.

Department of Health (1989) *An Introduction to The Children Act 1989*, HMSO, London.

Dixon, H. and Mullinar, G. (1983) *Taught Not Caught: strategies for sex education*, Learning Development Aids, Wisbech.

Donovan, C.F. (1988) Is there a place for adolescent screening in general practice. *Health Trends*, **20**, 64–5.

Dragone, M.A. (1990) Perspectives of chronically ill adolescents and parents on health care needs. *Pediatric Nursing*, **16**(1), 45–50.

Dryden, S. (1989) Paediatric medicine in the community. *Paediatric Nursing*, **1**(8), 17–18.

Dunphy, D.C. (1963) The Social Structure of Urban Adolescent Peer Groups. *Sociometry*, **26**, 230–46.

Erikson, E.H. (1963) *Childhood and Society*, Penguin Books Ltd, Harmondsworth.

French, J. (1984) Health Education and Youth: Whose Responsibility, in *Health Education and Youth* (ed. G. Campbell), Falmer Press, London.

Gibson, M. (1987) Developing what used to be 'the soft option'. *Health at School*, **2**(4), 116–17.

Graham, P. and Rutter, M. (1985) Adolescent Disorders, In *Child and Adolescent Psychiatry*, 2nd edn (eds. M. Rutter and L. Hersov), Blackwell Scientific Publications, Oxford.

Gray, E., Gammage, P. and Cottingham, M. (1987) *Smoking and Me*, Health Education Authority, London.

Gunn, S. (1987) Helping Parents to Cope with Adolescents. *Health at School*, **3**(3), 76–7.

Hersov, L. (1985) Adoption and Fostering, in *Child and Adolescent Psychiatry*, 2nd edn (eds. M. Rutter and L. Hersov), Blackwell Scientific Publications, Oxford.

Husson, R.N., Comeau, A. and Hoff, R. (1990) Diagnosis of human immunodeficiency virus in infants and children. *Pediatrics*, **86**(1), 1–9.

Jackson, R. (1988) Scoliosis in Juvenile and Adolescent Children. *Health Visitor*, **61**, 76–7.

Keating, D.P. (1980) Thinking Processes in Adolescence, in *Handbook of Adolescent Psychiatry* (ed. J. Adelson), Wiley, New York.

Kelly, J. (1991) Caring for Adolescents. *Professional Nurse*, **6**(9), 498–501.

Kolbe, L.J. (1984) Improving the Health of Children and Youth: Frameworks for Behavioral research and Development, in *Health Education and Youth* (ed. G. Campbell), Falmer Press, London.

Litt, I.F. and Cuskey, W.R. (1980) Compliance with Medical Regimens During Adolescence. *The Pediatric Clinics of North America*, **27**(1), 3–16.

Mackenzie, H. (1988) Teenagers in Hospital. *Nursing Times,* **84**(32), 58–60.
Mansfield, M.J. and Emans, S.J. (1989) Anorexia Nervosa, Athletics, and Amenorrhoea. *The Pediatric Clinics of North America,* **36**(3), 533–50.
Masterson, J. and Mordaunt, J. (1989) *Facing up to AIDS,* O'Brien Press, Dublin.
McClure, G.M. (1988) Suicide in Children in England and Wales. *Journal of Child Psychology and Psychiatry,* **29**(3), 345–9.
Moriaty, J. and Thomas, L. (1990) *Triple Jeopardy – Women and AIDS,* Panos Books, Washington DC.
Mussen, P.H., Conger, J.J., Kagan, J. and Huston, A.C. (1990) *Child Development and Personality,* 7th edn, Harper and Row, New York.
OPCS 1990 *Monitor* DH3 90/1 London Government Statistics Office.
Overton, W.F., Ward, S.L., Noveck, I.A. *et al.* (1987) Form and Content in the Development of Deductive Reasoning. *Developmental Psychology,* **23**(1), 22–30.
Pallikkathayil, L. and Tweed, S. (1983) Substance Abuse: Alcohol and Drugs During Adolescence. *The Nursing Clinics of North America,* **18**(2), 313–21.
Parry-Jones, W.L. (1985) Adolescent Disturbance, in *Child and Adolescent Psychiatry,* 2nd edn (eds. M. Rutter and L. Hersov), Blackwell Scientific Publications, Oxford.
Patrick, P. (1988) Sex Education, Homosexuality and the Law. *Health at School,* **3**(7), 201–2.
Reid, D. (1984) The Contribution of School Health Education Programmes to Health and Education, in *Health Education and Youth* (ed. G. Campbell), Falmer Press, London.
Russell, G.F.M. (1985) Anorexia and Bulimia Nervosa, in *Child and Adolescent Psychiatry,* 2nd edn (eds. M. Rutter and L. Hersov), Blackwell Scientific Publications, Oxford.
Schools Council/Health Education Council (1982) *Health Education 13–18,* Forbes Publications, London.
Scowen, P. (1988) AIDS Education in Schools: How to put the message across. *Health at School,* **3**(5), 142–5.
Simmons, R.J., Corey, M., Cowen, L. *et al.* (1985) Emotional adjustments of early adolescents with cystic fibrosis. *Psychosomatic Medicine,* **47**(2), 111–21.
Tauer, K.M. (1983) Promoting Effective Decision Making in Sexually Active Adolescents. *The Nursing Clinics of North America,* **18**(2), 275–92.
Thompson, J. (1990) The Adolescent with Cancer, in *The Child with Cancer – Nursing Care* (ed. J. Thompson), Scutari Press, London.
Tones, K., Tilford, S. and Robinson, Y. (1990) *Health Education: effectiveness and efficiency,* Chapman and Hall, London.
Vaughan, V.C. and Litt, I.F. (1990) *Child and Adolescent Development: clinical implications,* W.B. Saunders Company, Philadelphia.
Williams, T. (1986) School health education 15 years on. *Health Education Journal,* **45**, 3–7.

FURTHER READING

Campbell, G. (ed.) (1984) *Health Education and Youth,* Falmer Press, London.
Conger, J.J. (1991) *Adolescence and Youth,* 4th edn, Harper Collins.
Rutter, M. and Hersov, L. (eds.) (1985) *Child and Adolescent Psychiatry,* 2nd edn, Blackwell Scientific Publications, Oxford.
Vaughan, V.C. and Litt, I.F. (1990) *Child and Adolescent Development: Clinical implications,* W.B. Saunders Company, Philadelphia.

CHAPTER 7

The well and sick young adult

Miriam Rowswell

With the exception of women and their need for contraception and pregnancy-related care, the period of early adulthood is not part of the lifespan normally associated with particular health problems or health care needs. Attention is usually focused on the stages of childhood, adolescence and on the needs of the elderly and adult groups with special problems such as those with a disability or those from a different culture.

The healthy adult is an essential feature in the lives of all these vulnerable groups. It is the general adult population who conceive and rear children, cope with and care for the majority of the chronically sick, disabled and elderly, and work to finance the resources used by others. In turn they may well be future consumers rather than providers of health care, and demographic trends indicate that by the beginning of the 21st century there will be relatively fewer providers and a greater number of consumers. It is therefore essential that we preserve the potential of our young adults, maximizing opportunities to keep them healthier for longer.

In the early 1980s central government policy concentrated on personal responsibility for health and the need to convince individuals to change or avoid high-risk behaviours such as smoking or drug taking. Much of this activity was poorly organized, uncoordinated and did not achieve its aims. It was based on presenting messages about health threats and their causation, based usually on the most recent expert knowledge, and expecting behaviour modification to result. Recently, policy has been directed at developing a national strategy aimed at reducing premature deaths with established targets being set, e.g. a 40% reduction in death from strokes and heart disease in the under 65s by the end of the century (Department of Health, 1992). Impetus for this approach is partly a result of the Alma Ata Declaration and the subsequent establishment of European targets for Health for All (WHO, 1985).

Many of the conditions being targeted, such as heart disease and cancer, are chronic degenerative diseases that medicine is unable to cure and which are increasingly expensive to treat. As evidence has accumulated that their development can often be attributed to certain long-term patterns of behaviour such as smoking, or consumption of a high-fat and low-fibre diet, the need to promote healthy lifestyles has become more significant. It is therefore important that health education should be continued thoughout adult life in order to reinforce established healthy practices and counteract the multitude of anti-health pressures to which we are all exposed.

Current policy is to encourage and support the uptake of screening programmes and other preventive services. Revised contracts for general practitioners and dentists include preventive as well as curative responsibilities. Nurses will also inevitably be in the forefront of health promotion and education aimed at preventing disease at primary, secondary and tertiary levels. In order to meet this challenge it is important to understand the conflicts and dilemmas that exist when trying to facilitate greater individual responsibility for health within the wider social and environmental context in which individuals live.

It is envisaged that changes in nurse education introduced in Project 2000 programmes will better equip nurses to inform, advise, guide, assist and support their patients and clients to make and act on choices aimed at achieving and maintaining a higher level of physical, emotional, social and spiritual well-being. Rather than depending on the information giving, coercive and disease centred approach of the medical model it is anticipated that nurses will develop a range of strategies and approaches that will enable them to assist their patients and clients to make healthier choices and sustain changes aimed at improving health.

Legally deemed an adult at the age of 18, chronological age is only loosely related to biological and psychological maturation. It is generally accepted that the transitional phase of adolescence is completed by the nineteenth year, although psychological maturation and the process of becoming socially and financially independent may continue for several years longer. The phase of young adulthood spans the third and fourth decades of life. Precise parameters for this period vary according to the sources of data used.

Themes that dominate this phase of life are the transition to independent living, self-determination and the acquisition of personal autonomy. During this period, employment patterns are established and often some sort of career goals are set. The individual usually leaves the parental home and establishes his or her own home often in another location or region and may become exposed to new or different cultural influences. In addition, there is further exploration and development of relationships with others of the same sex and with those of the opposite sex that began during adolescence.

New patterns of daily living, communications with family and friends, sexual behaviour and a personal philosophy of life are developed and consolidated during this time. Decisions are made about jobs, about whether or not to commit oneself to one partner, about whether to have children or not. Contraceptive practices now facilitate the conscious postponement of reproduction, although this may generate new problems for women such as reduced fertility and a greater risk of obstetric complications. First births to women over 30 years of age increased by 4% between 1988 and 1989 according to the Chief Medical Officer's Report (1990) and these represented 23% of all first births within marriage compared with 14% in 1979.

The later part of this period of the lifespan is conventionally a period of consolidation when the focus is traditionally on work and family life. Social trends, however, suggest this may be changing. Many marriages are ending in divorce, increasing the numbers of one-parent families and 'single' people. Women have gained greater prominence in areas of work traditionally excluded to them and are often reluctant to relinquish the positions and financial independence they have gained for domesticity. Although more women are employed outside the home, the economic climate has resulted in us growing accustomed to the existence of a significant proportion of long-term unemployed.

The young adult is generally assumed to be in the 'prime of life' and is certainly likely to be at the peak of physical prowess. However, the acceptance of a broader concept of health suggests that other dimensions of health may be threatened by life events. There is evidence that physical as well as mental health may be put at risk by the stress induced by readjustment to a range of life events such as marriage, divorce, change or loss of job, change of residence, and even holidays (Holmes and Rahe, 1967; Theorell *et al.*, 1975).

Blaxter (1990), reporting on the results of a major health and lifestyle survey conducted in 1984/5, commented on the variations in expressed concepts of health with age. Young men generally defined health in terms of physical fitness and strength whereas young women focused on energy, vitality and an ability to cope. Older adults emphasized mental as well as physical well-being and the ability to function even in the presence of disease and disability. The young unemployed experienced more psycho-social malaise and those over 30 were less fit than their employed contemporaries. This finding appears to support others that have suggested that negative concepts of self worth and impoverishment resulting from long-term unemployment result in poor physical and mental health. This OPCS Longitudinal Study demonstrated a relationship between unemployment and suicide or attempted suicide. Understanding of the multidimensional concept of health is therefore essential when trying to establish with the client realistic goals.

ILL HEALTH IN THE YOUNG ADULT

Health statistics generally focus on negative aspects of health, e.g. mortality, morbidity and the incidence and prevalence of specific conditions and diseases.

After early childhood, mortality rates increase with increasing age. In the twenties it remains relatively stable at about 0.58 per thousand (OPCS, 1990a) but starts to increase in the thirties to a rate of about 1.0 per thousand for people aged 35–9. A gender difference in mortality is most pronounced in the 20–4 year old age group when the female mortality rate is less than half that of men. By the end of fourth decade the female mortality rate is approximately two thirds that of males (see Figure 7.1).

Examination of the causes of death in young adults demonstrates that injury and poisoning is the most frequent reason for death in those aged 20–30. This includes motor vehicle accidents which account for over half these deaths in both sexes. Over the age of 35 circulatory disease becomes the commonest cause of mortality in men, whereas in women of the same age it is cancer. Deaths from breast cancer and cervical cancer predominate over other malignant neoplasms.

Mortality trends in this age group have been highlighted as a cause of concern in the Chief Medical Officer's Report (1990) because of an increase in mortality rates since 1984. Reductions in deaths from cardiovascular disease appear to have been cancelled out by increased mortality due to injury and poisoning. Since motor vehicle accident deaths have also decreased, deaths due to suicide and injury whether accidentally or purposefully inflicted appear to account for this trend. For women there has also been an increase in the rate of suicide and undetermined injury fatalities in the youngest group and an increase in deaths from cancer in the over 30s.

Morbidity is determined from data derived from sources such as General Household Surveys (GHS) and Hospital In-patient Enquiries. As might be expected, young adults experience less ill health than other adult groups. Serious illness is commoner in men aged 21–5 than in women (Wadsworth, 1986) but in common with other age groups women consistently report more symptoms of physical and mental illness and use GP and hospital services more than their male counterparts.

Information from the General Household Survey (OPCS, 1989) suggests that young women are twice as likely to have been hospital

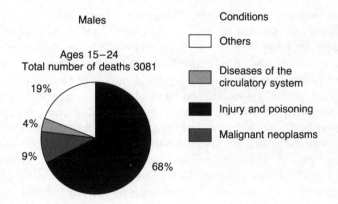

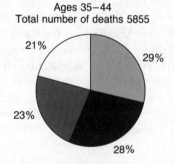

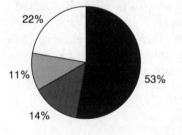

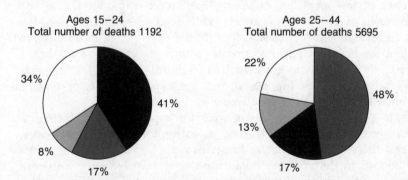

Figure 7.1 Selected causes of death by age-group, England and Wales 1988 (Source: Chief Medical Officer's Report (1990).

in-patients as men. This is largely attributable to pregnancy-related admissions. Women are also twice as likely to have consulted a doctor and to have had on average twice as many GP consultations. This applies to women whether they are working, unemployed or economically inactive. Commonly reported causes of long-standing illness were back problems, asthma and arthritis. Reasons for this greater apparent morbidity in women appear to be complex and cannot be explained just by the contribution of symptoms attributable to menstruation and pregnancy. Blaxter (1990) showed that exclusion of menstrual related symptoms still resulted in women reporting a greater prevalence of some of the commonest illness symptoms and a greater level of psycho-social malaise. Examination of patterns of admission for mental health problems demonstrate that young women are likely to be admitted for treatment of affective psychoses, neurotic disorders and depression. Men are more likely to be admitted for the treatment of schizophrenia, alcoholism and drug dependency.

Suggested explanations for these sex differences in morbidity include the possibility that patterns of socialization and cultural factors make it easier for women to admit to symptoms; that women experience a greater degree of stress that men in trying to fulfil the multiple roles of mother, housewife and employee or alternatively that social pressures encourage men to neglect their health and be selective in their use of medical services.

INFLUENCING THE HEALTH OF YOUNG ADULTS

The Black Report (Townsend and Davidson, 1982) demonstrated the existence of health inequalities between the social classes. Social class gradients in the mortality of young men were apparent for all the major causes of death except cancer. Whitehead's re-examination of the situation (Townsend *et al.*, 1988) found little evidence of differences in illness rates between socio-economic groups in young adults but a dramatic socio-economic gradient in the middle aged. This suggests that certain groups of the population are exposed to factors which differentially affect their health over a period of time.

Debate continues about the relative importance of social circumstances, such as occupation, income, housing, location, marital status, etc., and the effect of particular lifestyles and their associated patterns of behaviour in determining health and contributing to the apparent differences. As previously stated the importance of personal responsibility has been stressed in recent attempts to promote health. The public have been encouraged to participate in 'preventive behaviours'. The traditional preventive approach concentrates on information giving and assumes that the majority of people have an 'internal health locus of control'. Alternative methods used by health educators have focused on empowering individuals and communities by developing decision-making skills and presenting information about health-related issues in supposedly value-free ways. This may or may not result in the adoption of the 'appropriate' behaviour.

Whilst this strategy attempts to address and explore attitudes and beliefs about health it has been criticized along with the information-giving approach for ignoring the effects of external socio-economic factors over which individuals in reality have little control. For example there are many occupations where workers may be exposed to toxic substances, carcinogens and radiation; there is limited choice of housing in industrial areas where significant air pollution is associated with a high incidence of asthma and other respiratory conditions; families existing on a low income tend to have poor diets and occupy damp and cold accommodation which is not conducive to good health; and home-less families existing in bed and breakfast accommodation are likely to experience a variety of physical and mental health problems. All these situations are inherently unhealthy but the stress of enduring them may lead individuals concerned to adopt unhealthy behaviours, such as smoking, as coping mechanisms.

Evidence accumulated in the health and lifestyle survey (Blaxter, 1990) suggested that in fact social circumstances, which included social support, were more important in determining health than behaviour. It appeared that 'unhealthy behaviour does not reinforce disadvantage to the extent that healthy behaviour increases advantage'. The conclusion must be that policy focusing on changing personal attitudes and be-haviour should be combined with wider health promotion activities aimed at making 'healthier choices easier choices' through a variety of legal, fiscal, social, economic and public health measures. Use of this approach shifts attention from individual behaviour and directs it at the activities of, in the case of alcohol for example, the alcohol industry, advertisers and the licensing authorities whilst also seeking the co-operation of trades unions and employers in disseminating safer drinking guidelines.

This approach may also be criticized. It has been claimed to be educationally unsound because it restricts individual free choice such as whether or not to wear a seat-belt and where or when a cigarette may be smoked and whilst imposing behaviour change it does not necessarily result in 'healthier' attitudes. This may result in behaviour change being short lived, e.g. a no-smoking policy in the workplace may result in more cigarettes being smoked at home.

A current popular approach to promoting health is the community development or community participation approach where professionals act as facilitators enabling individuals to participate in collective action aimed at bringing about healthier environments and healthier lifestyles.

Examples of this approach include the work of organizations such as the Terrence Higgins Trust originally established by members of the gay community in response to the spread of AIDS amongst homosexual men. Its work has expanded enormously. As well as offering support to affected individuals and their carers, the Trust provides education and information about AIDS and HIV which is not just confined to the so-called high-risk groups. Other examples of this type of approach are the work of numerous self-help groups, established by those with common problems or needs, for example the Haemophilia Society, the National Childbirth Trust and The British Association for Cancer United Patients (BACUP) to name just three. Doctors and nurses are often involved in these organizations in an advisory capacity. At a local level health visitors may be involved in enabling small groups of clients in the community to establish mother and baby groups for mutual support.

Health careers

The concept of a health career (Dorn and Nortoft, 1982) suggests that health is determined through the way we interact and respond to environmental, cultural and social factors. Thus a lifestyle healthy or otherwise is a function of how and where we are brought up, our peer groups, the jobs we do and the people we work with and the social pressures on individuals and groups. Each individual has a health career that runs parallel to their occupational career. Careful assessment of a person's health career will yield valuable information to the professional seeking to positively influence that individual's health.

BEHAVIOUR PATTERNS IN EARLY ADULTHOOD

Tobacco use

Most individuals who smoke start to do so in adolescence, and their smoking habit is well established in early adulthood. Although in recent years the overall prevalence of smoking has declined at a rate of 1% per year this is due mainly to existing smokers giving up. In the 35–40-year-old age group equal numbers of men and women are ex-smokers (OPCS, 1983). The 1988 General Household Survey (GHS) quoted in the Chief Medical Officer's Report (1990) records a smoking prevalence in women aged 20–4 of 37% compared to 30% of all women and 32% of men and women. Up to a quarter of these women give up smoking by the age of 34. For men who are in manual employment it is the expense of smoking that appears to be the crucial factor that results in them giving up, rather than the fear of illness (OPCS, 1983). It is apparent that there is still a considerable way to go if the target of achieving a non-smoking environment for 80% of population is to be met (WHO, 1989).

Alcohol use

Alcohol consumption has been steadily increasing as price relative to disposable income has more than halved since 1960. Young people drink more heavily than other age groups. Dight (1976) found that in Scotland 30% of the alcohol consumed was drunk by 3% of the population who were predominantly young male working class men between 18 and 24 years of age. Blaxter (1990) found that in the Health and Lifestyle survey, 46% of men aged 18–39 reported a moderate or heavy alcohol consumption (11–50 units in the previous week). 28% of women claimed to be moderate or heavy drinkers (6–35 units). In addition to the effects on health of long-term chronic alcohol use there are problems caused by acute intoxication resulting in accidents, especially those involving motor vehicles, and crimes against people and property – the so-called 'lager lout' syndrome. The cost to industry alone in terms of sickness and absenteeism is in the region of £630 million a year. Alcohol education has aimed at promoting sensible drinking habits rather than promoting abstinence. Plant (1987) suggests that the majority of young people who drink excessively when young and single drastically reduce their consumption as they grow older or marry. Often a driving accident or dramatic incident triggers a change in behaviour, or other motivating pressures such as new friends,

Figure 7.2 Sensible drinking – limits to help you avoid damaging your health

For men: up to 21 units a week
For women: up to 14 units a week
Spreading out your drinks throughout the week is safer than concentrating it in bouts of drinking when you increase your chance of having an accident. Even one or two drinks may be dangerous if you are driving, operating machinery or taking certain types of medicine.

Damage to your health is likely if you are:
a man and drink 36 or more units a week;
a woman and drink 22 or more units a week.

If you are pregnant or planning to have a baby the less alcohol you drink, the better your chances of a successful pregnancy and a healthy baby.

1 unit of alcohol is equivalent to half a pint of ordinary beer/lager; a glass of wine; a single measure of spirits; a small glass of sherry.

interests, a partner or a job which depends on driving result in a different lifestyle.

Other forms of substance abuse

Upward trends in drug abuse amongst young people were noted in the Chief Medical Officer's Report (1990). Illicit drugs are generally used in a fairly limited way for a short period of time and tend to be a problem of the younger, unmarried adult. Legally prescribed mood-altering drugs such as the benzodiazepines have become less of a problem amongst the young adult age group as their ability to produce tolerance and dependence has been widely recognized.

Exercise

Regular vigorous physical activity is recommended as providing some degree of protection against coronary heart disease. Young adults exercise more and are on average fitter than older individuals. In the Health and Lifestyle Survey (Blaxter, 1990) 61% of men and 43% of women aged 18–39 claimed to participate in active sports and keep fit to keep healthy.

Figure 7.3 Summary of the major dietary recommendations

NACNE	*COMA*
Reduce total fat consumption (Fat intake should supply on average 30% of total energy intake with saturated fat supplying no more than 10%)	Reduce total fat consumption (Fat intake should be no more than 35% of total energy intake with saturated fat supplying 15% or less. Polyunsaturated fat should be substituted for saturated fat)
Reduce sugar consumption	No increase in sugar consumption
Increase fibre intake to at least 30 g a day by increasing intake of whole grain cereals, fruit and vegetables	Increase intake of fibre-rich carbohydrates to compensate for energy requirement previously met by fats
Reduce salt intake	No increase in salt consumption. A reduction would be advisable

54% of men and 59% of young women said they would like to take more exercise to keep themselves healthy. This trend obviously needs to be encouraged, put into practice and maintained. Balanced against a need to encourage greater levels of physical activity is the emerging problem of leisure accidents, especially sports-related injuries.

Diet

Dietary guidelines recommended by the National Advisory Committee on Nutrition Education (NACNE) and the Committee on Medical Aspects of Food Policy (COMA) reports are widely available and healthy eating policies have gradually been adopted by health and local authorities and other major employers. Media coverage of issues related to diet and health have also emphasized recommendations of these two reports. There is some evidence (OPCS, 1990b) to suggest that dietary habits have changed over the last decade. Sales of wholemeal bread and reduced fat milk in particular are indices of this change and the public has recently been submitted to a series of food safety scares (*Salmonella*; *Listeria*; bovine spongiform encephalopathy (BSE); etc.) which may have served to raise consciousness about food-related issues. Surveys suggest that women appear to eat more healthily and are more likely to intend to make healthier changes in their diets than men (Blaxter, 1990; Charny and Lewis, 1989). Young adults who change their diets appear to do so more commonly to change their appearance than on health grounds.

Sexual and reproductive behaviour

If they have multiple sexual partners sexually active young adults, both homosexual and heterosexual, are at risk of developing sexually transmitted diseases, including hepatitis B and HIV infections. Cervical cancer has also been associated with sexual behaviour in that a woman who first has intercourse before the age of 17, who has multiple sexual partners or whose partner has had other sexual relationships is at greater risk of developing the condition. As stated previously, although relatively few in number, when compared to the total number of women with cervical cancer, there has been a worrying increase in the incidence of young women with this form of cancer.

The spread of HIV infection in this age group is not known but from the increase in AIDS cases reported as being acquired through heterosexual intercourse it is likely that this will become a significant health problem for sexually active young adults. Efforts directed at limiting the spread of HIV infection through 'safer sexual practices' are also likely to reduce the incidence of other sexually transmitted conditions. This has been demonstrated to be the case amongst homosexual men where infections with gonorrhoea have decreased as the rate of infection with HIV has dropped. Unfortunately there is little evidence that this is so in the heterosexual population. As a result of government-initiated campaigns and media coverage, public knowledge about the AIDS problem is high (DHSS, 1987). Unfortunately evaluation of the effects of all the publicity on the behaviour of young adults suggests that behaviour change has been limited. This is mainly because individuals do not see themselves at risk especially if they are serially monogamous. There is often uncertainty about what constitutes 'safer sex' and difficulty adopting these practices due to a lack of confidence or assertiveness.

Road accidents

The behaviour of young people as road users has been identified as a cause for concern in view of the significant mortality resulting from road traffic accidents. Prevention of unnecessary deaths on the roads involves behaviour changes in addition to improvements in vehicle safety and road design. The main initiatives have been directed at reducing accidents caused by drinking and driving and using legislation to enforce the wearing of seat-belts. Since 1 July 1991 the law has now been extended to make compulsory the wearing of rear seat-belts by adults where these are fitted. It is worth noting that the combination of education and legislation appears to be relatively successful in encouraging parents to restrain their children adequately when travelling in cars (Baijal *et al.*, 1988).

OPPORTUNITIES FOR HEALTH PROMOTION AND PATIENT TEACHING

Primary prevention or health promotion aimed at encouraging young adults to adopt and sustain healthier lifestyles needs to be combined with secondary prevention aimed at identifying those at particular risk of developing a health problem, e.g. workers who are exposed to substances that might give rise to occupational asthma, individuals with raised cholesterol levels, or those in whom the disease process can be identified and treated at an early stage, e.g. asymptomatic hypertension, carcinoma *in-situ* of the cervix, etc. Also included in the approach are strategies aimed at informing people about symptoms that should be investigated at an early stage such as breast and testicular lumps, changes in warts and moles and unexplained bleeding. All screening activities need to be accompanied by information and education if they are to be effective and to avoid generating unnecessary anxiety. A problem in screening a young adult population is that of cost effectiveness because many of the conditions being screened for do not become apparent even at a very early stage until later life. If however the philosophy of prevention is encouraged by the judicious use of screening from an early age then it is more likely to be perceived as an acceptable and routine procedure as people get older.

With the exception of those young adults with chronic health problems such as diabetes most individuals by virtue of their better health have only limited contact with health professionals. It is therefore vital to maximize opportunities that arise.

For many young women the need for contraceptive advice offers a regular point of contact. While women should be encouraged to make choices about their contraceptive method, offered cervical smears, rubella screening, weighed regularly and have blood pressure monitored and be taught breast self-examination, etc., these activities are not always presented as being health promotion. Dietary information and advice on drinking or stress reduction techniques may be seen as irrelevant unless labelled as preconceptual counselling. This information, however, is relevant to all women whether they plan a pregnancy or not.

Antenatal care is another opportunity for promoting health with an almost literally captive audience. Antenatal clinic waiting times could be more effectively utilized for this purpose. Most women do accept the need for antenatal care and because of concern for their unborn child are perhaps more receptive at this time than any other to health advice.

There exists no equivalent point of contact for men of this age so it is important that male partners are encouraged to accompany women and welcomed at family planning and antenatal clinics, providing this does not result in compromising the woman's choice. Initiatives such as the 'Men Too' campaign tried to encourage men to attend family planning clinics, and are welcomed. Video demonstration of testicular self-examination techniques could be made available at relatively little extra cost and weight and blood pressure monitored easily.

Other contacts with health professionals which are available to both men and women are occupational health services and general practitioners. GP contracts now include specific responsibilities for monitoring health and offering health checks, although many are delegating these tasks to practice nursing staff. Roland (1989) claims that over 95% of the population have contact with their GP over a three-year period and thus there exists great potential for health education in general practice. Strategies used by general practitioners are reviewed by Roland and include waiting room displays, use of leaflets during routine consultations, audiotapes and videos. Some practices have established practice libraries and have facilitated health education groups and self-help groups. Whilst in reality health education plays a relatively small part in most doctor–patient interactions and is conducted in a traditional didactic way, practice nurses may become very effective health educators giving advice, health instruction, education and providing follow-up and support (Stilwell *et al.*, 1987).

Occupational health practitioners are becoming more active in promoting a holistic and proactive approach to health rather than concentrating just on the prevention of occupational related injury and ill health. Such an approach requires the co-operation and support of management who may need to be convinced of the benefits, for example, of a screening programme for hypertension. These may be both financial, in terms of less absenteeism or chronic sickness, as well as improved morale, motivation and therefore ultimately increased output. As workers spend up to a third of their waking hours in the workplace the occupational health practitioner has a large relatively captive audience. Many employers have been persuaded to participate in the 'Look After Your Heart' campaign (Crew, 1988), which now involves 3 million employees, with the emphasis on promoting a healthy diet, encouraging exercise, e.g. by running aerobic exercise classes at work, implementing smoking policies, offering support to smokers who wish to give up, educating people about the negative effects of stress and ways of managing stress and screening employees for coronary heart disease risk factors. Other health promotion initiatives that occupational health nurses may become involved in include 'Alcohol Education in the Workplace', which is aimed at reducing the cost of male alcohol-related sickness and absenteeism.

The role of the hospital nurse in health promotion

When young adults are admitted to hospital it is usually only for investigative procedures or for relatively minor surgery such as excision of benign lumps, treatment of haemorrhoids, varicose veins, gynaecological conditions and traumatic injuries. With the exception of the latter, these do not involve lengthy admissions. Nevertheless all admissions can be opportunities for promoting health and this should become an integral part of nursing care rather than an activity to be undertaken if the ward is quiet. Thorough assessment of each individual using a range of communication skills is essential. Promoting health may be about informing and counselling the patient in relation to their presenting condition or about giving appropriate advice about changing unhealthy behaviour. If any intervention is to be successful it must take account of the patient's own desire to acquire information and participate in decision making. Promoting health may also involve recognizing and responding to needs unrelated to the presenting problem. For example, a business man admitted for a haemorrhoidectomy may express concern about his lifestyle in view of a family history of hypertension or might mention the difficulties he experiences coping with jet lag when on foreign business trips. Teaching relaxation techniques or giving advice on coping with the effects of air travel would both be interventions aimed at enhancing his health. If the nurse is unable to provide the information required then a facilitatory role directing the patient to a resource will encourage active participation.

Young adults also often visit patients in hospitals. Rather than disappearing at visiting times, nurses may be able to use these as opportunities for health promotion. Ward resource 'centres' may provide written information for patients and visitors. Discussions may be initiated between staff, patients and their visitors. For example the daughters of a patient with breast cancer may welcome the opportunity to discuss the relative benefits of breast self-examination and breast screening.

The following case studies illustrate in more detail some of the situations where health education and patient teaching are integral parts of the health care a patient or client should receive. In each case the familiar nursing process framework of assessing planning, implementing and evaluating care is recommended as a systematic approach to undertaking health teaching and the promotion of healthier lifestyles.

CASE STUDIES

Case study 1

Consider the case of Phil who is 19 years old. He has been born and brought up in Liverpool and his parents and four brothers and sisters lived in a cramped and damp privately rented basement flat. As a child he always seemed to have a cough or cold and when he was 3 had a severe attack of bronchopneumonia. Eventually the family was rehoused in a block of council flats on an estate. Both his mother and father were unemployed and smoked heavily. There were frequent rows which often resulted in his father disappearing for weeks at a time. Phil smoked his first cigarette at 8, egged on by friends, and by 12 smoked regularly. Cigarettes were easily come by both at home, and from local shopkeepers. Sometimes Phil resorted to shoplifting to finance his smoking. He often played truant from school and would hang about the city centre where he occasionally experimented with glue sniffing and was introduced to a variety of drugs including heroin. At 16 Phil got a place on a YTS scheme and was placed with a small firm of electricians. Since completing the scheme he has been officially unemployed but has had a variety of light labouring jobs. Lunchtimes and most evenings are spent in the pub with his workmates. Phil gave up playing five-a-side football, preferring to watch sport on TV. He said he had grown out of the game but his increasing weight combined with smoking 20 or more cigarettes a day have made him breathless on exertion and in the winter he seemed to have a permanent chesty cough.

The reader may wish to consider whether or not Phil can be deemed healthy and identify the various factors that have influenced his health career to date. What opportunities exist that could have assisted Phil in developing a healthier lifestyle and how might his future health as a young adult be positively influenced?

Case study 2

Andrew is a 28-year-old man who works as a salesman for a small company manufacturing air filters. He is engaged to Val and they plan to get married in a few months time. Andrew has been hospitalized for several weeks following the diagnosis and treatment of an acute attack of ulcerative colitis which has subsided with a combination of rest, drug therapy and an elemental diet. A teaching plan is developed and implemented to take account of Andrew and Val's information needs throughout the admission. This would involve assessment of what Andrew and Val want to know about the condition; selection of information Andrew will need as the basis for making decisions about changes in his lifestyle that might be helpful in reducing the likelihood of recurrence and information on how to cope with exacerbations of the condition. This stage of the teaching process would also involve assessment of the appropriate timing of any intervention, e.g. Andrew and Val may be anxious about their children inheriting the condition or the possiblity of it developing into bowel cancer, but this would be unlikely to be a priority whilst Andrew is acutely ill.

Planning involves dividing the information into manageable amounts to be given at appropriate stages so that Andrew is not overwhelmed. Goals would need to be established with the couple, e.g. they would both demonstrate knowledge of the disease and be able to describe the treatment plan and medication programme. Understanding of the disease process would be demonstrated by Andrew reporting modifications that he could make to his patterns of work and his diet and his domestic and social activities in order to cope with frequent bowel motions.

Implementation involves the nurse selecting the most suitable teaching strategy and teaching aids. Initial information may be presented in a traditional didactic way with the assistance of written information in the form of booklets to which Andrew and Val can refer to reinforce or clarify details. At some point Andrew and Val will need an opportunity to explore and discuss their feelings with a doctor or nurse and to raise specific questions and anxieties. This participative approach would also be required to enable Andrew to identify factors in his life that might contribute to a recurrence and activities that he might be able to successfully modify. Provision of support and follow-up on discharge would need to be considered. Andrew and Val could also be put in touch with other individuals of a similiar age with the same condition and encouraged to contact the local group of the National Association for Colitis and Crohn's Disease.

Evaluation of the teaching plan would be undertaken in the light of the goals established by getting Andrew to explain what he understands about the condition and its treatment and to establish what changes Andrew intends to make when he is discharged. Achievement or progress towards his goals should ideally be reappraised with him at follow-up visits and changed if they are inappropriate.

Examples of goals for Andrew

---

1. Andrew will be able to describe dietary changes required and identify particular foods that exacerbate his symptoms. A high protein, high carbohydrate and low calorie diet may be recommended. Andrew may find that if certain foods are eliminated from his diet distressing symptoms may be relieved. Iced and carbonated drinks, fruits and vegetables, and dairy produce are often those best avoided.

2. Andrew will be able to resume a normal working and social life. Suggest that Andrew may acquire a disabled car sticker and use a 'Can't Wait' card to help him find a toilet quickly when away from home.

Case study 3

Rick is 22 years old and works on a building site. He is in hospital on traction for a badly fractured femur following a motorcyle accident in which his bike careered out of control on black ice. In conversation with nursing staff Rick often recalls drinking sessions in his local with all his mates and boasts about some of the close scrapes they have had with police over drinking and driving. His friends often come in after they have been in the pub and bring Rick cans of lager. Rick's drinking behaviour appears to be potentially harmful to himself and to others although it has not contributed directly to his current problem. An opportunity exists whilst Rick is in hospital to undertake some health education about alcohol and sensible drinking. A teaching plan will need to be devised that takes account of Rick's own beliefs and attitudes about drinking.

Much of the assessment process is likely to be undertaken informally, building up information about his drinking habits, when, where and how much Rick drinks; whether or not he perceives his drinking as a problem; whether or not he is aware of it being a problem for others in his circle of friends. From this information it may be possible to identify if Rick drinks excessively and whether this is due to lack of knowledge or due to 'inappropriate' attitudes towards drinking. It is important to establish if Rick is motivated to making any changes in his drinking habits.

The short-term goal of this exercise may be initially to enable Rick to think about his drinking activities and identify what the advantages and disadvantages are for him. Secondly, Rick may need some information about the physiological effects of alcohol on short-term performance and/or on future health and be able to assess his own drinking in the light of recommended limits. In the longer term if Rick expresses a desire to reduce or change his drinking habits, possibilities for achieving change can be explored with him and strategies developed to facilitate these changes. For example, how to avoid certain situations where Rick would be inclined to exceed his limits, how to reward himself for refusing 'one for the road' etc.

In order to implement such a plan, attention to the relationship between Rick and those undertaking the education is crucial. Good communication skills are essential and if Rick feels overtly or covertly criticized or pressurized he may well reject attempts to address this issue. It is likely that he will be more receptive to a professional he respects and likes and with whom he has already established a good relationship and perhaps who he perceives as sharing the same interests and values. This case illustrates the potential advantage of a system where primary nursing is used and an effective nurse–patient relationship established. Opportunities which arise spontaneously can be utilized to enable informal teaching to take place but within a structured overall plan.

Evaluation is likely to depend on establishing whether Rick has

Examples of goals for Rick

---

1. Rick will be able to calculate his weekly alcohol consumption and estimate whether it is within the advised limits.

2. Rick will describe strategies he could use to help him reduce his alcohol consumption from 40 to 20 units per week. For example:
   - drink something non-alcoholic to quench thirst;
   - avoid getting involved in rounds by buying his own drinks;
   - drinking more slowly and choosing half pints rather than pints;
   - decide how much he is going to drink and sticking to that limit by keeping count.

undergone any significant attitude change as demonstrated by an expression of interest in modifying his drinking. In the long term, effectiveness of the intervention will be advantaged if this can be maintained when Rick returns home.

Case study 4

Jenny is a 35-year-old supervisor in a high street store. She is married with three children. Jenny had a cervical smear taken at work by the occupational health nurse as part of a well woman screening programme. Jenny had been having regular smears at the family planning clinic up until six years ago but then her husband had a vasectomy and she never got round to seeing her GP, despite reminder letters. Jenny admitted that the absence of a female doctor in her practice had put her off attending and the local well woman clinics seemed to be at times which never fitted in with her family and work commitments. The occupational health nurse noted that Jenny's first baby had been born when she was just 18. The smear has been reported as being cervical intraepithelial neoplasia grade III (CIN III) and Jenny will need referral for a colposcopy. The term cervical intraepithelial neoplasia denotes a continuum of abnormalities of the epithelial cells of the cervix ranging from mild dysplasia, CIN I, through to severe dysplasia or carcinoma *in-situ*, CIN III. CIN III is considered to be a pre-malignant condition, and the risk of it progressing to become invasive carcinoma of the cervix if left untreated is believed to be high. A teaching plan implemented for Jenny at this point should be developed based on information and advice given prior to the smear.

Assessment at this stage would have established what Jenny understood about the purpose of the test. It is particularly important that women understand that the smear is intended to detect changes in cells of the cervix before they have become malignant. A positive result indicates some abnormality of the cells that requires further investigation and possibly minor treatment to eliminate the possibility of cancer developing in the future. Many women are unaware that up to 1 in 10 may be recalled for a repeat smear and that the incidence of a positive result is in the region of 1 in 50 women.

Despite adequate preparation and explanation, notification of a positive smear with changes observed suggestive of severe dysplasia or carcinoma *in-situ* is likely to cause considerable anxiety. As there is often some delay in obtaining an appointment for a gynaecological opinion and for colposcopy it is important that Jenny is reassured that having opted to be screened for a potentially malignant condition, effective treatment is available. Screening alone does not promote health but must be complemented by a planned programme of education and support.

In Jenny's case this is likely to involve explanation of the referral process and discussion about possible treatment options. Opportunities to ask questions and seek further clarification of information are likely to be important for Jenny as part of her decision-making process. Jenny should be offered support and information as soon as she is made aware of the smear result. She will probably appreciate follow-up on either a formal or informal basis and be reassured by the knowledge that she can contact a particular individual for further information and support.

Jenny should choose who this person is and there needs to be close liasion particularly with her GP. Continuing support may be required until and after Jenny has been seen and given appropriate treatment. As there has been considerable media coverage of cervical cancer and links to sexual behaviour it is important to provide an opportunity to discuss Jenny's feelings and attempt to alay any misconceptions that she may have. For further information about cervical smears and their meaning various sources of information are available such as the Women's National Cancer Control Campaign; Women's Health and Reproductive Rights Centre; and books written for women (Barker, 1987; Quilliam, 1989; and Posner, 1987).

In the long term Jenny needs to be reassured that she will be carefully followed up and that after treatment she will need regular smears probably at yearly intervals. Liaison will be required to ensure that this is undertaken either by the gynaeocologist or by the GP or by the occupational health department.

As Jenny smokes about 10–15 cigarettes a day she may wish to consider giving up smoking in the long term to eliminate a further risk factor associated with the development of cancer of the cervix and this option can be discussed with Jenny when she is less anxious (see Figure 7.4).

Examples such as these typify difficulties that might arise when attempting to fulfil the role of health promoter and patient educator. Andrew's case is an example of tertiary prevention and is likely to be one where the professional's input is welcomed because of the need to learn to adjust to an existing health problem. Jenny's case illustrates some of the issues associated with screening or secondary prevention. Screening programmes can only be effective when individuals can be reassured of effective treatment and support if they should be found to be at risk or if they have the early stages of a potentially serious condition. Primary prevention in the form of promoting a change in lifestyle is illustrated by Rick's case. In reality this is probably the most difficult intervention to implement and evaluate as the message may be rejected or not retained. It is important that opportunities such as this are not ignored however challenging or daunting they may seem. In

Figure 7.4 *Smoking – giving it up*: a strategy to help the smoker

Step 1 Think about stopping
Identify the reasons why you smoke.
Be aware of how giving up smoking may improve your health, e.g.
    reduced risk of coronary heart disease and cancer; fewer coughs and
    chest infections, etc.
Identify other advantages to you of giving up, e.g. more money to
    spend; better tasting food; clothes no longer smell stale.

Step 2 Prepare to stop
Identify where and when you usually smoke as you will need to avoid
    these situations as much as possible.
Plan new activities to replace smoking and distract yourself, such as
    going for a walk after a meal instead of smoking a cigarette.
Decide on a day to stop. Choose a day when you expect to be fairly
    relaxed.
Get rid of cigarettes, lighters, etc. the day before.
Identify family and friends whose support you will need. Tell them your
    plans in advance and enlist their help.

Step 3 Stop
Plan a reward for yourself at the end of the day.
Change your routine to avoid situations that give you the urge to
    smoke.
When you feel the urge to smoke do something else.
Keep reminding yourself that any unpleasant side-effects – stomach
    upsets, bad cough, irritable feelings, etc. – will pass off.

Step 4 Staying stopped
Take each day one at a time.
For the first few weeks give yourself plenty to do.
Don't be tempted to smoke any cigarettes at all.
Put aside the money you are saving.
Keep reminding yourself of the benefits you are gaining.
Make contact with local support groups. Your GP, health visitor or
    health promotion unit will be able to put you in contact with these if
    you feel they help.

combination with other multidisciplinary efforts aimed at promoting safer drinking, modification of an individual's drinking habits may eventually occur.

The benefits of promoting health through education, screening, patient teaching on an individual level and through influencing policy and practice on a societal level with not be appreciated overnight but must be a goal worth persuing if the young adults of today are to avoid being the patients of tomorrow.

REFERENCES

Baijal, E., Carter, H., Jones, I.G. and Walkingham, I.W. (1988) The role of infant car seats in road safety. *Journal of the Institute of Health Education*, **26**(4), 176–81.

Barker, G. (1987) *Your smear test*, Adamson Books, London.

Blaxter, M. (1990) *Health and lifestyles*, Tavistock/Routledge, London.

Charny, M. and Lewis, P.A. (1989) Eating patterns in a randomly selected population: current behaviour and trends. *Journal of the Institute of Health Education*, **27**(I), 34–9.

Chief Medical Officer, Department of Health (1990) *On the state of the public health*, HMSO, London.

Crew, V. (1988) *Look after your Heart: A six months Report*. The Health Education Authority, London.

Department of Health (1992) *The health of the nation: a strategy for health in England*. Cm 1986, HMSO, London.

Department of Health and Social Security (1987) *AIDS. Monitoring response to the public education campaign February 1986–February 1987*, HMSO, London.

Dight, S. (1976) *Scottish drinking habits*, HMSO, Edinburgh.

Dorn, N. and Nortoft, B. (1982) *Health careers: Teachers manual*, ISSD, London.

Holmes, T.H. and Rahe, R.H. (1967) The social maladjustment rating scale. *Journal of Psychosomatic Research*, **II**, 213–18.

Office of Population Cersuses and Surveys (1983) *Smoking attitudes and behaviour*, HMSO, London.

Office of Population Censuses and Surveys (1989) *General Household Survey 1987*, Series GHS no. 17, HMSO, London.

Office of Population Censuses and Surveys (1990a) *1988 Mortality Statistics*, Series DH I no. 21, HMSO, London.

Office of Population Censuses and Surveys (1990b) *The dietary and nutritional survey of British adults*, HMSO, London.

Plant, M. (1987) *Drugs in perspective*, Hodder and Stoughton, London.

Posner, T. (1987) *An abnormal smear – what does it mean? A woman's guide to the medical investigation and treatment of abnormal cells*, Women's Health and Reproductive Rights Information Centre, London.

Quilliam, S. (1989) *Positive smear*, Penguin Books, Harmondsworth.

Roland, M.O. (1989) What is the GP's role in health education? *Journal of the Institute of Health Education*, **27**(4), 173–8.

Stilwell, B., Greenfield, S., Dury, M. and Hull, F.M. (1987) A nurse practitioner in general practice: working style and pattern of consultation. *Journal of the Royal College of General Practitioners*, **37**, 154–7.

Theorell, T., Lind, E. and Floderus, B. (1975) The relationship of disturbing life changes and emotions to the development of myocardial infarction and other serious illnesses. *International Journal of Epidemiology*, **4**, 281–93.

Townsend, P. and Davidson, N. (1982) *Inequalities in health: the Black Report*, Penguin Books, Harmondsworth.

Townsend, P., Davidson, N. and Whitehead, M. (1988) *Inequalities in health and the health divide*, Penguin Books, Harmondsworth.

Wadsworth, M.E.J. (1986) Serious illness in childhood and its association with later life achievments, in *Class and Health: research and longitudinal data* (ed. R.G. Wilkinson), Tavistock, London.

World Health Organization (1985) *Targets for health for all 2000*, Regional Office for Europe, Copenhagen.

World Health Organization (1989) First European Conference on tobacco policy. *Journal of the Institute of Health Education*, **27**(I), 42–3.

FURTHER READING

British Medical Association (1990) *Guide to living with risk*, Penguin Books, Harmondsworth.

Quilliam, S. (1990) Positive smear: the emotional issues and what can be done. *The Health Education Journal*, **49**(I), 19–20.

Smith, A. and Jacobson, B. (1989) *The Nation's health: a strategy for the 90s*, King Edward's Hospital Fund for London, London.

CHAPTER 8

Teaching those in
middle age

Dinah Gould

In contrast to the young and elderly, the middle-aged have attracted comparatively little attention from health care professionals, although those few authors who have made detailed examination of this stage in the life cycle agree that it is a time of increasing awareness of physical limitations, when interest in health becomes more prominent (Hunter and Sundel, 1989).

Perhaps one of the greatest drawbacks to health promotion aimed at those in mid-life is lack of clear boundaries for entry to and exit from middle age. Some authors, like Levinson (1978), believe that middle age must logically commence at 35 in a society where life expectancy is still often quoted as three score years and ten. But the few studies investigating the general health and life concerns of a middle-aged population draw samples from those between 40 and 60 (Musgrove and Mennell, 1980). In contrast, Hunter and Sundel (1989) believe that individuals arrive at the middle period of their lives at slightly differing chronological ages, depending on the time at which they completed full-time education, entered a stable relationship and became parents. This more liberal definition is perhaps the better one as chronological markers are likely to become rapidly out-dated with ever increasing life expectancy.

Riley (1984) points out that in 1900 members of both sexes could expect to live for approximately 50 years. By 1980 the average male was estimated to live for 70 years, females for 78 years. As the stretch of time between birth and death increases, the number of years spent in mid-life also lengthen, giving men and women greater opportunities for personal and career development once children have become independent.

The traditional view of middle age is not optimistic. The typical middle-aged couple is depicted as bored with life and with one another. He is swamped under the responsibilities of a demanding job and providing financial support for adolescent children in the throws of completing expensive education. She is fretfully experiencing the menopause with attendant depression, physical discomfort and fears of waning attractiveness. Confidence is reduced after years devoted to home and family and self doubts arise as one by one children leave home, giving rise to the 'empty nest syndrome', first described by the feminist author Bart (1974). Parents too, are growing older and provision for their care falls upon their offspring in mid-life.

To describe changes in outlook and the major re-examination of life goals believed to occur at this time, psychologists coined the term 'mid-life crisis', believing it to represent an era of disillusionment and despondence at unfilled ambitions and unrealised dreams.

This view is not, however, supported by research data. Until very recently the few authors prompted to study middle life restricted themselves to interviewing white, middle class people, usually men, using cross sectional rather than longitudinal research designs not permitting them to compare personality factors for the same individual on more than one occasion. Actual changes over time could not, therefore, be examined. Theory, when used at all in these studies, rested heavily on Freudian psychoanalytic perspectives. Drawing together the results of more recent longitudinal studies in their edited book, Hunter and Sundel (1989) refute the numerous myths which have come to surround mid-life.

Personality can continue to develop in positive ways as maturity is reached and, contrary to long-established popular opinion, intelligence does not decline until the 60s in the absence of organic dysfunction. Sexual performance need not decline: for women freed of worry about unwanted pregnancy and the inconvenience of menstruation, interest in sex may be enhanced. The menopause is not necessarily a difficult time (Bungay, 1980). Those who experience problems will probably have responded to previous life crises with anxiety and depression more likely to be generated by disadvantaged living conditions (Greene and Cooke, 1978). Where genuine physical problems exist, the judicious use of hormone replacement therapy is likely to alleviate many of the troublesome symptoms.

Women today do not mourn loss of fertility and menstruation, even when these are induced relatively early by hysterectomy (Webb, 1983). Parents may look forward to the time when the last child leaves home, because it marks the beginning of an era when they have more time to invest in companionship, shared interests and more free time. Although education for children and paid care for elderly relatives are expensive, people in mid-life are likely to be at the peak of their earning capacity and for men and women, paid employment brings interest and enhanced self-esteem in addition to financial reward. Hunter and Sundel (1989) draw upon epidemiological evidence to support their case. They argue that although depression is a widely acknowledged problem among women (Weisman and Paykel, 1974), its incidence does not suddenly peak in mid-life among those with no previous experience of mental health problems. Major emotional upheavals are at least as common in younger age groups when the tasks of completing education, meeting a partner and raising a family are accomplished. Although divorce, alcoholism and suicide are problems of middle age, they do not, according to epidemiological data, occur exclusively or even primarily at this time.

Despite an emphasis on positive changes, it is apparent that the individual who gradually perceives that he or she is no longer quite so young, must accept that less time remains for living. The years may not exactly be running out, but fewer of them are left and there are physical reminders. Women will have a menopause, but some changes are common to both sexes, e.g. presbyopia (stiffening of the lens so that the visual near point recedes) indicated by a need to wear spectacles for reading and other close work. These are normal physiological changes, but they may be unwelcome reminders that fitness is not quite all it formerly was. Morbidity and mortality, especially from cardiovascular and malignant conditions, also increase during middle life. Coronary heart disease remains the greatest single health problem in the UK, killing 1 man in 11 and 1 woman in 40 before the age of 65 (National Forum for Coronary Heart Disease Prevention, 1988).

Cancer is primarily a disease of older people, yet it still claims too many victims during their middle years (Cancer Research Campaign, 1987). Increasing concern with health and promotion of fitness is natural ar d appropriate among men and women experiencing middle age and could be capitalized upon by health care workers, whether the aim is to avoid a health problem in an individual who so far has no existing deficit (primary prevention); to avert a potential health problem or avoid deterioration (secondary prevention); or to help an individual towards maximal levels of functioning where illness is already established (tertiary prevention).

PRINCIPLES OF PATIENT TEACHING FOR PEOPLE IN MIDDLE LIFE

The principles of patient teaching for people in middle life do not differ greatly from methods applicable at any other stage in the life cycle, but to kindle interest, promote motivation and secure compliance, a number of points need emphasis.

Seeing the patient's point of view

The first, and most obvious point is that for middle-aged people health-related behaviour, potential and established health problems have gradually been accruing against a background of habits, beliefs and attitudes endured over 20 or more years. Gradually, these ideas and behaviour resulting from them will have contributed towards current health status and will be difficult to challenge because they have become entrenched. The overweight, sedentary male who stead-fastly eats too much saturated fat, smokes and avoids exercise has cultivated this pattern of behaviour over many years because he perceives the benefits (convenience and enjoyment) to outweigh the disadvantages (new, less comfortable habits which have to be learned). In this situation it could be difficult for a doctor or nurse to feel sympathetic and all too easy to apportion blame when cardiovascular problems supervene. To empathize with the patient as a first step towards health promotion, it is necessary to re-create the predicament from his point of view, remembering the extent to which ideas of illness, health and health-promoting behaviour have altered over rela-tively recent years.

The patient in our example, now well advanced in middle life, grew up during the early 1940s, in a community where war-time rationing kept in short supply many of the food commodities widely available and taken for granted today. Eggs, butter and meat were limited, though at the time firmly regarded as vital constituents of a healthy diet in view of their high protein content. Restriction was followed by a more prosperous era in the 1950s, when dairy produce was again abundant.

Our patient was earning a good wage and ate plenty of saturated fat to compensate for the deprivations of his youth. Proud of his ability to provide all the best things for his family, he encouraged his children to follow the same diet, so that a second generation, now entering middle life, has also been brought up to believe in the virtues of meat, milk and eggs eaten without restriction. Cardiovascular disease in the UK has thus reached an incidence almost unparalleled throughout the rest of Europe (National Forum for Coronary Heart Disease, 1988), but not surprisingly, our patient and his children have been slow to alter their perceptions of 'healthy eating' because the recommendation of advisory groups such as NACNE and COMA fly in the face of values promoted when they were young.

Building on existing knowledge and dispelling myths

To be successful, new information must build on what is already known and accepted and this prior knowledge must be sound, not misconceptions engendered through prejudice. An assessment of exist-ing knowledge, attitudes and motivation to learn and change behaviour must, therefore, be undertaken before teaching can begin. Health care professionals can be surprised at the knowledge as well as the ignorance shown by lay people in relation to health, their bodies and disease.

For example, the Welsh Heart Health Survey (Welsh Heart Programme Directorate, 1985), derived from a study of 22 000 people aged 12–64, showed that knowledge of risk factors for cardiovascular disease was comprehensive among more than two thirds of the population with minimal differences between age, sex and social class, although incidence of the disease remains high in Wales. Evidently telling people the facts about cigarettes, saturated fat and sedentary lifestyle, then exhorting them to adopt better ways is only part of the story. The survey provided clues that manual social groups were more likely to cite unfavourable environment circumstances as important contributory factors, while eating food rich in animal fat was most often mentioned by non-manual groups.

Because higher social class is so often linked with better educational attainment, members of the professions are often regarded as better-informed about health or automatically more intelligent; a form of stereotyping that may do injustice to individuals who do not fit the mould.

Gould (1984), interviewing a sample of 85 women during their recovery from hysterectomy, observed that 1 patient, wife of a clergy-man (social class I), had probably under-estimated the length of time required to return to her previous levels of functioning because she failed to comprehend the extent of surgical intervention. Believing 'the womb to be the size of a nut', she had been astonished by the size of her incision. The researcher was aware of the explanations and advice given to some of the women by the experienced ward sister. This patient denied receiving information, attributing this omission to the sister's reluctance to discuss sex with a woman married to a vicar. Women included in this sample had heard many 'old wives' tales' in relation to hysterectomy and in contrast to previous studies, rejected these although they still felt hurt when they heard horror stories from relatives and appreciated opportunities for reassurance with a health care professional (Webb, 1983).

In a later interview study conducted among predominantly younger women, Gould (1986) noted that interest in antenatal education did not necessarily reflect social class. The wife of a postman (social class IV) rated the conveyor belt classes provided by the local hospital as less informative than an author whose books about pregnancy are believed to appeal to a predominantly middle class audience, a salutary warning to health visitors responsible for organizing antenatal education, who had assured the researcher that their typically working class clientele would be too apathetic to discuss health promotion during pregnancy. In fact, of the 141 women approached, most were articulate and many had thought-provoking recommendations to make on the antenatal care that they received. None demonstrated lack of interest in health during pregnancy, although many were disillusioned with the quality of the information they had received and poor facilities in clinics, making attendance a chore.

These anecdotes may be useful to health visitors, community nurses and general practitioners as they emphasize the dangers of stereotyping more vividly than statistics, which mask the individuality of the people who are reduced to numbers in surveys. The value of getting to know the individual, discovering their needs, outlook on the world and their view of the service offered during feedback becomes evident. Also worth remembering is the value of life experience among mature patients. Women interviewed by Gould and Webb in the studies cited above were grateful to be relieved of menstrual disorders by hysterectomy. They did not regret loss of fertility or periods, and nearly a year after the operation, still had no regrets. In the words of the clergyman's wife, initially disappointed with her rather slow recovery, 'I'm happy. I've got four children. Babies are nice and the possibility (to have another) would be nice, but I think I could live without more'.

Avoiding stereotypes

Stereotypes are the products of attitudes, providing a 'shorthand' mechanism of rapidly forming first impressions, then extending them to judge the whole person. Health care professionals who meet large numbers of patients, often with similar complaints and in rapid succession, may find they tend to expect them all to behave in the same way and to have similar concerns. To teach effectively, however, more time must be spent with the individual and as patient and professional become more closely acquainted, stereotyping should be less marked, although it is still a cause for concern among those examining interpersonal relationships between doctors and nurses and their clients (Moss, 1988; Jeffry, 1979).

Researchers themselves are guilty of biased views. Gould, in her study of hysterectomy patients, was surprised that a woman in her 40s with one child, who had experienced numerous miscarriages, should accept surgery so willingly, especially as she belonged to a faith and culture in which fertility is highly prized. She told the researcher that she had experienced so many disappointments with each unsuccessful pregnancy that she was now grateful that she could no longer be 'expected' to have more pregnancies. In contrast, an older patient, already a grandmother and closely involved in the upbringing of her grandchildren, made the following comment, 'I'm too old now (to have more children), but my husband and I love children. I've said to him only the other day that we should have had more and spread them out more'.

Clearly regret at loss of fertility is a complex issue to which the individuals concerned react in very different ways. To predict that a woman who has had obstetric problems will feel wholehearted regret and that another will be thankful by virtue of her grandchildren and her age is too simplistic. Such predictable stereotypes belong in textbooks, not the real world, justifying research to determine the many ways in which different people feel and behave when confronted with the same issue.

Just as health care professionals may judge patients on the basis of a brief encounter, so patients in turn may dismiss the service they receive as typical of the 'average' doctor or nurse. In the hysterectomy study, women were not systematically asked about their experiences in the outpatient clinic. When they returned six weeks after the operation for a follow-up appointment, many raised this topic spontaneously because they were so disappointed at seeing only a junior doctor, especially as they had usually waited a long time and the appointment itself was quickly over. Not only did they feel too rushed to ask questions, they believed that to do so would have been inappropriate in view of the perceived lack of experience and understanding on the part of the doctor. The two people whose advice and information were most highly rated before discharge were the consultant and ward sister – perhaps because they were regarded as more experienced and therefore more reliable. Many research studies have been conducted to evaluate the effect of a teaching intervention on patients' recovery from surgery, usually producing beneficial effects (Hayward, 1975; Boore, 1978). However, in these classic studies, information has usually been provided by a senior and experienced professional. The value of teaching supplied by house officers and staff nurses has been less closely examined and more time may need to be spent providing these groups with teaching skills and opportunities for increasing confidence to educate patients. The experience of teaching someone old enough to be a parent can be potentially threatening for a junior member of staff, especially when difficult questions are asked.

Choosing an effective approach

Group teaching for a number of patients facing the same operation has been demonstrated to be effective (Lindeman and van Aernam, 1971), and is often advocated for people with the same condition on the grounds that they can provide mutual support. The education of diabetic patients is commonly approached in this manner. However, there are a number of disadvantages which seem especially relevant when this method is contemplated for use with a group which will include mature people who may not have encountered a structured teaching session for many years. Finding the situation reminiscent of school, some may fail to participate because they feel threatened, others may lose interest through resentment or imagined patronage, while a third group, harkening back to school days, try to ensure 'good marks' by monopolizing the discussion. The atmosphere may not be conducive for learning by the under-confident, for lonely patients who regard the session as an opportunity for a pleasant chat, or for those accustomed to autonomy and greater responsibility at work and who cannot adapt to a different pace.

Health care professionals involved in group teaching must be able to differentiate clearly between the aims of androgogy and pedagogy and constantly remind themselves that the principles of adult teaching differ sharply from those applicable to the teaching of children (Redman, 1984).

Patients are not obliged to comply with instructions. They may do so in hospital but lapse on discharge through lack of motivation or because they were never sufficiently persuaded to learn at all. When the goal of teaching is to enable the individual to pass an examination the worst possible outcome is failure of that examination. Though disappointing, this need not be serious, as there are nearly always opportunities to resit. If, however, the goal is to teach the newly diagnosed diabetic patient about the appropriate care of his feet, there is no 'second chance' if the information is misunderstood or ignored. Neglect to examine the feet and ignorance of how to recognize and act upon early signs of infection and ulceration could have tragic consequences.

Group teaching can provide patients with a great deal of support and reassurance that they are not alone with their problems, as well as being economic of health care professionals' time. It may be extremely successful for those in middle-life, but more difficulties may be encountered than immediately meet the eye. For patients of any age, there is, of course, a need to provide opportunities for discussion and questions in private.

Ensuring the main points are remembered

One of the stereotypes that we have already explored is the mythological decline of intelligence as soon as middle life begins. There is no need to make information easier for the mature patient than for a younger one, but as with any individual, learning is likely to be reduced by fear, illness and the unfamiliar hospital environment. Information needs to be paced slowly, repeated often, and as at any age, written information provides a good supplement to verbal instructions, although one should not supplement the other (Steele and Goodwin, 1975).

Although intelligence remains intact in the absence of organic dysfunction, approaches to teaching and the type of material included routinely during general education at school have changed over the years. Today we hear much in the media of the declining standards of education amongst young people, especially in relation to science, but today's school leavers are more likely to have taken formal examinations. Opportunities to undergo higher education are greater, and anyone working in the health care field has almost certainly encountered scientific concepts and methods of measurements at some stage. Thus the dietician may show a patient recovering from a recent myocardial infarction tables of the amount of fat and cholesterol in different kinds of food. A good cookery book, such as the *Readers' Digest Complete Guide to Cookery* (Willan, 1989), is useful for this purpose, as it shows a range of foods giving cholesterol, carbohydrate, fat, protein and fibre content (when applicable), in addition to suggested methods of preparation. The patient, all too aware of the pain and fear accompanying his recent heart attack, is anxious to comply with a low cholesterol diet and to learn about foods best avoided, yet is bewildered by the units of measurement – after all a milligram of cholesterol is not very much! A more carefully planned approach, listing foods in ascending order of their cholesterol content and writing the cholesterol value alongside each item, may be more helpful. Relative values thus become apparent, giving a better picture of what may be safely eaten and what is best avoided.

Lay people are often confused about cholesterol, especially what it is and where it comes from: facts easy to overlook in a busy cardiology ward or health centre, but which if ignored may lead to confusion and disillusionment later on. If the patient is under the misapprehension that cholesterol is only another type of dietary fat, he may make the mistake of following a low calorie diet. Some delicious foods, including many seafoods, are low in calories and suitable for slimmers, yet contain relatively high proportions of cholesterol. Failure to realize that the body manufactures cholesterol and is particularly likely to do so under conditions of stress may lead to worry when blood levels are found to be high. More stress results, setting up a vicious circle and the diet is dismissed as ineffective and unhelpful.

To sum up this section: nobody can be bombarded with information and remember all of it; and to be remembered and, more importantly, acted upon, information must be provided in sufficient detail and make sense.

ACHIEVING COMPLIANCE

In order to teach patients effectively, health care professionals must have a fund of knowledge to impart and the ability to communicate, picking up verbal and non-verbal cues to identify appropriate times to provide information (Macleod Clark, 1983). Simply giving information, even when the patient appears to be receptive, does not guarantee compliance, however. In this section we will examine some of the barriers to motivation as they apply to the middle-aged patient.

Of the many theories of motivation which exist, probably that most widely known specifically in relation to health teaching is Becker's Health Belief Model (1974). According to Becker, the individual's own perceptions are crucial to his or her motivation to learning about health or illness and acting on advice. Five major influences are seen to affect the level of motivation.

1. The individual must believe he is susceptible to a disease. The middle-aged man who has smoked all his life and eaten a diet rich in saturated fat may still not accept that he is at risk of undermining his health, especially if he knows other people who have smoked all their lives and apparently come to no harm.
2. The individual must believe that the acknowledged condition will have serious consequences. The cardiovascular diseases and malig-nancies which tend to affect middle-aged and older people are generally viewed by the public as very serious, although there are some exceptions. For example, it may be difficult to regard hyper-tension as much of a risk if it has been identified during a routine medical without producing any symptoms. Similarly, the individual whose Type II (adult onset) diabetes has been identified during routine urinalysis may find it difficult to accept the need for edu-cation and dismiss arguments for changing lifestyle.
3. The individual must believe that action to counter the disease will be effective. Some people in middle life may feel that they have now reached a stage in the lifespan when they are too old or it is too late for changes in lifestyle to be very effective. Someone who has always smoked may not believe that by giving up cigarettes his or her general health will improve, although evidence suggests that many of the deleterious effects of smoking are reversible. Mild diabetes in middle life may be controlled very effectively by diet, but the patient who associates diabetes with a regime of insulin may not accept this less stringent approach with much faith.
4. To be motivated, the individual must believe not only that action is possible: barriers to taking action must not be perceived as too great. The demands of a new diet may defeat some people even though many of the high fibre foods recommended for patients with high blood cholesterol or elevated blood glucose levels are much cheaper than meat or convenience foods containing large quantities of fat and sugar. Taking more exercise may not fit in easily with a busy work schedule or the 'image' the individual has cultivated over the years.

5. Even when all four criteria described above have been fulfilled, there often still needs to be a cue for action. A prompt or added persuasion can be provided by a partner, friend or relative. The diabetic may be more willing to follow a diet if his wife is complimentary about his weight loss. Willingness of a friend to play golf may persuade someone to take more exercise. As people grow older, members of their acquaintance may become ill or even die: a friend's diagnosis of lung cancer may provide a sudden, powerful deterrent to the inveterate smoker. Symptoms experienced by the patient himself may alert the individual to change his ways: for example, breathlessness or the development of a morning cough in the smoker or angina in the individual with arterial disease. Unfortunately, some of the diseases which have their onset in mid-life begin insidiously, with very little in the way of symptoms. The classic example is hypertension. Compliance with drugs used to treat this condition may be low, as many have marked and unpleasant side-effects, so that by taking them the patient actually feels less well than he did before. Denial and refusal to 'own' the problem of silent asymptomatic hypertension may consequently follow.

Perhaps one of the greatest threats to motivation and one of the main reasons for denial at any age is anxiety. For people conscious that they are advancing in years, anxiety may become more marked, firstly because common sense suggests that the types of illness to which an individual is prone become increasingly serious with age, recovery when possible proceeding more slowly than in youth, and because middle life brings a multitude of responsibilities at home and at work, which are not easily put aside for protracted treatment or lengthy hospital admission.

Levels of motivation can be assessed by asking patients directly: an open-ended question may yield more information. Questions may be put when a course of action is suggested, then again later, to establish how patients feel with experience. Encouragement to try a diet or to take their drugs for a trial period may be beneficial because this breaks down treatment into small stages and prevents the individual rejecting it out of hand, especially when changes in lifestyle seem overwhelming. Giving positive feedback enhances motivation, so progress should always be emphasized and praised, however small. The help of partners, friends and relatives can be enlisted where appropriate. It is possible to find out details of the patient's lifestyle from them, giving further estimation of the likely impact of their illness and the changes it will bring. Other people can be included in teaching. This is of particular benefit when a practical skill is taught, such as urine-testing or giving injections, as it provides contingency when the patient feels unwell and is not inclined to bother. Where a wife always cooks the meals, teaching is more effectively aimed at her, even though it is the husband whose diet needs changing.

Experience with patients suggests that most appreciate being made to feel a little 'special' and when genuine difficulty is encountered following instruction, individuals like to feel the doctor or nurse can see things from their perspective. The best advice is realistic and the best information is relevant: studies have repeatedly demonstrated that patients want precise information rather than the vague general guidelines they so often receive, especially when they leave hospital (Wilson-Barnett, 1980). Women in Gould's study (Gould, 1984) were told not to lift 'heavy' weights without definition of 'heavy' (vague advice). Others were told not to lift anything as heavy as a kettle filled with water (unrealistic advice for someone who would be at home alone all day). Specific problems which might arise following hysterectomy were not discussed and there were some indications that the same traditional advice was given routinely by doctors, irrespective of need. For example, women were always told to avoid intercourse until after they attended the outpatient appointment six weeks later, but they were never given any reason for this advice. A few women who disregarded the instruction encountered no problems, but another bled heavily following intercourse months after the operation. Granulation tissue in the vaginal vault had been traumatized. The woman had not been told of this possibility, although the delicate nature of granulation tissue is widely recognized. Health care professionals do not always know all the answers and even when communication is good, with attention paid to verbal and non-verbal cues, they may not be able to anticipate all the questions that will arise during longer term recovery at home.

Trust has been identified as a necessary component of effective health care relationships, especially when the illness is of an on-going nature (Thorne and Robinson, 1988). In this qualitative study, the informants described relationships with health care professionals as evolving to a predictable pattern: distinct stages with transitions linked to the amount of trust felt for those in charge of their care. When the condition was first diagnosed, absolute trust was the norm, based on the assumption that all the answers to existing problems would be forthcoming. There was a naive belief that treatment and advice would be provided on a shared understanding of the patient's best interests. However, straightforward solutions seldom presented themselves for the chronic conditions which these people suffered and at the same time it quickly became apparent that doctors and nurses did *not* generally understand or even care about the patient's perspective of his best interests: professional decisions were based upon a distinct set of values, often contradicting with those of the patient. Anger, suspicion and vulnerability were then experienced. In a later resolution stage, trust was reconstructed based on a more informed, less naive expectation of what health care could provide. Blind faith never returned, especially when chronically ill people realized that doctors and nurses would be unlikely ever to know as much about the problems of living with the condition as they did themselves. In fact, relationships were described as particularly good when health care professionals acknowledged the patient as the authority on his illness. Dissatisfaction continued when the patient's competence was under-estimated. The authors of this study do not provide any information on the age of their informants, but given the long term nature of their illnesses it is reasonable to suppose that many of them must have entered middle life. Their message has clear implications for anyone involved in teaching this age group: experience of illness (and probably life experience) must be acknowledged and much will be gained by attending to the patient's perspective, planning goals and evaluating care with him. Little will be achieved by devising aims which he does not share and refusing to believe in barriers to compliance which seem very real to him.

ABSOLUTE RELUCTANCE

Throughout this chapter ways of involving patients in their care and of enhancing understanding of illness and treatment have been discussed, and possible barriers to motivation and ways of removing these have been described. Using this knowledge, supportive presence, counselling and information-giving have all been incorporated into patient care, often with the assumption that more knowledge is bound to be a good thing, irrespective of any demonstrable change in behaviour (Wilson-Barnett and Batehup, 1988). Where teaching provides reassurance and aids compliance, it is indeed beneficial, but the enthusiastic doctor or nurse must bear in mind those situations where knowledge is too threatening and the individual may steadfastly reject the truth even when it seems obvious to outsiders. McIntosh's ethnographic study (1977) of communication in a cancer ward suggested that some patients steadfastly denied the nature of their illness despite strong evidence of its nature, appearing to collude with the medical staff when diagnosis and treatment were discussed in euphemistic terms.

As medical technology advances and increases in sophistication, it has become possible to diagnose many diseases with serious and potentially fatal outcome at an earlier stage, making them more amenable to treatment. Although most people would agree that to preserve life of good quality is advantageous, this situation also means that more people are living under the shadow of the threat posed by disease and for longer. Sometimes the decision of whether to treat and tell or to treat but not provide the whole truth unless it is actively sought becomes a major dilemma of medical ethics. This is exemplified by the severe genetic disorder, Huntingdon's disease, which results through deficiency of the neurotransmitter GABA (gamma-aminobutyric acid). Neurons in the extrapyraminal nervous system progressively degenerate, culminating in antisocial behaviour, severe mental deterioration and distressing, uncoordinated movements of the head and body. Huntingdon's disease is autosomal dominant, so that every child of an affected parent has a 1 in 2 chance of developing the disease (assuming only 1 parent has the defective gene) in middle life, the time when symptoms manifest. By this time the individual is likely to have married and already had children, who in turn, have a 50% risk of inheriting the gene.

Predictive testing for Huntingdon's has recently become possible, but many people who initially approached the medical genetics service, aware that they might be affected later, withdrew before the test was performed (Cranford *et al.*, 1989). In such a very threatening situation, knowing the course of the illness, which at the present time remains untreatable, would be too stressful irrespective of any help the results might give when planning for the future or deciding whether to have children.

Even in more everyday situations some people may be reluctant to collaborate in their care. A small scale exploratory study (Waterworth and Luker, 1990) indicates that some patients are more concerned about doing what is expected of them by pleasing the doctor or nurse, than in participating in decisions about their care. Although they acknowledge their small sample ($n = 12$), the authors stress that more thought should be given to involving patients in their care than the naive assumption that any involvement must necessarily be good for its own sake. This conclusion, though thought-provoking, is not new. For example, Davis and Morobin (1977) pointed out that the patients in their hospital study tried to manage their fear and pain in order to present a façade of co-operation and motivation.

Every so often a patient will be encountered who remains the passive recipient of treatment, ignoring all offers of education about his condition and unmoved by messages of health promotion, irrespective of efforts to interest and motivate him. When patient teaching falls upon such stony ground, the right of the individual must, in the last resort, be respected.

CONCLUSION

By the time they enter middle life, many people have developed a real interest in promoting and preserving their health and fitness and are excellently motivated towards their health care professional who seeks to actively involve them in their own care. Drawing on their life experiences, they make good partners in the teaching process and their accounts, when shared with doctors and nurses, provide valuable insights into ways of coping with health and illness. From these encounters it is not only the patient who will learn. Others need more encouragement to participate in care, sometimes understandably, in view of the stereotypes and misconceptions often held by the public and by health care workers towards middle age. To persuade the individual to change behaviour at this stage in the lifespan is perhaps one of the major challenges of the educator: middle age is a comfortable time when habits are established but the dangers associated with them have yet to become apparent. People are individuals and by the middle years idiosyncrasies have had time to mature, hence no single teaching approach is suitable for all. The flow chart below summarizes the main points in this chapter and should be regarded as a guide when meeting the health needs of people in middle life.

GUIDELINES FOR TEACHING THE PATIENT IN MIDDLE LIFE

1. Be optimistic. Middle age is *not* a time of decline.
2. Beware of myths about middle age, e.g. mid-life crisis – your own false impressions and your patient's.
3. Try to see the patient's point of view. Ideas about health have changed considerably in recent years and people are understandably confused by contradictory messages from the media.
4. Build on existing knowledge by careful assessment. Anticipate myths your patient is likely to have encountered and provide a supportive atmosphere in which ideas not anticipated could be raised.
5. Be alert to the pitfalls of stereotyping – of your patient and yourself and the service you represent. By treating people as individuals you can get to know them better and avoid the mistakes of presuming knowledge or ignorance.
6. Choose your teaching approach with care based on acquaintance with the individual. Remember the merits of written as well as verbal information and acknowledge need for privacy when discussing some topics.
7. Select information that is relevant, consider the detail required carefully and be prepared to present it in different, imaginative ways.
8. Remember the barriers to motivation which may specifically affect the individual at this stage in his/her lifespan and explore ways of overcoming these. Realistic aims and prompt feedback help.
9. Treat the patient as a person worthy of acquaintance in his/her

own right. Promote trust by sharing ideas and listening to their point of view.

10. People in mid-life have much to gain by adopting health-promoting behaviour – and much to lose, as their long-established and prized attitudes and habits are threatened. Their views will colour any changes they make and their experiences of health and illness provide a rich source of information for the health care professional. Be prepared to learn from patients too.

REFERENCES

Bart, P.B. (1974) Depression in middle-aged women, in *Women in Sexist Society* (ed. V. Gomick and B.K. Moran), Basic Books, New York, pp. 99–117.

Becker, M.H. (1974) The health belief model and sick role behaviour. *Health Education Monographs*, **2**, 409–19.

Boore, J. (1978) *Prescription for Recovery*, Royal College of Nursing, London.

Bungay, G.T. (1980) Study of symptoms in middle life. *British Medical Journal*, **2**, 181–3.

Cancer Research Campaign (1987) *Facts about Cancer*, Cancer Research Campaign, London.

Cranford, D., Dodge, A., Kerzin-Storrary, L. and Harris, R. (1989) Uptake of pre-symptomatic predictive testing for Huntingdon's Disease. *The Lancet*, **1**, 603–5.

Davis, A. and Morobin, G. (1977) *Medical Encounters: The Experience of Illness and Treatment*, Croom Helm, London.

Gould, D.J. (1984) Patient's Perception of Recovery from Hysterectomy, MPhil Thesis, London University.

Gould, D.J. (1986) Locally organised antenatal classes and their effectiveness. *Nursing Times Occasional Paper*, **82**(12), 59–62.

Greene, J.G. and Cooke, D.J. (1978) Life stress and events at the climacteric. *British Journal of Psychiatry*, **136**, 486–91.

Hayward, J. (1975) *Information – Prescription Against Pain*, Royal College of Nursing, London.

Hunter, S. and Sundel, M. (1989) *Midlife Myths: Issues, Findings and Practice Implications*, Sage, London.

Jeffry, R. (1979) Normal rubbish: deviant patterns in casualty departments. *Sociology of Health and Illness*, **1**, 98–107.

Levinson, D.J. (1978) *The Seasons of a Man's Life*, Knopf, New York.

Lindeman, C.A. and van Aernam, B. (1971) Effects of structured and unstructured pre-operative teaching. *Nursing Research*, **20**, 310–32.

Macleod Clark, J. (1983) Nurse–patient communication – an analysis of conversations from surgical wards, in *Nursing Research: Ten Studies in Patient Care* (ed. J. Barnett), John Wiley and Sons, Chichester, pp. 25–6.

McIntosh, J. (1977) *Communication and Awareness in a Cancer Ward*, Croom Helm, New York.

Moss, A.R. (1988) Determinants of patient care: nursing process or nursing attitudes? *Journal of Advanced Nursing*, **13**, 615–20.

Musgrove, B. and Mennell, Z. (1980) *Change and Choice: Women and Middle Age*, Peter Owen, London.

National Forum for Coronary Heart Disease Prevention (1988) *Coronary Heart*

Disease Prevention. Action in the UK 1984–1987, Health Education Authority, London.

Redman, B.K. (1984) *The Process of Patient Education*, Mosby, St Louis.

Riley, M.W. (1984) Women, men and the lengthening life course, in *Gender and the Life Course* (ed. A. Rossi), Aldine, Chicago, pp. 333–47.

Steele, S.J. and Goodwin, M.F. (1975) A pamphlet to answer the patient's questions before hysterectomy. *The Lancet*, **2**, 492–3.

Thorne, S.E. and Robinson, G.A. (1988) Reciprocal trust in health care relationships. I. *Journal of Advanced Nursing*, **13**, 782–9.

Waterworth, S. and Luker, K.A. (1990) Reluctant collaborators: do patients want to be involved in decisions concerning care? *Journal of Advanced Nursing*, **15**, 971–6.

Webb, C. (1983) Hysterectomy – dispelling the myths. *Nursing Times Occasional Paper I*, **79**(47), 52–4; II **79**(48), 44–6.

Weisman, M. and Paykel, E. (1974) *The Depressed Woman: A Study of Social Relationships*, University of Chicago Press, Chicago.

Welsh Heart Programme Directorate (1985) *Welsh Heart Health Survey – Heartbeat Report No 2*, Heartbeat, Cardiff.

Willan, A. (1989) *Reader's Digest Complete Guide to Cookery*, Dorling Kindersley, London.

Wilson-Barnett, J. (1980) Keeping patients informed. *Nursing*, January.

Wilson-Barnett, J. and Batehup, L. (1988) *Patient Problems. A Research Base for Nursing Care*, Scutari Press, London.

CHAPTER 9

Enhancing health and function in late life

Jan Dodge and Patricia Knutesen

All parts of the body which have a function, if used in moderation and exercised in labours to which each is left idle, they become liable to disease, defective in growth and age quickly. (Hippocrates)

CHANGING DEMOGRAPHICS

The number of people living beyond age 60 is increasing to significant proportions in all developed countries. For example, the proportion of people aged 60 and over in Europe has increased from 12.9% in 1950 to 16.7% in 1970 and is expected to increase to 19.5% by the year 2000. The number of Europeans aged 60 and over is projected to increase from 81 million in 1980 to over 101 million in the year 2000 (WHO, 1983).

In 1950, 1 person out of 9 was 60 years or over; however, by the year 2028, 1 person out of 4 will be 60 years or over. Within this elderly population, different groups of older persons are increasing at various rates. The oldest-old, those 80 years and over, are the fasted growing sector of the ageing population (Golini and Lori, 1990).

The majority (67%) of non-institutionalized older persons live in a family setting. Recent data in the UK, Canada, Australia and the USA show that approximately one-third of those over 60 years live alone. Significant among this group are the oldest-old and widowed women (Ageing International, 1990).

The elderly, in general, live in older buildings with poor facilities when compared to the rest of the population. Not surprisingly, the elderly run a higher risk of accidents in the home than those under 60 years of age. There is a rate of 5 accidents per 100 elderly resulting in fractures in 26–7% of these accidents (Golini and Lori, 1990). While many countries provide funds for repairs or improvements, older persons may be unaware of how to obtain this assistance (Ageing International, 1990).

The rate of institutionalization of the elderly remains relatively stable in most countries. The rate varies from 4% in Germany to a rate of 10.9% in the Netherlands. Among those who live in institutions, the highest proportion are composed of unmarried and very old women with high levels of functional impairment (Ageing International, 1990).

The level of education of the elderly is lower than that of the younger population. For example, of the older persons in Italy, 34% have no educational qualifications, 47% have a grade school diploma and only 7% have a high school diploma. In general, older women have a lower level of education than older men (Ageing International, 1990). Older persons often experience lower income levels in relationship to the rest of the population. In fact, as age increases, pension incomes often continue to decrease relative to inflation (Golini and Lori, 1990).

Older persons are much more likely than younger persons to have multiple chronic and disabling illnesses. Of those over 60, 80% have 1 or more chronic conditions, and approximately 50% are somewhat limited in an activity of daily living. However, the majority of elderly are able to adjust to their functional impairments and remain independent in the community (Ouslander and Beck, 1982).

RECONCEPTUALIZING OLD AGE

Growing old was once believed to be associated with inevitable decline in function and frailty. Researchers in gerontology (the study of ageing) and geriatrics (health care of the elderly) have challenged this universal acceptance of decline with age and offer more positive images and expectations via concepts such as the compression of morbidity (Fries, 1980), active life expectancy (Katz *et al.*, 1983), productive ageing (Butler and Gleason, 1985), and successful ageing (Rowe and Kahn, 1989). The premise of each one of these concepts is that decline in overall function can be forstalled until late in the ageing process allowing older adults to live with greater independence and autonomy, thereby experiencing improved quality of life (Omen, 1990).

Longitudinal studies on ageing subjects demonstrate wide variability in physiological, psychological and social function, thus highlighting the heterogeneity of the elderly (Williams, 1986). The losses attributed to ageing appear more modest than once expected and are more directly related to disease and extrinsic factors such as health behaviours (smoking, diet, exercise) and lifestyle (Rowe, 1991).

Through modification of health behaviours and lifestyle it has been estimated that 50–80% of health problems in late life could be prevented or postponed (O'Brien and Vertinsky, 1988; Dychtwald and Zitter, 1988).

Goals of health promotion in the elderly

- Maintain functional capacity;
- prevent premature institutionalization;
- maintain informal network of care (e.g. family caregivers);
- maintain quality of life.

Such estimates as these warrant attention to health promotion and disease/disability prevention in older adults (Institute of Medicine, 1990). Recent longitudinal studies searching for predictors of healthy and successful ageing demonstrate that older persons without hypertension, cardiovascular disease, and arthritis continue to function at a very high level, even among the oldest-old (Roos and Havens, 1991; Guralnik and Kaplan, 1989; Harris *et al.*, 1989). Additionally, health behaviours such as being a non-smoker, having moderate body weight, and consuming moderate amounts of alcohol were predictors of high functioning (Guralnik and Kaplan, 1989; Harris *et al.*, 1989).

Developed countries are acknowledging the need for broadened health care and social service strategies in response to the 'greying of the nations', a phrase coined by Dr Robert Butler. Groups such as the World Health Organization (1983) and United States Health Services (Healthy People 2000, 1990) are calling for health promotion and disease prevention objectives specific to the older population. The goals of health promotion emphasize the need for enhanced function of physical, mental, social and environmental status of older adults. Recognizing that ageing is frequently associated with chronic disease (e.g. cardiovascular disease, arthritis, hypertension, cancer) and chronic conditions (e.g. sensory loss, urinary incontinence, foot disorders), the Institute of Medicine (1990) also calls for attention to disability prevention in order for older persons to be spared the progression of dependency and diminished function due to illness. Thus, the aim of this chapter will be to overview potential health promotion and disease/disability prevention measures for the elderly.

BARRIERS

Before beginning health promotion and screening activities for the elderly it is important to recognize potential barriers. These barriers, outlined in Figure 9.1, identify unique aspects to both the health professional and the older person.

Health professionals may possess negative attitudes regarding ageing often due to insufficient knowledge of the normal ageing process and lack of exposure to 'healthy' older adults. Consequently, health promoting activities may be viewed as both unnecessary and costly.

Health professional
- Negative attitudes regarding ageing;
- lack of knowledge regarding benefits of screening;
- limited screening standards specific to the elderly;
- increased time spent with older patients.

Older person
- Fatalism regarding own health;
- limited access (e.g. transportation, convenience, lack of facility, etc.);
- misperception of information regarding benefits of screening;
- reliance on physician to make screening recommendations;
- emotional concerns (e.g. fears, embarrassment);
- cost of screening programme.

Figure 9.1 Potential barriers to screening.

Similarly health professionals may believe that older persons are unable or unwilling to learn new behaviours (Pastorino and Dickey, 1990) despite evidence that older persons are more likely to engage in healthy behaviours (Day, 1990).

Because health promotion and screening for disease are relatively new activities for the elderly, lack of consistent guidelines and screening standards specific to the elderly exist (Institute of Medicine, 1990). Therefore, professionals may not possess current information needed to promote the health of the elderly.

Time constraints are a reality for most health professionals. Health promotion, screening and health education may necessitate increased time spent with older patients (Stults, 1984). With this in mind, it is imperative to collaborate with team members in delegating or implementing those activities (Day, 1990).

Older people often possess inaccurate knowledge about ageing and may under-report symptoms as they believe those symptoms are attributed to 'normal' ageing (Matteson *et al.*, 1988). This fatalism regarding health may prevent participation in screening activities, resulting in presentation of advanced stages of disease/disability rendering interventions less effective (Stults, 1984). Older persons are more likely to rely on the advice of their physicians in both recommending screening and lifestyle changes despite a desire for a healthy lifestyle (Day, 1990; Pastorino and Dickey, 1990).

Access to health promotion activities is a major consideration and often a limitation (Pastorino and Dickey, 1990). Lack of transportation is a common problem for the elderly. For example, elders residing in rural areas or high crime urban areas experience frequent transportation barriers. It has been noted that approximately 25% of persons over 75 were unable to use public transportation in the UK because of physical difficulties (*The Nation's Health*, 1988). Thus, travelling to a doctor's appointment or going out for increased socialization becomes a challenge. Elderly residing in rural areas may need to travel long distances for services not rendered in their area. Long waits in physicians' offices and other ambulatory settings may fatigue and further discourage participation in health-promoting activities.

Emotional concerns must also be kept in mind when working with older persons (Day, 1990). Fear of confirming an illness via screening is often a worry to many older persons especially when coupled with fear of institutionalization. Embarrassment and loss of dignity may prevent participation in procedures such as pelvic examination, sigmoidoscopy, and mammography.

Finally, the cost of screening for preventive health care may limit participation as most older persons live on fixed incomes and may not perceive the benefits of screening in relation to out-of-pocket expenses.

Knowledge of the multiple barriers to health-promoting activities is useful as health professionals assess their own need for more information. Similarly, health professionals will benefit from exploring with elderly clients their attitudes, knowledge and expectations of health promotion, screening, and health education in order to achieve mutual goals.

HEALTH PROMOTION AND DISEASE/DISABILITY PREVENTION

Providing preventive health care to the elderly must be a major concern of health professionals and the health care system. While much is still not known about the benefits of health promotion in the elderly, some research has shown that certain programmes have improved or maintained elderly persons' health and functional abilities, such as smoking cessation and exercise programmes.

Prevention of health problems in the elderly means anticipating and averting problems or discovering them as early as possible in order to minimize possible disease or disability (Spradley, 1990). The three levels of prevention are primary prevention, secondary prevention and tertiary prevention. Figure 9.2 lists some potential geriatric preventive health measures as suggested by Stults (1984). Primary prevention keeps the health problem from occurring at all, 'It precedes disease or dysfunction and is applied to a generally healthy population' (Shamansky and Clausen, 1980). Primary prevention interventions include health promotion and specific protection, such as immunizations, to achieve the optimal health for individuals. Specific examples in the elderly include: health behaviour such as diet, exercise, and smoking cessation; accident prevention; and immunization. Secondary prevention seeks to detect and treat existing health problems at the earliest possible stage. Pathology is now involved. Secondary prevention attempts to discover a health problem so that interventions may lead to

Primary Prevention
Health Promotion
  Nutrition
  Exercise
  Smoking Cessation
  Accident Prevention
Immunization
Secondary Prevention
Cancer
Hypertension
Medication
Mental Health
  Depression
  Dementia
  Social Support
Urinary Incontinence
Tertiary Prevention
Comprehensive Functional Assessment

Figure 9.2 Guidelines for geriatric preventive health measures (Adapted from: Stults, 1984, with permission).

its eradication and control. Specific examples in the elderly include hypertension and cancer screening. Tertiary prevention attempts to minimize the effects of disease and disability by preventing complications and deterioration. If function cannot be restored, the goal is to help prevent or forestall increasing dependency or placement in an institution (Stults, 1984). In the elderly, screening programmes that detect symptomatic but unreported disease are considered tertiary prevention. Screening programmes targeted toward maximizing functional status (tertiary prevention) are particularly appropriate for the elderly 'where long-term survival is less important than maintaining an independent life' (Day, 1990, p. 14). For example, glaucoma screening could reveal the findings of increased ocular pressure before visual problems (secondary prevention) or screening could detect glaucoma after a person complains of vision loss (tertiary prevention). The treatment in the latter situation would be the prevention of further progression of the disease and the maintenance of the usual activities of daily living.

Approaches to health promotion and disease/disability prevention require broad and comprehensive strategies in order to reduce morbidity and enhance physical, psychological and social function in older age (Institute of Medicine, 1990). Since enhanced function and quality of life are the goals of any preventive health measure, it follows that the cure or treatment for the problem must have a positive effect on the quality or quantity of an older person's life. Additionally, acceptable methods of treatment must be available (Frame and Carlson, 1975).

Therefore, if an older person cannot withstand treatment due to another comorbid condition or if there is no effective therapy to offer, screening may not be justified. 'Adding life to years' not 'adding years to life' should be kept in mind throughout all prevention measures.

Primary prevention

Healthy lifestyles which include sound nutrition, moderate alcohol intake, regular exercise, not smoking, and adequate amounts of sleep are becoming recognized as effective primary prevention strategies in avoiding disease as well as reversing the effects of disease in older adults (Guralnik and Kaplan, 1989; Omen, 1990). Many studies report that compliance with health behaviours improves with age (Belloc and Breslow, 1972; Breslow and Enstrom, 1981; Prolaska *et al.*, 1985). In fact, not only are older adults more likely to practise health-promoting activities, but many also report the need for more emphasis on prevention (Prolaska *et al.*, 1985).

Health education is an integral part of primary prevention. Health professionals who are planning health education programmes need to consider changes associated with the normal ageing process. In addition to the general principles of health promotion, special strategies can improve the quality of health education for the elderly. Table 9.1 offers some specific teaching strategies for working with the elderly.

Table 9.1 Special teaching strategies for the elderly

Intervention	Rationale
Use deep tone of voice.	Loss of ability to hear high-frequency sounds.
Speak distinctly.	Decreased ability to distinguish words with S, Z, T, F, and G.
On printed materials use non-glossy paper and contrasting colours (black on white, red on white, etc.).	Decreased visual acuity.
Avoid using blue, green and violet in printed materials.	Decreased ability to see blues, greens, and violets. Lens become thickened and yellow.
Use adequate lighting.	Pupils smaller with less light reaching retina.
Keep environment as free of distractions as possible.	Decreased ability to concentrate.
Slow pace of teaching.	Slowed cognitive functioning.
Present one idea at a time using short, concrete words and practical applications.	Decreased ability to think abstractly.

Nutrition

Dietary guidelines and accommodations for the elderly have not been clearly defined as scientific data is lacking. It has been noted that approximately 30% of community dwelling elderly consume diets deficient in at least one major nutrient (Forciea, 1989). Undernutrition is not uncommon for the 'at-risk' elderly, i.e. the chronically ill/disabled, alcoholics, persons living alone or having limited retirement incomes. Functional problems such as low vision and ill-fitting dentures also impair nutrition (Morley *et al.*, 1986).

On the other hand, obesity is more common in the elderly than is undernutrition. Obesity in older adults contributes to hypertension and diabetes and is associated with increased risk of cancer of the colon, breast and uterus (Sutnick, 1988; Forciea, 1989). A weight loss programme should be encouraged for the grossly obese (40% or more above ideal body weight) or those who are having complications from their obesity.

Dietary assessment and recommendations should be individually determined eliciting the elder's perception of obstacles to improving nutrition.

The nutritional evaluation of the elderly should include the following: ability to pay for food; ability to procure food; ability and willingness to prepare food; and ability to eat food. Stults (1984) suggests that detailed nutritional assessment programmes be focused on the elderly at risk for nutritional deficiencies. For those seeking education regarding a healthy diet, the following simple principles may be applied:

1. eat a variety of foods;
2. maintain a desirable weight;
3. avoid too much fat and cholesterol;
4. eat foods with adequate starch and fibre;
5. avoid too much sugar;
6. avoid too much sodium; and
7. drink enough water (about 8 glasses/day) (Sutnick, 1988).

Strategies
- Provide an ongoing nutrition education class for older adults and offer certificates to those who attend.
- Establish a library or resource centre of books, articles, brochures and audiovisuals regarding nutrition.
- Prepare a nutrition education column for local publications that have a high elderly readership.
- Include the physician as a means for education, for studies have shown the physician as the preferred source of information.
- Recognize the importance of mealtime as a time for socialization and organized small group meal programmes (e.g. lunch club).

Exercise

Exercise is consistently identified as one of the most significant health interventions in the lives of the elderly. A physically active older woman is likely to be physiologically one to two decades younger than a sedentary contemporary (O'Brien and Vertinsky, 1991). Positive effects of exercise include lowering of blood pressure, decreasing cholesterol level and decreasing bone loss (Grisso and Mezey, 1990). In addition, a regular exercise programme can enhance physical, social, and emotional well-being. Another important outcome of exercise is stress reduction which is linked to better sleep, muscle relaxation and improved self-concept (Berger, 1989).

Many physiological changes that have been attributed to ageing are similar to losses that occur from inactivity. If loss of function in the elderly is due to inactivity, exercise programmes for the elderly may prevent or restore some of the functional loss (Stults, 1984).

Prior to starting an exercise programme, it is essential to determine an elder's capacity to exercise and to develop an appropriate exercise programme. The American Heart Association recommended a physical examination and exercise stress testing for sedentary men over 45 years of age and for sedentary women over 50 years of age. The Royal College of Physicians advises a physical examination but minimal use of special testing (Pastorino and Dickey, 1990).

The appropriate intensity level of exercise and the type of activity will vary for each person depending on their present status. Even the slowest pace of walking has been shown to be sufficient to provide significant benefits to extremely frail individuals who usually remain sitting (Gueldner and Spradley, 1988). Although lower-level activity programmes probably have more appeal to a larger segment of the older population, some healthy older subjects are able to receive great health improvements in high-intensity exercise programmes, such as running, swimming, and calesthenics (Gorman and Posner, 1988). Most health-promoting exercise specialists recommend that 20–30 minutes of continuous exercise three to four times each week is necessary for most individuals (O'Brien and Vertinsky, 1991). Listed below are specific recommended measures for a physical fitness programme (Stults, 1984).

- Educate older persons about the types of exercise (i.e. stretching, strengthening, aerobic, relaxation) and benefits
- Obtain physician approval prior to initiating an exercise programme (a physical examination or other testing may be required)
- Assess the older person's history of exercise, particularly likes and dislikes
- Prescribe an exercise programme based on functional abilities, individual needs, and interests. (Remember, even performing activities of daily living is a form of exercise in frail elderly)

- Gradually increase the frequency and/or duration of the exercise programme
- Monitor progress and offer positive feedback
- Arrange for qualified supervision of exercise if needed
- Set an example for those around you by following your own exercise programme

Strategies
- Educate the elderly in your community that it is never too late to start an exercise programme.
- Encourage programmes that include a variety of exercises to improve co-ordination, muscle strength, flexibility, and endurance.
- Encourage elderly persons to capitalize on the exercise of everyday activities, such as walking to post a letter or gardening (see Case study 1, p. 184).

Smoking cessation

Smoking remains prevalent among those over 65 (Forciea, 1989). Smoking has been identified as the single most preventable cause of disease and premature death. An estimated average of 5½ minutes is lost for each cigarette smoked (Fielding, 1985). Smoking is a primary factor associated with lung cancer and other lung diseases, cardio-vascular diseases, as well as cancer of the larynx, pharynx, oral cavity, oesophagus, pancreas and bladder. Cigarette smoking is a stronger predictor of stroke mortality than high blood pressure (Institute of Medicine, 1990). In addition, passive smoking, the exposure of non-smokers to tobacco smoke, has been shown to have harmful effects on the non-smoker (Gambert and Gupta, 1989). Finally, older smokers may be fire hazards in their own homes or in congregate living sites (Forciea, 1989).

People who stop smoking at any age show an immediate improve-ment in lung function. Smokers who are able to stop smoking reduce coronary heart disease mortality to nearly the levels of non-smokers within 1 to 5 years of cessation. Reduction in the rate of lung cancer is seen after smoking stops (Forciea, 1989).

Public attitude surveys have indicated that the majority of smokers have either tried to stop smoking or would like to do so. Elderly persons may not be aware of the physiological improvements achieved by smoking cessation. Additionally, smokers may be physically or psychologically addicted to nicotine (Forciea, 1989).

Most people who have stopped smoking do so on their own. Physician advice and counselling have been associated with a signi-ficant increase in the rate of smoking cessation. The rate improves more significantly with educational material and, for some, nicotine gum

(Sachs, 1986). Formal smoking cessation classes, such as group counselling, and aversion techniques, such as rapid smoking and hypnosis, are successful for some smokers. Health care professionals can play an important role in helping older persons to stop smoking. Ockene and Ockene (1982) have developed important strategies for health care professionals to help reduce the incidence of smoking.

Strategies

- Emphasize the value of cessation at any age and no matter how long the person has smoked when urging the smoker to stop.
- Foster the smoker's belief in an ability to stop as you maintain a positive attitude.
- Educate the smoker regarding various smoking cessation methods available.
- For those smokers who are unable or unwilling to quit smoking, encourage cutting down on cigarettes.

Accident prevention

Accidents are the fifth leading cause of death in the elderly (Rubenstein *et al.*, 1988). Falls, motor vehicle accidents, fires and contact with hot substances account for 85% of all injury deaths (Stults, 1984).

Falls are the most common cause of accidents in people over 60 and are the cause of a half of all accidental deaths. Over the age of 75, the frequency of falls increases dramatically (Stults, 1984). Complications associated with falling include soft tissue injuries, fractures, especially of the hip and femur, subdural haematomas and hot water burns subsequent to falling in the bathtub (Kay and Tideiksoar, 1990). Death associated with falls in the over 65 age group is more common in: women; urban populations; persons who live alone; persons with multiple medical problems; and persons receiving multiple medications (Brody and Persky, 1990). Factors that contribute to the risk of falling are listed below (Grisso and Mezey, 1990; Rubenstein *et al.*, 1988).

- Postural hypotension blood pressure decline;
- medications (e.g. sedatives, antihypertensives, neuroleptics);
- alcohol use;
- diminished vision and/or hearing;
- decreased mobility/gait disturbances (e.g. Parkinson's disease, post stroke);
- decreased mental status;
- previous history of falls;
- decreased ability to perform ADLs (activities of daily living);
- cardiovascular or neurological disorders (e.g. arrhythmias, chronic heart failure (CHF), dementia).

Strategies to prevent falls require not only identifying the factors that cause the falls but also an assessment of environmental factors. Persons at risk of falling and their families should be made aware of the home hazards listed in Figure 9.3 and be reminded that most falls occur in the bathroom and bedroom. Balance and gait abnormalities are often associated with falls. Rehabilitative strategies include muscle strength training, motor co-ordination exercises for persons with balance problems and gait training for those with gait imbalance. Proper use of assistive devices, if appropriate, needs to be taught (Institute of Medicine, 1990). Attention to minimizing environmental hazards and identifying and treating medical conditions and risk factors can potentially decrease the incidence of falls in the elderly (Rubenstein *et al.*, 1988).

Motor vehicle accidents are another major area of injury in the elderly. Elderly persons with impaired vision, mental illness (e.g. dementia), or major neuromuscular impairment should be counselled to limit or discontinue driving. Pedestrian deaths generally occur at junctions and have been related to the elderly person's slow rate of walking (Stults, 1984). A Swedish study demonstrated that 205 persons over age 75, living in the community, were unable to cross a junction in the time allocated between traffic signals (Lundren-Lindquist *et al.*, 1983).

Burn injuries result mainly from scalds due to hot tap water, from contact burns and from flame injuries. Scalds from hot water in the bathing area are most common and most preventable by setting hot water heaters at a lower temperature (Stults, 1984).

Research in the UK has shown that a low indoor temperature can cause disease or death as well as discomfort. Deaths related to cold temperatures are estimated to be responsible for 40 000–75 000 deaths in the UK every year. A national study in the UK showed that elderly

Home
Inadequate lighting, especially in bathroom and stairs
Low-lying objects, such as foot stools, low tables, toddlers, toys and pets
Slippery surfaces and spills
Loose rugs
Faulty flooring
Rickety stairs and/or loose banisters
Temperature control
  Water too hot
  Environment too cold
Personal
Improper shoes, especially worn slippers
Trips to bathroom at night, especially if lighting inadequate

Figure 9.3 Hazards associated with falls in the elderly (Source: Grisso and Mezey, 1989).

living alone, having no central heating/unheated bedrooms or having no community services, were at highest risk from cold-associated diseases or deaths (The Nation's Health, 1988).

Education is an essential element in the prevention of accidents. Health professionals working with the elderly have the opportunity to reduce falls and injury through preventive measures.

Strategies
- Educate the elderly and the community to assess homes for potential hazards related to falls and fires.
- Teach the elderly methods to prevent falls by reducing or eliminating hazards, staying physically active and using assistive devices when necessary.
- Educate the elderly and the community about the risk of pedestrian injuries at junctions, especially at night.
- Educate the elderly and their families about the need to maintain an indoor temperature of 21°C, as recommended by WHO.

Immunizations

The elderly are at risk from certain infectious diseases. Influenza, pneumococcal pneumonia and tetanus are all diseases that are potentially preventable by immunization. These diseases can have serious effects, especially among the elderly who have chronic debilitating illness or who live in institutions. Old age itself appears to be a risk factor for becoming severely ill from infectious disease. Generally speaking, the number of elderly who get the disease and any complications is significantly reduced through appropriate immunizations (Powers and Sears, 1987). The recommended schedule for the immunizations is included in Table 9.2.

Strategies
- Check the influenza, pneumococcal and tetanus immunization status of all elderly.
- Educate the elderly about the importance of immunizations.
- Distribute printed educational literature about the 'why and how to get' immunizations.
- Keep a record of immunization status of elderly clients.

Secondary prevention

Routine health screening of the elderly has been a subject of controversy largely due to limited guidelines regarding screening of healthy older adults (Wolf-Klein, 1989). Given our present knowledge of common disease in the elderly such as hypertension and cancer, screening is a vital role in the early diagnosis and treatment of disease. Outcomes

Table 9.2 Suggested preventive health care for persons 60 and over without symptoms

Examination/test	Frequency
Physical examination	Every 1–3 yrs until 75 yrs old; then annually
Pelvic examination	Annually
Pap smear	At least every 3 yrs after 2 negative examinations 1 year apart
Breast self-examination	Monthly
Breast examination by physician	Annually
Mammogram	Every 1–2 yrs until at least age 85
Rectal examination	Annually
Stool for occult blood	Annually
Sigmoidoscopy	Every 3–5 yrs after 2 negative examinations 1 year apart
Prostate examination	Annually
Blood pressure	Every six months
Eye examination	Every 2 yrs
Glaucoma testing	Every 2 yrs
Medication review	Annually
Dental examination	Yearly
Hearing test	Every 2–5 yrs
Immunizations	
Flu vaccine	Annually
Pneumonia vaccine	Once after age 65
Tetanus booster	Every 10 years
Comprehensive functional assessment	Baseline data before age 80, then every 1–2 yrs or upon any significant change in condition

Sources: Ebersole and Hess, 1990; Robie, 1989; Spitzer *et al.*, 1979.

of this secondary level of prevention may include 'cure' or, of equal importance to the elderly, the prevention of complications or further disability (Turner and Chavigny, 1988; Wolf-Klein, 1988). Table 9.2 represents a computation of screening guidelines.

Cancer screening

Cancer is commo in the elderly. In fact, just growing older is cited as the single greatest risk factor for the development of cancer (Welch-McCaffrey and Dodge, 1988). Over 57% of all cancers occur in the over

65 population (Crawford and Cohen, 1987) and unfortunately a third to a half of new cancers are diagnosed at advanced stages (Warnecke *et al.*, 1983). Most older adults are unaware or misinformed about the risk of cancer. Symptoms often viewed as 'normal ageing changes' by the elderly such as constipation, anorexia, weight loss and malaise may go unreported, further negating the likelihood of early diagnosis and treatment (Welch-McCaffrey and Engelking, 1992).

Robie (1989) believes the two major functions of cancer screening in the elderly are, first, early detection and 'cure' of symptomatic localized cancers, and second, time to provide necessary health education to persons in order to alter health habits which may increase cancer risk (e.g. primary prevention via health education and smoking cessation).

The effectiveness of cancer screening and risk factor modification in the elderly is unknown at this time due to lack of scientific data (Robie, 1989; Institute of Medicine, 1990). Recent guidelines suggested by groups such as the American Cancer Society (1984) and Canadian Task-Force (Spitzer *et al.*, 1979) outline the need for routine screening of breast, colorectal, prostrate and uterine cancers in the elderly (see guidelines in Table 9.8). Screening high-risk elderly in this population has been suggested as the most realistic approach. However, since ageing is a primary risk factor, narrowing the scope of those screened may cause a large number of cases to be missed (List, 1987). Consideration of patient preference, ability to withstand both screening and any needed treatment and improving quality of life may be useful as guides for health professionals to further tailor screening. For example, one may not choose to perform sigmoidoscopy in an elderly man with advanced dementia. Therefore, when cancer screening and detection occur, it is necessary to consider assessment of improved quality of life and functional status, as well as decreased mortality (Robie, 1989).

Strategies
- Educate the elderly about their increased risk of cancer and the need for routine screening to detect cancer in early stages.
- Teach signs and symptoms of most common cancers in the elderly (see Figure 9.4).
- Teach the elderly techniques which aid in early detection (e.g. breast

Men	Women
Prostate	Breast
Lung	Colon
Colon	Lung
Bladder	Uterus
Rectum	Rectum

Figure 9.4 Leading cancer sites in the elderly (Source: Baranovsky and Myers, 1986).

self-examination, reporting changes in skin lesions, fecal occult blood screening).
- Consider cancer screening 'outreach' clinics as a means of screening rural or economically disadvantaged elderly.
- Individualize cancer screening for specific patients considering patient preferences, functional status and presence of comorbid disease.

Hypertension

High blood pressure is estimated to affect 30–50% of the elderly (Applegate, 1989). Both diastolic hypertension (diastolic pressure ≥90 mmHg) and isolated systolic hypertension (systolic pressure ≥160 mmHg and diastolic pressure ≤90 mmHg) are known to be predictive of future cardiovascular and cerebrovascular disease in the elderly. Not surprisingly, cardiovascular disease is the most common cause of morbidity and mortality in persons over 75 years while cerebrovascular disease is the third most common cause (Institute of Medicine, 1990; US Bureau of the Census, 1988). In the elderly, isolated systolic hypertension carries greater risk of morbidity and mortality than diastolic hypertension (Kannel *et al.*, 1971; Rowe, 1982).

In developed countries, systolic blood pressure increases with age due to an increase in vascular resistance. Diastolic pressure rises with age, but generally stabilizes after 60. While some increase in blood pressure may be acceptable, high blood pressure should not be considered normal ageing (Kane *et al.*, 1984). Rowe (1991) cautions that not counselling older patients with slightly elevated blood pressures to exercise and reduce weight/sodium intake will increase their risk of adverse cardiac events and strokes.

Blood pressure screening in a physician's office, ambulatory or home setting is effective (Rosner and Polk, 1983; Sumner, 1991) and has been predictive of future cardiovascular events. Of all preventive screening measures, blood pressure examination is performed most routinely. In fact, older persons often self-initiate blood pressure checks at health fairs, community shopping centres, etc. (Omen, 1990).

Non-pharmacological therapy (i.e. weight loss, salt restriction, relaxation/biofeedback and exercise) may be useful initially in patients with borderline elevations (Stults, 1984). Pharmacological treatment of moderate to severe hypertension is often warranted. Monitoring the elderly for common side-effects such as postural hypertension, electrolyte imbalance, glucose intolerance, and depression is essential to prevent adverse effects on the person's quality of life (Mosner, 1982).

Strategies
- Monitor blood pressure, checking for orthostatic changes as part of all routine examinations in the elderly.

- Educate the elderly about the benefits of diet, exercise, not smoking and relaxation in the prevention of hypertension.
- Consider non-pharmacological interventions in treatment of borderline blood pressure elevations.
- Teach patients on drug therapy to report potential side-effects such as fatigue, mental status changes, incontinence and sexual dysfunction.

Medication

Due to an increase in health problems and chronic conditions associated with ageing, polypharmacy is a common phenomenon in the elderly. It has been noted that persons over 60 years consume 30–40% of all prescription drugs in Canada, the UK, and the USA (Nolan and O'Malley, 1988; Safe use of medications: A consumer issue, 1990). Given this current level of drug use by the elderly, it has been predicted that usage could increase to 50% by the year 2000 (Lamy, 1986). Non-institutionalized older adults take approximately 3.8 drugs daily while those in chronic care facilities and nursing homes receive an average of 6.1 drugs daily (Thomas and Price, 1987; Chien *et al.*, 1978). The most common prescription drugs include diuretics, digoxin, antihypertensives, antiarthritis medications and anxiolytics (Stults, 1984; Kurfees and Dotson, 1987; *The Nation's Health*, 1988).

The elderly are the largest consumers of over-the-counter (OTC) medications such as analgesics, vitamins, antacids, hypnotics and laxatives (Guttman, 1977). Traditional medications such as folk medicine, herbs and homeopathic remedies may also be utilized. Most older persons are unaware that OTC medications are indeed drugs and can interfere with the use of prescription drugs.

Approximately 30% of community dwelling elderly experience adverse drug reactions resulting in up to 10% of hospital admissions (Carty *et al.*, 1985; *The Nation's Health*, 1988). Multiple factors may contribute to the increase in adverse drug reactions in the elderly and include: altered pharmacokinetics and pharmacodynamics; multiple chronic illnesses often requiring multiple medications; types of drugs prescribed; and poor compliance with drug regimen (Nolan and O'Malley, 1988). Bigby *et al.* (1987) have estimated that 50% of hospital admissions due to adverse drug reactions could be prevented by more judicious prescribing by physicians.

As many as a third of older persons do not receive counselling or education from their health care professionals about how to use medications correctly. Many are additionally uncomfortable questioning professionals about drug therapy (Safe use of medications: A consumer issue, 1990). Poor vision and inability to read prescription labels, misunderstanding instructions, inability to get to a pharmacy or afford

1. Establish a diagnosis and consider nonpharmacological methods of treatment if possible.
2. Take a careful drug history, including OTC drugs, alcohol use and other home remedies.
3. Know the pharmacology of the drug(s) prescribed.
4. Dose carefully, utilizing the rule 'start low and go slow' to achieve desired response.
5. Simplify the medication regimen by reducing unnecessary drugs whenever possible.
6. Provide necessary information to patient/caregiver including reason for drug, expected benefits, possible side-effects, possible food/drug interactions.
7. Be sure patient can read prescription labels and can open containers.
8. Regularly review the need for continued drug therapy.

Figure 9.5 Principles for prescribing for the elderly (Source: Stults, 1984; Rousseau, 1987; O'Brien and Kursch, 1987).

medications further impede the effectiveness of drug therapy (Stults, 1984). Care in prescribing medications (see Figure 9.5), periodic review of medications, adequate instruction of the patient and/or caregiver can serve as essential preventive measures in minimizing adverse drug reactions (O'Brien and Kursch, 1987).

Strategies
- Educate the elderly to take medication properly (utilize written materials, memory aids, pill dispenser, etc.).
- Educate the elderly regarding their responsibility to memorize or carry a list of current medications (including OTC medication) and supply this information to health professionals.
- Teach the elderly and/or caregivers common symptoms that may indicate adverse drug reaction.
- Encourage the elderly to ask questions regarding medications.
- Invite local pharmacists to give talks on proper use of medication.

Mental health

Screening for mental health problems such as depression and dementia in old age is imperative in order to enhance the psychological well-being of the elderly. Unfortunately, mental health needs are often overlooked and thus unmet (Ebersole and Hess, 1990). Better understanding of depression and dementia in the elderly, as well as their social support system, will equip health professionals in meeting mental health needs in this population.

Depression
Depression is the most common mental illness in the aged population. The incidence of depression varies in the elderly, with higher rates

Symptoms of depression in the elderly

- Somatic complaints/body preoccupation;
- deny dysphoric mood;
- loss of interest in usual activities;
- apathy and withdrawal from contact with others;
- disturbed sleep patterns;
- agitation or psychomotor retardation;
- loss of self-esteem;
- inability to concentrate;
- recurrent thoughts of death/suicide.

Sources: Ebersole and Hess, 1990; Kane, Ouslander and Abrass, 1984.

associated with physical illness and disability. The elderly dwelling in nursing homes experience high rates of depression often related to illness and disability causing loss of autonomy and control. Approximately 25% of those with dementia also suffer from major depression (Institute of Medicine, 1990).

Although depression is prevalent among the elderly, diagnosis and treatment are often delayed (Heckheimer, 1989). Older people often find seeking help for emotional problems taboo, and are more likely to present with somatic complaints. Some may believe their problems are part of normal ageing and consequently believe nothing can be done. Health professionals may also fail to recognize depression due to lack of knowledge of depression and atypical presentation in the elderly. The most serious consequence of depression is the risk of suicide, particularly in men aged 75 and over (Kinsella, 1990).

Risk factors for depression in late life are multiple and often relate to loss. Common losses may include: physical limitations due to loss of health; sensory losses; death of spouse, family, and friends; unplanned retirement; loss of a confidant; and residential relocation. A family history of depression or a history of having been depressed earlier in life also serves as a risk factor (Gottlieb, 1988; Blazer and Maddox, 1982). The elderly are thought to be more vulnerable to depression due to decreased production of mood-controlling neurotransmitters (Ebersole and Hess, 1990). Medical illnesses may present with signs and symptoms of depression (e.g. malignancies, endocrine disorders). Medications can also cause symptoms of depression in the elderly (Levenson and Hall, 1981).

In general, older persons respond very favourably to treatment. Effective treatments include psychosocial, pharmacological and electro-convulsive therapies. Given the prognosis of treatment, the primary objective should be to identify depression in this population.

Strategies
- Consider periodic screening of elderly patients for depression utilizing an established screening instrument.
- Be alert for depression factors.
- Assess patient's ability to cope with stressors or losses.
- Encourage the bereaved or grieving patient to find a confidant.
- Discuss treatment options for depression with patient and/or family members.
- Educate the elderly to recognize that depression is not considered a normal part of ageing.

Dementia

The exact prevalence of dementia is unknown; however, it is thought to affect over 5% of persons over 65 years with rates up to 20% in the oldest-old group. Alzheimer's disease accounts for 70% of all dementing illnesses (Schneck *et al.*, 1982). Sadly, dementia is an illness which affects the entire family and is the leading cause of institutionalization (Arie, 1984).

While there are few beneficial treatments for most dementias, rigorous attention must be given in the medical evaluation in order to detect reversible causes of dementia which may be present in up to 15% of demented older patients (Larson *et al.*, 1984). Health professionals play an essential role in dementia care in the areas of symptom management, adapting the environment and supporting the caregiver. Screening these three areas are important secondary prevention methods in attempting to maximize patient function while delaying dependency on the caregiver, prevent premature institutionalization and enhance well-being of the patient and family. Periodic evaluation of the patient and caregiver by various team members is recommended and demonstrated in Case study 2 (p. 185).

Strategies
- Educate family about dementia and suggestions for management.
- Provide anticipatory guidelines to caregiver to prevent premature disability, i.e. never do for patients what they can do for themselves.
- Educate caregivers to keep the environment quiet and structured.
- Assess caregiver need for support, home help and respite care. Provide resources whenever possible.
- Perform an environmental assessment and adapt environment to enhance safety and function.
- Remain alert to a sudden change in function, indicating the presence of a secondary medical process/illness.
- Monitor for side-effects of medication.

(Sources: Dwyer, 1987; Heckheimer, 1989.)

Social support

Social support and maintenance of the social network throughout the lifespan is an essential element to successful ageing. Antonucci and Akiyama (1991) suggest that 'social relations influence how individuals experience their lives, how they feel about the experience – in essence, whether or not they age well' (p. 42).

Recent studies recognize the importance of social support to the overall health and well-being of individuals. A decrease in immunological function is reported in people who are socially isolated or lonely (Kiecolt-Glaser and Glaser, 1988). The lack of family and community support is associated with higher mortality rates (Berkman and Symes, 1979; Blazer, 1982). Benefits of social support that are 'health protective' range from improved rehabilitation and recovery to sustaining good health in old age secondary to strong social support (Wortman and Conway, 1985; Langlie, 1977). It is believed that individuals with strong social networks will practise health-promoting behaviours thus achieving better health. For example, family or friends may intervene to assist in making medical appointments, provide transportation, etc.

Screening for social support is an important secondary prevention measure. It is at this stage when older persons may require additional help or support, particularly in those requiring long-term assistance, secondary to illness/disability. In general most older persons receive the informal help they need from family and friends (Herzog and House, 1991). However, with the growing number of elderly being cared for in their homes by family members (usually wives, daughters or daughters-in-law), caregivers must also be questioned regarding their support needs (*The Nation's Health*, 1988). The goal in screening is to provide needed services, prevent social isolation, and maintain meaningful relationships for both the elderly and their caregivers (Rook, 1984). Matching patient health and social needs to resources is a challenge for health professionals working with the elderly. Services available to the elderly may be home or community based or institutional. Figure 9.6 demonstrates the continuum of care which may provide services to the elderly which are diagnostic, preventive, therapeutic, rehabilitative, or supportive. Knowledge of services available to elderly patients and caregivers within the continuum is necessary so that patients and families may be directed to appropriate resources. Meeting health and social support needs via the continuum of care may postpone institutionalization and increase quality of life for the elderly and caregiver.

Strategies
- Assess social support available to 'high-risk' elderly patients (e.g. elderly with chronic illness, impairments in self-care and/or domestic tasks, recent widowhood, homebound and family caregivers).

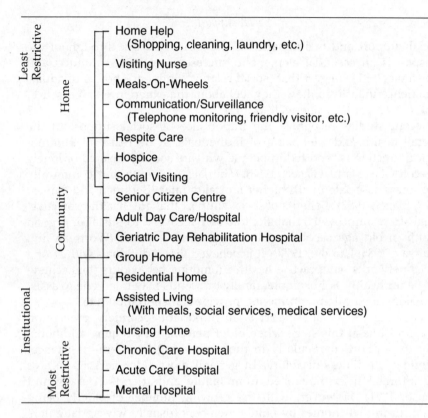

Figure 9.6 Continuum of care: services for the elderly (Adapted from: Brody and Masciocchi, 1980).

- Identify potential community resources available for elderly patients (see Figure 9.6).
- Initiate community resources and home help in a timely manner in order to prevent/postpone institutionalization.
- Educate the elderly and their families about the importance of social needs.
- Provide information to the elderly and/or caregivers about available resources.

Urinary incontinence

Urinary incontinence, as defined by the International Continence Society, is the involuntary loss of urine causing social and/or hygienic consequences (Bates *et al.*, 1979). Studies citing the incidence of incontinence among the elderly are raising public awareness of this problem. It has been estimated that 15–30% of community-dwelling elderly and 50–70% of nursing home residents suffer from some degree of urinary incontinence (National Institute of Health, 1988).

Consequences of incontinence are significant and include social isolation, lowered self-esteem, depression and related health problems such as infection and skin breakdown (Noelker, 1987). Family members caring for an incontinent elder report that incontinence care is a difficult task and often determines the need for institutionalization (Mohide, 1986; Ouslander, 1981). The financial implications of incontinence care are staggering when factoring in diagnostic and evaluation costs, treatment pads, labour costs and consequences related to incontinence (e.g. falls, urinary tract infection, etc.) (Hu, 1986).

Many older persons fail to report incontinence to health professionals as they consider it a normal part of ageing for which nothing can be done (Mittness, 1988). Health professionals also lack knowledge about incontinence. Brocklehurst (1988) cites curriculum and clinical experience dedicated to urinary and faecal incontinence is lacking in both medical and nursing education. This lack of knowledge may further reinforce lay beliefs that little can be done to treat incontinence.

While the natural history and risk factors of urinary incontinence remain relatively unknown, tremendous progress is being made in the assessment, diagnosis and management of incontinence. Treatments vary according to the type of incontinence and include pelvic muscle exercise, behavioural therapies, drug therapies and surgical interventions. Although treatment of incontinence may not result in a 'cure', it can be significantly improved even in frail elderly.

The UK has taken a lead in incontinence care by producing materials for professional education (*Action on Incontinence*, 1983) and establishing nurse continence advisors to assist both patients and health professionals in the management of incontinence (Norton, 1986). As other countries follow this example, it is hoped that those with incontinence will come forth sooner for evaluation and treatment.

Strategies

- Obtain or update health professional's knowledge of assessment, evaluation and treatment of urinary incontinence.
- Query adult and elderly patients about signs and symptoms of incontinence (see Figure 9.7).

- Do you have trouble making it to the toilet on time?
- Do you lose urine when you have a strong urge to urinate?
- Do you lose urine when you lift heavy objects?
- Do you lose urine when you cough or sneeze?
- Do you lose urine when you walk, run, or exercise?
- Do you wear protective pads or garments?
- When you lose urine, how much do you lose?
- How frequently do you lose urine?
- Have you ever talked to a health professional about urine loss?

Figure 9.7 Questions regarding presence of urinary incontinence.

- Individualize evaluations and treatment considering the patient's functional and cognitive status.
- Provide patients and families accurate information on the management of incontinence.
- Educate the public that incontinence is not a normal part of ageing and that most cases can be cured or improved.

Tertiary prevention

Comprehensive functional assessment is considered the cornerstone of tertiary prevention in the identification and subsequent minimization of existing disability (Johnson and Mezey, 1989; *The Nation's Health*, 1988). This multidemensional assessment attempts to sort through the effects of normal age-related changes, acute and/or chronic illness(es), and the demands of the social and physical environment. The interactions among these variables have a dramatic effect on the ability of the older person to perform the functional tasks needed to live independently. This assessment can provide valuable information to health professionals working with the elderly, often determining the elder's overall health, well-being, ability to function and potential service utilization (Kane *et al.*, 1984). Additional benefits may include diagnosis and treatment of previously unrecognized conditions, more

Table 9.3 Comprehensive functional assessment of health in old age

Components	*Domain*
Physical Health	Evaluates health status by history and physical, self-rated health, etc.
Mental Health	Evaluates cognitive, behavioural and emotional status.
Social Economic Status	Evaluates support network, cultural and ethnic values, and economic resources.
Functional Status Activities Activities of Daily Living (ADL)	Evaluates self-care activities such as bathing, dressing, toileting, feeding, continence, and mobility.
Instrumental Activities of Daily Living (IADL)	Evaluates performance in activities such as meal preparation, shopping, housekeeping, transportation, financial management, etc.
Environmental Characteristics	Evaluates patient's physical environment to determine safety and access to services.

Sources: Solomon, 1988; Kane and Kane, 1981.

appropriate and decreased use of medications and potentially lower rates of institutionalization (Solomon, 1988).

Components of comprehensive functional assessment include physical, mental, socio-economic, functional and environmental status (see Table 9.3). Particular attention is given to functional status, i.e. the older person's ability to carry out activities of daily living (ADL) and instrumental activities of daily living (IADL). Completion of this assessment adds to the health professional's database, often shifting the emphasis from curing diseases to improving function and preventing further decline. Maintaining or improving even small increments of function can contribute to improving an elder's quality of life. For example, increasing strength in an older person to allow for independent transfers will promote self-care in toileting, thus avoiding episodes of incontinence, need for additional caregiver assistance and potential nursing home placement.

Since the rate of functional disability increases with age, comprehensive functional assessment warrants special attention in those over 80 years. A team approach is often the best method for assessing the elderly. Numerous screening scales and instruments have been developed to measure function. Those instruments which are most useful are easily administered, and detect slight changes in function. Direct observation of an elder's performance in ADLs and IADLs generally yields more reliable information, as elderly patients tend to overestimate their abilities while family caregivers underestimate abilities.

When working with the elderly who have disabilities, it is important to focus on what individuals can do and build on those functional abilities rather than to focus on deficits. Lawton (1991) notes that with frailty, the elderly may selectively retain or cultivate special skills as a mechanism to adapt and therefore maintain a sense of competence. Health professionals need to support and/or facilitate such adaptive abilities in elders so that successful ageing may be achieved.

Strategies

- Establish a programme of comprehensive functional assessment.
- Select appropriate assessment instruments consistent with purpose of assessment, patient population and setting.
- Utilize team members to assist with comprehensive functional assessment.
- Match patient function/needs to desired services.

CONCLUSION

The advances of science and public health in conquering life-threatening communicable diseases has increased the average life expectancy from

47 years in 1900 to 75 years in 1987 (Institute of Medicine, 1990). This ageing of the population and the focus from communicable to chronic disease directs the health professional to encompass the essential elements of health promotion. The aim of geriatric health promotion/ disease prevention efforts is to reduce morbidity and increase function in older persons. For health promotion strategies to be effective, health professionals in all fields, including social, behavioural, biomedical and pharmacological, must work in collaboration with the elderly.

An increasing amount of evidence indicates that older people can benefit from health promotion and disease prevention efforts. Until recently, research has focused on younger populations with little documentation on special risks among the 50-and-older age group. Progress made in prolonging functional independence in the elderly is dependent on research in the biology of ageing and the genetic determinants of age and predisposition to disease (Institute of Medicine, 1990).

Health professionals need to be aware of policy issues that affect the future, including legislative issues, public health and self-responsibility. Curricula in schools for health professionals need to focus on the ageing process, rationing of care and the prevention of disease and promotion of health philosophy. Ageing *per se* and the inevitable end of life cannot be avoided but, preventive strategies can potentially help us reach old age in good health. Ageing is an issue that affects all of us. Hopefully, we will all have an opportunity to be old – and in good health.

CASE STUDIES

Case study 1

Arvel H., an 83-year-old male with a history of arteriosclerotic heart disease and hypertension, and Dorothy C., a 73-year-old female with diet-controlled diabetes and osteoarthritis, are enrolled in an Adult Day Care programme, attending three days a week for socialization and health monitoring. Both Arvel and Dorothy express an interest to participate in a fitness programme. Arvel's goal is to increase his endurance and distance in walking. Dorothy has an additional goal of weight loss.

The Adult Day Care Centre has a fitness programme called 'Walk around the World'. Travel posters from cities around the world are strategically placed on walls around the centre. Distances between the posters are measured and assigned 'kilometres' to represent distance from one country to another. Chairs for participants to rest are located throughout this walking course, thus encouraging rest periods when necessary. Participants record the distance walked on a monitoring log located at the beginning of the course. Participants are measured at baseline for distance walked (in metres), blood pressure and pulse. The nurse at the centre assists the participants in setting reasonable goals and monitors progress on a weekly basis.

At baseline, Arvel is able to walk 200 metres, has a blood pressure of 154/86 with a pulse of 82. His goal is to achieve a distance of 800 metres. This distance will allow him to walk to and from his home to the corner market. Arvel and the nurse set a plan for him to increase his distance by 50 metres per week with one short stop of approximately two minutes. Over the next twelve weeks Arvel achieved his goal and maintained his blood pressure and pulse at acceptable levels.

Dorothy was able to walk 600 metres at baseline with a blood pressure of 136/78, pulse 76, and weight of 68 kg. Her goal was to increase her distance to one kilometre and decrease her weight to 61 kg. (Dorothy is following a 1200 kcal reducing diet prescribed by her physician.) Dorothy and the nurse set the goal for her to walk one kilometre and lose 7 kilograms over 14–16 weeks. Dorothy weighed in once a week and had her blood pressure and pulse monitored after each walk. She was able to achieve her goal after 17 weeks.

Case study 2

A newly designed community programme has been implemented to assess newly diagnosed persons with Alzheimer's disease and their family/caregivers. Referrals may be made by health professionals, family members, etc. A nurse trained in geriatrics visits the home to assess family needs and potential caregiving resources, performs a functional assessment of the person with Alzheimer's disease, assesses the environment for safety, and identifies community resources that may enhance caregiving. A second visit is scheduled for a social worker or trained volunteer to review the assessment with the family. Suggestions are given about environmental changes, dealing with identified difficult behaviours (e.g. wandering, incontinence, etc.), how to obtain community services and support groups that are available. Education is a central theme as information about the disease is given to family members.

Ethel is an 82-year-old female diagnosed with Alzheimer's disease approximately two months ago, although her husband reports 'memory problems' for the past three years (since she had gallbladder surgery). Her husband, George, is 84 years old and has hypertension and arthritis. He has gradually taken over all of the household duties. The functional assessment reveals: Ethel needs assistance (verbal cueing) with bathing and dressing, and is independent in feeding, grooming and ambulation. Ethel is unable to assist with instrumental activities with the exception of setting the table. The environment is without

186   *Enhancing health and function in late life*

hazards but since Ethel is prone to wandering out of the home, adding locks may be necessary. George believes his primary needs are for assistance in bathing Ethel and time away from home to socialize with his former co-workers.

A follow-up visit was made by the social worker. Recommendations were made to install deadbolt locks to prevent Ethel from leaving the home. Discussion of home help for assistance with bathing and other home chores resulted in obtaining on-going assistance. George was encouraged to enrol Ethel in an Adult Day Care programme two times per week to allow him an opportunity for respite and time to visit his friends. He was also encouraged to join a support group for his own mental health and to receive additonal information about Alzheimer's disease. The social worker encouraged him to call her for any additional information. As part of tertiary prevention, this couple will receive an annual re-evaluation to determine further needs.

REFERENCES

Action on incontinence. Report of a working group (1983) King's Fund Project Paper No. 65.
American Cancer Society (1984) Publication 84–20 m – No. 5005.04.
Antonucci, T. and Akiyama, H. (1991) Social relationships and aging well. *Generations*, **15**, 39–44.
Applegate, W.B. (1989) Hypertension in elderly patients. *Annals of Internal Medicine*, **110**, 901–15.
Arie, T. (1984) Prevention of mental disorders of old age. *Journal of the American Geriatric Society*, **32**, 460–5.
Bates, P., Bradley, W.E., Glen, E. *et al.* (1979) The standardization of terminology of lower urinary tract function. *Journal of Urology*, **121**, 551–4.
Belloc, N.B. and Breslow, L. (1972) Relationship of physical health status and health practices. *Preventive Medicine*, **1**, 409–21.
Berger, B.G. (1989) The role of physical activity in the life quality of older adults, in *The academy papers: Physical activity and aging* (eds. W.W. Spirduso and H.M. Eckert), Human Kinetics Publishers, Champaign, IL, pp. 42–58.
Berkman, L.F. and Symes, S.L. (1979) Social networks, host resistance and mortality: A nine-year follow up study of Alameda County residents. *American Journal of Epidemiology*, **109**, 186–204.
Bigby, J., Dunn, J., Goldman, L. *et al.* (1987) Assessing the preventability of emergency hospital admissions. *American Journal of Medicine*, **83**, 1031–6.
Blazer, D.G. (1982) Social support and mortality in an elderly community population. *American Journal of Epidemiology*, **115**, 684–94.
Blazer, D. and Maddox, G. (1982) Using epidemiology survey data to plan geriatric mental health services. *Hospital & Community Psychiatry*, **33**, 42–5.
Breslow, L. and Enstrom, J.E. (1981) Persistence of health habits and their relationship to mortality. *Preventive Medicine*, **9**, 469–83.
Brocklehurst, J.C. (1988) Professional and public education. Paper presentation at NIH Consensus Development Conference, Bethesda, MD.
Brody, J.A. and Persky, V.W. (1990) Epidemiology and demographics, in *Merck Manual of Geriatrics*, Merck & Co, Rahway, NJ, pp. 1115–27.

Brody, S.J. and Masciocchi, C. (1980) Data for long-term planning by health systems agencies. *American Journal of Public Health*, **70**, 1194–8.

Butler, R.N. and Gleason, H.P. (eds.) (1985) *Productive aging: Enhancing vitality in later life*, Springer Publishers, New York.

Carty, M., Avorn, J., Everitt, D.E. *et al.* (1985) Physician–patient communication and geriatric medication use. *Gerontologist*, **25**, 33.

Chien, C.P., Townsend, E.J. and Townsend, A.R. (1978) Substance use and abuse among the community elderly: The medical aspect. *Additive Diseases*, **3**, 357–72.

Crawford, J. and Cohen, H.J. (1987) Relationship of cancer and aging. *Clinics in Geriatric Medicine*, **3**, 419–32.

Day, S. (1990) Principles of screening, in *Practicing prevention for the elderly* (eds. R. Lavizzo-Mourey *et al.*), Hanley & Belfus, Philadelphia.

Dwyer, B.J. (1987) Alzheimer's Disease: Providing a meaningful existence in the absense of definitive management. *Focus on Geriatric Care and Rehabilitation*, **1**, 1–10.

Dychtwald, K. and Zitter, M. (1988) Medical information is key to treating older citizens. *Modern Healthcare*, **18**, 38 ff.

Ebersole, P. and Hess, P. (1990) Mental health and cognition, in *Toward Healthy Aging* (eds. P. Exersole and P. Hess), 3rd edn., CV Mosby Company, St. Louis, pp. 603–58.

Fielding, J.E. (1985) Smoking: Health effects and control. *New England Journal of Medicine*, **313**, 491–8.

Forciea, M.A. (1989) Nutrition, alcohol, and tobacco in late life, in *Practicing prevention for the elderly* (eds. R. Lavizzo-Mourey *et al.*), Hanley & Belfus, Philadelphia.

Frame, P.S. and Carlson, S.J. (1975) A critical review of periodic health screening using specific screening criteria. *Journal of Family Practice*, **29**, 29 ff.

Fries, J.F. (1980) Aging, natural death and the compression of morbidity. *New England Journal of Medicine*, **303**, 130–5.

Gambert, S.R. and Gupta, K.L. (1989) Preventive care: What it's worth in geriatrics. *Geriatrics*, **44**, 61–71.

Golini, A. and Lori, A. (1990) Aging of the population: Demographics and social changes. *Aging*, **2**, 319–36.

Gorman, K.M. and Posner, J.D. (1988) Benefits of exercise in old age. *Clinics in Geriatric Medicine*, **4**, 181–91.

Gottlieb, G.L. (1988) Optimizing mental function of the elderly, in *Practicing prevention for the elderly* (eds. R. Lavizzo-Mourey *et al.*), Hanley & Belfus, Philadelphia, pp. 153–66.

Grisso, J.A. and Mezey, M.D. (1990) Preventing dependence and injury: An approach to sensory changes, in *Practicing Prevention for the Elderly* (eds. R. Lavizzo-Mourey *et al.*), Hanley & Belfus, Philadelphia.

Gueldner, S.H. and Spradley, J. (1988) Outdoor walking lowers fatigue. *Journal of Gerontological Nursing*, **14**, 6–12.

Guralnik, J.M. and Kaplan, G.A. (1989) Predictors of healthy aging: Prospective evidence from the Alameda County study. *American Journal of Public Health*, **79**, 703–8.

Guttman, D. (1977) *A Survey of drug taking behavior of the elderly*, National Institute on Drug Abuse, Rockville, MD.

Harris, T., Kovar, M.G., Suzman, R. *et al.* (1989) Longitudinal study of physical ability in the oldest-old. *American Journal of Public Health*, **79**, 698–702.

Heckheimer, E.F. (1989) Coping with depression and dementia, in *Health promotion of the elderly in the community* (ed. E.F. Heckheimer), W.B. Saunders Company, Philadelphia, pp. 299–319.

Herzog, A.R. and House, J.S. (1991) Productive activities and aging well. *Generations*, **15**, 49–54.

How do older women fare in the European Community? (1990) *Ageing International*, June, 38–42.

Hu, T.W. (1986) The economic impact of urinary incontinence. *Clinics in Geriatric Medicine*, **2**, 673–81.

Institute of Medicine (1990) *The second 50 years: Promoting health preventing disability*, National Academy Press, Washington, DC.

Institutionalization rates in cross-nation perspective (1989) *Ageing International*, December, 33–5.

Johnson, J.C. and Mezey, M.D. (1989) Functional status assessment: An approach to tertiary prevention, in *Practicing prevention for the elderly* (eds. R. Lavizzo-Mourey *et al.*), Hanley & Belfus, Philadelphia.

Kane, R.A. and Kane, R.L. (1981) *Assessing the elderly*, Lexington Books, Lexington, MA.

Kane, R., Ouslander, J.G. and Abrass, I.B. (1984) *Essentials of Clinical Geriatrics*, McGraw-Hill, New York.

Kannel, W.B., Gordon, T. and Schwartz, M.J. (1971) Systolic vs. diastolic blood pressures and risk of coronary heart disease. *American Journal of Cardiology*, **27**, 335–46.

Katz, S., Branch, L.G., Branson, M.H. *et al.* (1983) Active life expectancy. *New England Journal of Medicine*, **309**, 1218–24.

Kay, A.D. and Tideiksoar, R. (1990) Falls and gait disorder, in *Merck Manual of Geriatrics*, Merck & Co, Rahway, NJ, pp. 52–68.

Kiecolt-Glaser, J.K. and Glaser, R. (1988) Psychological influences on immunity: Implications for AIDS. *American Psychologist*, **43**, 892–8.

Kinsella, K. (1990) Suicide at older ages: An international enigma. *Ageing International*, Winter, 36–9.

Kurfees, J.F. and Dotson, R.L. (1987) Drug interactions in the elderly. *Journal of Family Practice*, **25**, 477–88.

Lamy, P. (1986) Adverse drug reactions and the elderly: An update, in *Geriatric Medicine Annual* (ed. R.J. Ham), Medical Economic Books, Oradell, NJ.

Langlie, J.D. (1977) Social networks, health beliefs and preventive behaviors. *Journal of Health and Social Behaviors*, **18**, 244–60.

Larson, E.B., Reifler, B.V., Featherstone, H.I., *et al.* (1984) Dementia in elderly outpatients: A prospective study. *Annals of Internal Medicine*, **100**, 417–23.

Lawton, M.P. (1991) Functional status and aging well. *Generations*, **15**, 31–4.

Levenson, A.J. and Hall, R.C.W. (eds.) (1981) *Neuropsychiatric manifestation of physical disease in the elderly*, Raven Press, New York.

List, N.D. (1987) Perspectives in cancer screening in the elderly. *Clinics in Geriatric Medicine*, **3**, 433–45.

Lundgren-Lindquist, B., Grimbly, G. and Landahl, S. (1983) Functional studies in 79 year olds: Performance and climbing capacity. *Scandinavian Journal of Rehabilitation Medicine*, **15**, 109–15.

Matteson, M.A., McConnell, E.S., Calhoon, M. *et al.* (1988) Context of services – Network of care, in *Gerontological nursing: Concepts and practice* (eds. M.A. Matteson and E.S. McConnell), W.B. Saunders Company, Philadelphia, pp. 651–86.

Mittness, L.S. (1988) Knowledge and beliefs about urinary incontinence in adulthood and old age. Paper presentation at NIH Consensus Development Conference, Bethesda, MD.

Mohide, E. (1986) The prevalence and scope of urinary incontinence. *Clinics in Geriatric Medicine*, **2**, 639–55.

Morley, J.E., Silver, A.J., Fiatarone, M. *et al.* (1986) Geriatric Grand Rounds: Nutrition and the elderly. *Journal of the American Geriatric Society*, **34**, 823–32.

Mosner, M. (1982) The management of cardiovascular disease in the elderly. *Journal of the American Geriatric Society*, **30**, 20–9.

National Institutes of Health Consensus Development Conference Statement (1988) *Urinary Incontinence in Adults, National Library of Medicine* **7**, 1–32.

Noelker, I.S. (1987) Incontinence in elderly cared for by family. *Gerontologist*, **27**, 194–200.

Nolan, L. and O'Malley, K. (1988) Prescribing for the elderly. *Journal of the American Geriatric Society*, **36**, 142–9.

Norton, C. (1986) *Nursing for Continence*, Beacons Field Publishers Ltd, Beaconsfield, pp. 295–99.

O'Brien, J.G. and Kursch, J.E. (1987) 'Healthy' prescribing for the elderly. *Postgraduate Medicine*, **82**, 147–57.

O'Brien, S. and Vertinsky, P. (1988) Unfit survivors: Exercise as a resource for aging women. *Gerontologist*, **31**, 347–57.

Ockene, J.K. and Ockene, I.S. (1982) *Your patient and cancer*, Dominus Publishing Co, NY, pp. 55–6.

Omen, G.S. (1990) Prevention and the elderly: Appropriate policies. *Health Affairs*, **19**, 80–93.

Ouslander, J.G. (1981) Urinary incontinence in the elderly. *Western Journal of Medicine*, **135**, 482–91.

Ouslander, J.G. and Beck, J.C. (1982) Defining the health problems of the elderly. *Annual Review of Public Health*, **3**, 55–83.

Pastorino, C.A. and Dickey, T. (1990) Health promotion for the elderly: Issues and program planning. *Orthopaedic Nursing*, **9**, 36–42.

Powers, D.C. and Sears, S.D. (1987) Influenza, pneumonia, tetanus: How effective is vaccination? *Geriatrics*, **42**, 81–90.

Prolaska, T.R., Levanthal, E.A., Levanthal, H. and Keller, M.L. (1985) Health practices and illness cognition in young, middle-aged and elderly adults. *Journal of Gerontology*, **40**, 569–78.

Robie, P.W. (1989) Cancer screening in the elderly. *Journal of the American Geriatrics Society*, **37**, 888–93.

Rook, K.S. (1984) Promoting social bonding: Strategies for helping the lonely & socially isolated. *American Psychologist*, **38**, 1389–407.

Roos, N.P. and Havens, B. (1991) Predictors of successful aging: A twelve-year study of Manitoba elderly. *American Journal of Public Health*, **81**, 63–8.

Rosner, B. and Polk, B.F. (1983) Predictive values of routine blood pressure measurements in screening for hypertension. *American Journal of Epidemiology*, **117**, 429–42.

Rousseau, P. (1987) Pharmacologic alterations in the elderly: Special considerations. *Hospital Formulary*, **22**, 543–5.

Rowe, J.W. (1982) Altered blood pressure, in *Health and Disease in Old Age* (eds. J.W. Rowe and R.W. Bedsine), Little, Brown, Boston, pp. 211–22.

Rowe, J. (1991) Reducing the risk of usual aging. *Generations*, **15**, 25–8.

Rowe, J. and Kahn, R.L. (1989) Human Aging: Usual and successful. *Science*, **237**, 143–9.

Rubenstein, L.Z., Robbins, A.S., Schulman, B.L. *et al.* (1988) Falls and instability in the elderly. *Journal of the American Geriatric Society*, **36**, 266–78.

Sachs, D.P. (1986) Cigarette smoking: Health effects and cessation strategies. *Clinics of Geriatric Medicine*, **2**, 337–62.

Safe use of medications: A consumer issue (1990) *Perspectives in Health Promotion and Aging*, **5**, 1.

Schneck, M.K., Reisberg, B. and Ferris, S.H. (1982) An overview of current concepts of Alzheimer's disease. *American Journal of Psychiatry*, **139**, 165–73.

Shamansky, S. and Clausen, C. (1980) Levels of prevention: Examination of the concept. *Nursing Outlook*, **28**, 104–8.

Solomon, D. (1988) NIH Consensus Development Conference Statement: Geriatric assessment methods for clinical-decision-making. *Journal of the American Geriatrics Society*, **36**, 342–7.

Spitzer, W.O., Bayne, R.D., Charron, K.C. *et al.* (1979) Task Force report: The periodic health explanation. *Canadian Medical Association Journal*, **121**, 1193–254.

Spradley, B.W. (1990) *Community Health Nursing* (3rd edn), Scott, Foresman & Co., Glenview, IL.

Stults, B.M. (1984) Preventive health care for the elderly. *Western Journal of Medicine*, **141**, 832–45.

Sumner, J. (1991) Screening the elderly. *Nursing Times*, **87**, 60–2.

Sutnick, M.R. (1988) Dietary guidelines for the elderly. *Clinics of Geriatric Medicine*, **4**, 193–201.

The Nation's Health: A strategy for the 1990's (1988) King Edward's Hospital, Fund for London, London.

Thomas, B. and Price, M. (1987) Drug review. *Journal of Gerontological Nursing*, **13**, 17.

Turner, J.G. and Chavigny, K.H. (1988) *Community Health Nursing*, J.B. Lippincott, Company, Philadelphia.

US Bureau of the Census (1988) *Statistical abstract of the United States* (108th edn), US Government Printing Office, Washington DC.

US Department of Health and Human Services (1990) *Healthy People: National Promotion and Disease Prevention Objectives*, US Government Printing Office, No. (PHS) 91-50213, Washington DC.

Warnecke, R.B., Havlicek, P.L. and Manfredi, C. (1983) Awareness and use of screening by older-aged persons, in *Perspectives in Prevention and Treatment of Cancer in the Elderly* (eds. R. Yancik *et al.*), Raven Press, New York.

Welch-McCaffrey, D. and Dodge, J. (1988) Planning breast self-examination programs for elderly. *Oncology Nursing Forum*, **15**, 811–14.

Welch-McCaffrey, D. and Engelking, C. (1992) Position paper on cancer and aging: The mandate for oncology nursing. *Oncology Nursing Forum*, **19**, 913–33.

Williams, T.F. (1986) Geriatrics: The fruition of the clinician reconsidered. *Gerontologist*, **26**, 345–9.

Wolf-Klein, G. (1988) Screening examinations in the elderly: Which are worthwhile? *Geriatrics*, **44**, 36–47.

World Health Organization Regional Office for Europe (1983) *Protecting the health of the elderly*, World Health Organization, Denmark.

Wortman, C.B. and Conway, T.L. (1985) The role of social support in adaption and recovery from physical illness, in *Social Support and Health* (eds. S. Cohen and S.L. Syme), Academic Press, New York, pp. 281–98.

FURTHER READING

Professional

Butler, R.N. and Gleason, H.P. (eds.) (1985) *Productive aging: Enhancing vitality in later life*, Springer Publishers, New York.

Institute of Medicine (1990) *The second 50 years: Promoting health and preventing disability*, National Acadamy Press, Washington, DC.

Lavizzo-Mourey, R., Day, S.C., Diserens, D. and Grisso, J.A. (1990) *Practicing prevention for the elderly*, Hanley & Belfus, Philadelphia.

Self-help

Burgio, K.L., Pearce, K.L. and Lucco, A.J. (1989) *Staying dry*, Johns Hopkins University Press, Baltimore, MD.

Mace, N.L. and Rabins, P.V. (1981) *The 36-hour day*, Johns Hopkins University Press, Baltimore, MD.

Zgola, J.M. (1987) *Doing things*, Johns Hopkins University Press, Baltimore, MD.

PART THREE

Groups with Specific Needs

CHAPTER 10

Working with black and minority ethnic groups

Kathy Elliott

To achieve effective health education we, as health professionals, need to understand the client's perspective about the health issue being discussed. This is the case whether working with an individual in a consultation, a family or in a group. It might involve exploring a range of aspects of a health issue: knowledge, attitudes, beliefs, behaviour, reasons for a health choice and future intentions. In much of our health education we don't achieve these goals but our lack of success becomes even more evident when we look closely at the health education we do give to people who come from a different culture from our own or who speak another language. There is little, if any, evidence to suggest that national or local health education initiatives are achieving cross cultural success.

The purpose of this chapter is to explore the special issues raised when we aim to achieve high-quality health education for all the population. Often it is assumed that 'ethnic minority groups' will always have problems and will therefore need special health education initiatives. This may not be the case. At other times we continue, almost blindly, using resources and approaches which have not been developed with the needs of a range of cultures in mind, hoping that they will meet everyone's needs. They rarely do. All health professionals must ensure that they are making appropriate, effective and non-racist judgements when they are examining this aspect of their work.

A MULTICULTURAL SOCIETY

Britain, like most other countries, is made up of a range of ethnic groups. Historically there have always been movements of people between countries whether it be for political, economic, religious or other reasons. Since World War II there have been a significant number of people from other countries settle in Britain. The data available to describe the size of these groups is limited. Current national estimates are based on the 1981 census data (OPCS, 1982). In England and Wales, the population of 48 million includes around 3 million people who were born in the Indian subcontinent, the West Indies or Africa. By having only asked questions about place of birth the data leaves out many important groups, for example black and Asian young people born in England. The next census will ask more detailed questions which will hopefully give a more complete and useful picture. The information being collected will include the person's assessment of their ethnic group as well as the country of birth.

Statistics published in 1991 (Haskey, 1991), based on the annual Labour Force surveys and information gained from the census, show that almost 1 in 20 people living in Britain, a total of 2.57 million, belongs to an ethnic minority. The largest ethnic minority groups are from the West Indies, the Indian subcontinent and China. In addition there are smaller groups from many countries including Turkey, Vietnam, Poland and Greece.

These statistics provide only a starting point to help you understand the black and minority ethnic group population in the country and the geographic district in which you work. There are many other factors you will need to know if you are to develop effective health education initiatives. Within each black and minority ethnic group there may be a range of social class groups, languages spoken, religious beliefs, education levels, literacy rates and of course health knowledge, attitudes, beliefs and values.

They also shouldn't be seen as permanent or unchanging groups. The accounts of why and how people have come to settle in this country are worth investigating and will provide you with valuable background information as you begin your health education with individuals, families and groups.

Being precise about the terms we use in planning health education initiatives for black and minority ethnic groups helps to clarify issues which can result in more effective practice.

- An **immigrant** is a person who has recently moved from one country to live in another country. It is not an appropriate way to describe someone who has lived for many years in one country.
- **Culture** has been defined as 'that complex whole which includes knowledge, beliefs, art, morals, law, custom and any other capabilities and habits acquired by man as a member of society'. It is shaped by education, the media, family and friends, economic development and the rules and regulations of the society in which we live (Fuller and Toon, 1988).

- **Ethnic groups** refers to any group with a shared culture. This term is interpreted and measured in many ways. For example, in the 1981 census, it was measured by place of birth. This is a very simplistic way to describe and classify cultural groups. It can lead to generalizations which are not accurate.
- **Black and minority ethnic** groups or ethnic minority groups are terms frequently used. It is important not to assume that the group being referred to is always in a minority or that they can be grouped together.
- **Race** is used in a variety of ways to describe genetic differences between people, differences in physical appearance, especially the colour of skin and in a political sense as a way to bring people together to fight discrimination.

Health educators have often not thought deeply enough about these terms when planning their work. Generalizations have been made about ethnic groups which are based on a lack of information. For example some programmes aimed at 'Asians' haven't taken into account the fact that people from the Indian subcontinent can come from a wide range of places geographically with differing languages and customs. Other initiatives have assumed that people have immigrated recently, when in fact they have lived their whole lives in England.

In order to help people to make positive health choices there has to be good communication and understanding. Issues related to migration, culture, religion, beliefs and language can affect the quality of the support you provide. Understanding and coping with racism adds an extra dimension to the work done with ethnic groups.

The development of health education initiatives has, almost always, been done from a Western point of view. The public health or medical diagnosis of the problem, the research on links between the health problem and behaviours, the views of the target group and the preparation of resources, such as leaflets and videos, have rarely been done from a cross cultural perspective. The centrality of a Western perspective is interwoven into all our working practices. If we are to provide an effective service for all the population many ways of working and assumptions will need to be examined.

In developing cross cultural, non-racist health education practice we need to put efforts in a broader perspective. Members of black and ethnic minorities experience racism as both patients and employees within the NHS. Equal opportunities policies have been an important step in tackling racism but there still is much to be done (Potrykus, 1991). Your clients will respond to your efforts with past experiences, some racist, still very much in their minds. By taking the time to understand their perspective, and at times their anger, you will build confidence and also contribute to wider efforts to undermine racism. You will want to look at a copy of your Health Authority's Equal Opportunity Policy and link to training and implementation initiatives. You should be able to obtain this information from your manager or the Human Resources Department in your Health Authority or Trust.

KNOWING YOUR PATIENTS AND COMMUNITY

The first step is to gather information about the community you work in and your patients or clients. It is now a statutory duty for the Director of Public Health in each Health Authority to produce an annual Public Health Report. In this report information is published about the population of the Health Authority, including black and minority ethnic groups, causes of death and the results of any special studies carried out during the past year. Increasingly, both in District and Regional Annual Reports, sections are being included on black and minority ethnic groups. Other sources of information include the Local Authority information department, community groups, Councils for Racial Equality and the Community Health Council. From this information you should be able to list the black and minority ethnic groups in your locality and the key health problems.

The next step is to find out how your particular part of the health service is responding to the needs of black and minority ethnic groups. What proportion of your patients are from these groups? Does this reflect an over or under use of services? Have the reasons for this been debated? Are their health problems as identified in reports such as the Annual Public Health Report, being addressed? Are consumer satisfaction surveys and quality initiatives taking into account black and minority ethnic group needs? This type of information should be available through your manager, projects and staff developing quality initiatives, the Health Education Department or the local Community Health Council. Unfortunately the relevant data is not always available.

Through reading, your experience and small studies you can begin to build up a more accurate picture of how your service is used by black and minority ethnic groups. This will help you make wiser decisions about what information should be collected through the newly developing NHS information systems and what your health education priorities should be.

LISTENING

One of the keys to successful health education is listening. Without the information gained through listening we can easily fall into the trap of 'telling people what to do' without knowing if the information is appropriate or helpful. There are good guidelines available describing how to develop effective listening skills in health conversations (Health Education Authority, 1989a).

It is useful to think about listening at two levels, one with individual patients and their families and the second with population or patient groups. New studies and evaluations of past health education programmes targeted at ethnic groups show why it is essential that we do listen. The following examples show this clearly.

Immunization

Many inner city areas, with large black and minority ethnic populations, have low uptake rates for childhood immunizations. Health professionals have sometimes linked low uptake rates with particular ethnic groups but often there has been little data available to substantiate these claims (Bhopal and Samin, 1988). A small study carried out in one inner London district helped to clarify the issue with one minority ethnic group, the Turkish community (Atun and Jenkins, 1990). Parents attending a local child health clinic, staffed by Turkish speaking health professionals, were asked about what they knew about immunization and their child's immunization history. The results showed a high uptake and good knowledge levels of the triple vaccine (DPT) which was a vaccine widely used in Turkey, but a low uptake of mumps, measles and rubella (MMR). This vaccine had only recently been introduced in the UK and the initial publicity was not made available in Turkish or targeted at the Turkish community. Listening, in this case through a small study, helped to define the health education priority. It could be argued that a more cross cultural approach to health promotion related to immunization would have prevented this need from developing.

Smoking and young people

There are many assumptions made about young people from black and minority groups and smoking. Some people feel that because there are low (or high) smoking rates amongst specific groups, the pattern of smoking amongst the young people will be similar. Recent research is beginning to present a clearer picture. In one study carried out by the Health Education Authority the answer to the question 'have you ever tried a cigarette', was analysed by ethnic groups. The results showed no significant difference between the white (33%) and Afro-Caribbean group (31%), a higher proportion of smokers in the Irish (40%) and south eastern European group (40%) and a lower proportion in the Asian group (22%) (Health Education Authority, 1989b). In this study the sample sizes for each ethnic group were too small to break the categories down further. This data shows the need to include discussions about smoking and health with all young people. Research on adults and smoking points out the similarities between ethnic groups in information and cessation needs and the gaps, such as relevant information for community group leaders.

Other health education initiatives

Without listening it is easy to develop approaches and resources which cause offence. Early HIV/AIDS resources presented a picture of AIDS 'coming from' specific countries. The offence and racist practices which developed from this unclear and unnecessary health education set back health education about HIV and AIDS with black and minority ethnic groups by years. Through proper pre-testing and listening this could have been overcome. A wide range of health promotion organizations, both in the statutory and voluntary sectors, have been working to develop more effective approaches and resources (such as black HIV/AIDS network – see Appendix for their address).

Evaluations of the Asian Mother and Baby Campaign point out that the initiative would have been more successful '. . . if it hadn't assumed that all Asian adults require more information and the same information on pregnancy and care of the baby, irrespective of sex and their social and cultural background' (Rocheron and Dickenson, 1990).

Developing your listening

Increasingly there is more population data to use as we develop our cross cultural health education skills. But often we have to make decisions about how to lead health conversations and groups without adequate population data. In the absence of good data (and sometimes alongside of it) the first step is to ask the person or group their views and experience. As we do this with black and minority ethnic groups there are two special dimensions which have to be taken into account: language and the cultural perspective, particularly if the person is from a culture different to our own.

When there is a cultural divide between you and the client it is useful to have found out as much as you can about their culture. There are short and useful descriptions available (Henley, 1982). The references given in 'Further reading' give information on many black and minority ethnic groups. It is important though, not to stereotype people. You may find that your client has different views from the cultural norm. Leave yourself enough time to explore properly the patient's perspective. You need to be open to both similarities and differences. A combination of open and closed questions should help you explore the person's knowledge, attitudes, current behaviours, reasons for their health choice, future intentions and need for support.

It is important not to make assumptions and to respect the patient's views. As with all health education we're bound to fail if we work against these beliefs as it is the client who will be making the final choices, not the health professional.

The inability to speak the same language inevitably leads to much greater difficulties. Health beliefs and reasons for health actions are even more difficult to explore across a linguistic divide. Guidelines presented for medical consultations apply equally to health education conversations. The following is a list taken from *Medical Practice in a Multicultural Society* (Fuller and Toon, 1988).

When using an interpreter, look for someone who:

- is *fluent* in both languages;
- has some training in interpretation;
- has some medical knowledge;
- has a good knowledge of how the health service works;
- is available every time the patient is seen;
- is accepted and trusted by the patient and the health worker;
- is sensitive to the needs of the patient and health worker;
- will not allow his or her own beliefs to override those of the patient or health professional;
- puts the patient at ease;
- has a good memory and pays attention to detail;
- can translate fine shades of meaning;
- is able during the interaction to tell the health worker when there are problems and why;
- is aware of the cultural expectations of both patients and health worker and can explain them to both;
- is the same sex as the patient;
- is able to carry the responsibility.

There are a range of ways health professionals arrange for interpretation. Although services are often not adequate, it is important to know all the local resources available and to keep up-to-date. In many health authorities services are slowly improving, but you may not hear of new resources, particularly if they are being funded through a different part of the organization. This information should be available through your manager. If not, the local Community Health Council, Council on Racial Equality or Health Education Department may be able to help find local resources.

PROVIDING INFORMATION AND SUPPORT

Many of the issues raised in relation to listening also apply to providing information. The need for a translator and time to ensure understanding and cultural appropriateness are examples. As in all health conversations it is important to make sure the information you give is clear, correct and understandable. Most important, it must be useful to the person you're talking with whether it gives them an answer to a question, fills a knowledge gap or helps them make a decision about what to do in the future. The information given will vary depending on the amount of time you have for the health conversation and whether you are challenging the person or group to think about a health issue or supporting them in seeing through a health decision.

Improving the quality of health conversations, whether it be related to listening and assessment or providing information and support, is often quite difficult. Until recently very little training in health education skills was linked to good communication skills. Evaluation techniques have focused on data from notes or patient interviews. Although potentially useful these don't always give the depth of information required and often aren't a practical way for health professionals to feedback on their work. A few studies have chosen audio-recording to analyse the health education content of consultations and this may be a useful tool (MacLeod *et al.*, 1990; Farquhar and Bowling, 1990). Listening by yourself or preferably with a trusted colleague to a conversation can give valuable insight into how you are listening and providing information.

Although it sounds more difficult doing it with a colleague it usually ensures you look at the positive sides of your practice instead of what you interpret as the problems. Issues you might like to discuss could include:

- what was important to the client?
- did you use your opportunity to question constructively?
- did the questions lead you into interesting or key health areas?
- did you ascertain the client's questions or interests?
- what issues were discussed?
- did you link your concerns with the client's?
- was the information given correct and useful?

There is no research which documents and analyses cross cultural consultations in this way so it is even more important to develop ways to support and improve your practice.

Translation or advocacy?

As you think about how you will provide information and lead conversations about health choices, it is useful to learn from the experiences of two styles of projects which have been developed during the 1980s with minority ethnic groups: linkworker and advocacy schemes. The Asian Mother and Baby Campaign, launched in 1984, combined publicity, the production of resources and the appointment of linkworkers with appropriate language skills. The campaign grew out of experiences from the Stop Rickets Campaign, which highlighted problems of access to services and lack of sensitivity within services to minority groups. Full details about the campaign and how it was implemented are available (Bahl, 1987).

Some schemes have gone beyond a translation and information-giving role to provide advocacy for patients. This includes explaining options to the patients, raising issues thought to be racist with the health care professionals and educating staff about cultural differences and requirements (City and Hackney Community Health Council, 1991). A bilingual health advocacy course has been developed jointly by a London FHSA and Academic Department of General Practice (Fuller, pers. comm.). It is 6 months long and covers a wide range of issues which link to health promotion: concepts of health and disease, informed decision making, interviewing skills, health promotion in general practice, communication skills, discrimination in the health service and how it affects health care, assertiveness and personal management. Practitioners completing this training will take forward valuable initiatives within a general practice setting.

It is important to make use of these schemes, if they exist in your area, either to help in individual or group health education or to give advice on how to solve problems or approach issues. As you work with linkworkers, interpreters or advocates you will need to think through your views on the issues raised by these projects. Is the cultural knowledge of the worker useful? Could it add to the health conversation? Does an advocacy role help to empower the patient to use services and make positive health choices? As a health professional you will want to use all the resources available to you to improve the quality and effectiveness of your health education.

HEALTH EDUCATION RESOURCES

Health professionals turn to a variety of health education resources to support them in their work. Traditionally this is a leaflet but can also include other audiovisual aids such as 35 mm slide presentations, posters or videos. The first step is to ensure that the health education resource adds to the quality of the health conversation. All too often we turn to the use of a particular resource, mostly leaflets, without questioning their value. A leaflet or other resource should be a valuable addition to a consultation, not a substitute for a personal conversation. It can never help to identify the specific learning needs of a client.

If you have decided a health education resource is appropriate and adds to the effectiveness of the consultation you will need to take into account the needs of black and minority ethnic groups. Are the materials culturally sensitive and appropriate to use with your client? Are they in the correct language? There are a number of sources of translated health education resources in England. Unfortunately there is no complete collection and so it does mean checking a number of different places. The first to try is your local health promotion or education unit. With the recent organizational changes in the NHS you may find health promotion units with either the purchasers or the providers. They should also be concerned about the needs of local groups and should have ideas about what translated resources exist and how they can be obtained. Another useful publication is the Resource List *Health Education for Ethnic Minorities* which is prepared by the Health Education Authority (1990). The list provides details about suppliers. Many items can be viewed at the HEA's library in London. The Resource Lists are free from the HEA and may also be available from your local health promotion/education unit. Other sources may include specialist organizations such as self-help groups and local libraries.

The production of translated health education resources is relatively recent and there are still many problems with the materials. A recent day organized in London to review materials available in Bengali high-lighted many of these problems: unsatisfactory translation standards, inaccurate graphics, cultural mistakes and poor overall quality. Often materials have been produced without sufficient pretesting and check-ing. Before you use 'bought in' leaflets or other resources check that they are appropriate to use with your clients and that they will be understood and helpful. It would be useful to look at the leaflet or resources with people who know the language or the targeted group.

In a number of health education initiatives with black and minority ethnic groups other audiovisual aids, usually videos, have been used. One example is an initiative in Leicester City to increase the uptake of cervical smear tests amongst Asian women (McAvoy and Raza, 1991). The research linked to the project compared the effectiveness of three different health education resources and methods: written materials by post, personal intervention and personal intervention with a videotape. Personal intervention with the videotape and fact sheet was nearly three times as effective as sending the leaflet and fact sheet by post. It is important, though, to guard against thinking that this level of contact is only appropriate or necessary with black and minority ethnic groups. It may be that it would improve outcome for all groups.

Even after doing a thorough search for the health education resources you need, you may find they are not available. Local health profes-sionals are still often in the position of having to produce translated information. There is regularly a debate about whether members of a minority ethnic group can read their own language. Views differ and health professionals are often in a position of not having the right information to make a decision. One study in the early 1980s with the Bangladeshi and Pakistani people in Oldham showed that a significantly higher proportion could read their mother tongue than could read English (Learmonth, 1980). In making your decision it is important to find out as much as you can about the community with whom you are working. Think about your target group as there may be differences between age groups and between men and women. Ask your patients, translators and advocates, and local community groups for their views. Usually, if we are to ensure equal access to health information to all population and client groups there is a need for translated materials. There will be circumstances when, to ensure equal access, new resources will need to be developed. Recent research has highlighted the need to think beyond leaflets to other health education resources (e.g. posters, community radio, newspaper articles) but getting started often means the local production of leaflets and handouts. An excellent guide to producing health information for non-English-speaking people has recently been produced (Lovell, 1990). It gives valuable ideas about getting the message right and how to produce and distribute the material. It reinforces that the principles of producing information for ethnic groups are the same as for the production of all materials. They must be:

- attractive;
- relevant and culturally appropriate;
- non-patronizing;
- easy to understand;
- persuasive;
- clear and acceptable to the target audience;
- accurate.

The ideas are practical and sensitive to the lack of resources often facing health professionals. For example, they suggest multilingual productions instead of many single-language leaflets, and give advice on producing high quality photocopied information sheets when professionally designed and printed material cannot be produced. Many of the same issues arise as in the translation versus advocacy debates. Straight translations from English may be meaningless and, at worst, cause offence. It is very worthwhile involving community groups or representatives from the minority ethnic group in the development of the material. This can also help to ensure the materials or content aren't racist or stereotyped. Good translation and rigorous proof reading are both essential to the eventual production of a good-quality resource. This guide, taken from *Health in Any Language* (Lovell, 1990), offers an excellent checklist for translation.

A CHECKLIST FOR TRANSLATION

- Use recognized translators wherever possible.
- Translation is a skill which includes adapting messages to cultural needs. You cannot ask just anyone to do it.
- The cost of translation needs to be worked into the overall budget for a project.
- Decisions, such as whether to translate place names on maps and telephone numbers, will have to be made. Consultation with the relevant community group should establish which form is acceptable.
- Text can take up more- or less-space after translation. Allow for this in the overall design of the publication.
- Select the translator or translation agency through personal recommendation if possible. You will need to research this, as for any other service you might use.
- It is less time-consuming to use an agency, and the agency will often guarantee to check the material for you after typesetting and artwork stages.
- Voluntary groups often have expertise in this area.
- Payment allows for a more accountable and efficient delivery of a translation service.
- Check and negotiate that colloquial rather then 'PhD' language is used.

Health professionals should be aiming to produce and use materials of high quality with black and ethnic minority groups which stand up to the same scrutiny as all health education materials. This very useful guide gives practical and useful tips to achieve high standards, including a stage-by-stage guide to production which can be a valuable checklist. To carry out these steps you'll need access to the names of local community groups, local translators, typesetters and printers. If your budget allows, a designer with experience of producing translated materials is also useful. Local contacts should be available through your health promotion unit, Local Authority services or community groups.

The same issues apply to the use or production of other types of health education resources: videos, films, slide/tapes and packs. The Resource Lists and ideas for finding resources also cover these types of material.

DEVELOPING MULTICULTURAL HEALTH PROMOTION – CURRENT INITIATIVES AND FUTURE DIRECTIONS

Partnerships

By creating partnerships and joint projects with black and minority ethnic groups many new and positive health promotion initiatives are developing. As with most health promotion, when people are involved in interpreting messages for themselves, more effective initiatives emerge. For many health promoters it has often been a quite slow process of getting to know local groups and people. Many small and hard-pressed umbrella organizations representing groups have given their time and expertise. From the other side health promoters have been willing to respond to requests and discuss problems and concerns. Some health education/promotion units have a specialist health promotion officer for minority ethnic groups. A recent study showed specialist posts in 13 Health Authorities. Many units have been keen not to isolate the work with black and minority ethnic groups but to ensure that all programme areas and methods are taking into account cross cultural needs. A survey of initiatives with minority ethnic groups showed work on a wide range of topics (women's health, smoking, heart disease, immunizations and many others) and through a variety of methods (training courses, health days, group work, resource production, research and many others) (Rocheron, 1991). These first steps have begun to result in more innovative and larger projects. The following are examples of the types of initiatives currently being developed.

An HIV/AIDS Community Grant Scheme

One example is an HIV/AIDS Community Grant Scheme being run in one Inner London Borough. Much of the original health education material on HIV/AIDS caused great offence to many black and minority ethnic groups. The portrayal of 'where AIDS comes from', which to many health educators was unnecessary and incorrect, left many groups angry and not prepared to participate in HIV/AIDS education programmes. After careful consultation with a range of community groups, the Health Promotion Officers in Hackney overcame much of this mistrust and launched a community grants scheme. A small grant was offered to any community group who would undertake a health promotion initiative related to HIV/AIDS. The response was very positive, with a number of groups being successful and receiving grants. Projects being done include a theatre production and video in Turkish, translation of health leaflets in Greek, discussion groups and a photography exhibition.

The Health Promotion Officers are working closely with the groups to provide support and guidance but the groups are developing approaches which fit with the needs of their community. It is hoped that the results of the projects will point the way forward, either for the wider distribution of materials within the community or the identification of new needs or approaches.

A health education resource

A number of health promotion units have developed health promotion resources in collaboration with local ethnic groups. These partnerships have resulted in the production of videos on a wide range of topics, leaflets and teaching packs.

One example is a video, 'Getting Older, Keeping Well' (Bloomsbury and Islington Health Promotion Department, 1991) made after extensive consultation with members of the Cantonese-speaking community and with Chinese and English health professionals. Production involved a Health Promotion Department and a Chinese video production company.

Linked through the account of a Cantonese-speaking health advocate, the video follows several different older Chinese people through use of various services such as chiropody, physiotherapy, GP and dental services, which can enable them to be healthier and more comfortable in their later years. The older people themselves speak about diet, exercise and the importance of getting out of the house and staying active.

Health campaigning

Increasingly health campaigning organizations are being started by black and minority ethnic groups or long-standing health organizations are addressing their needs. Two examples are the work of BHAN: the Coronary Prevention Group's Response to Asians and Heart Disease, and the Food Commission.

BHAN have produced a multilingual range of posters and videos on HIV/AIDS. As well as the resource being useful, the organization provides an important contact point for ideas, workshop and training leaders, examples of good practice and training.

The second example is that of a health organization responding to the needs of a particular group, in this case the increase rate of coronary heart disease in the Asian community. The proceedings of a conference (Coronary Prevention Group and the Confederation of Indian Organisations, 1991a) held to discuss the issue gave a useful overview of the medical evidence, and the problems that exist in understanding the reasons for the high rates. A video and accompanying booklet *Action on Coronary Heart Disease in Asians* is a valuable resource (Coronary Prevention Group and the Confederation of Indian Organisations, 1991b). The videos are available in five Asian languages. The booklet provides information on mortality statistics, risk factors associated with the prevalence of coronary heart disease among the Asian communities, culturally relevant health messages, ideas for health promotion activities with Asian communities, advice on strategies for effective health promotion and useful resources.

The Food Commission has produced a detailed and useful resource to support people doing nutrition education and implementing food policies (Hill, 1990).

Empowering and providing skills

There are many ways health professionals, community group leaders and others increase their health promotion skills. Many health promotion units have, as part of the implementation of equal opportunities policies, worked to recruit and promote health promotion officers from black and minority ethnic groups. For many health professionals and community group leaders the aim is to improve their health promotion skills, not to become full-time health promotion officers. Training such as the Certificate in Health Education provides a useful one-day release course, is nationally available and results in a recognized qualification. Other local initiatives are being developed which also help to point the way forward. One example is the training of bilingual Look After Yourself tutors. The Look After Yourself Programme trains tutors who in turn lead local health groups. In a recent pilot project bilingual tutors, speaking a wide range of languages, have been trained. These tutors, who come from community groups, primary care teams, community nursing and local authorities, will run groups in languages other than English as well as with the English-speaking community. In addition, the training provides valuable skills which will improve the other aspects of their health promotion work (D'Aguilar).

Research

The development of new approaches and more effective programmes needs to be shaped by research. Improved information about health needs will help to decide the health focus of initiatives. Outcome studies are also essential to show the effectiveness of health education initiatives with all communities as well as black and minority ethnic groups. The difficulties of adapting scientific methodologies to evaluate health education activities continue to make this a challenge. Of more immediate relevance to most health educators is having access to more in-depth information about the knowledge, attitudes and behaviour related to a range of health issues in these groups, plus their views on specific health education methods. A series of research projects which have recently been commissioned by the Health Education Authority provide useful examples. Development research related to the pregnancy book (Health Education Authority, 1989c) pointed to the needs of older members of the family who have an influence on health decisions, the importance of diagrams, the problems raised by pictures of the birth which were too explicit, the different interpretations given to photographs, the lack of cultural sensitivity and problems with understanding cartoons. Another study on smoking pointed to new ways of distributing health information, for example, community newspapers (Health Education Authority, 1990) and radio, posters and new venues such as shops, coffee shops and community centres. The research on HIV/AIDS (Health Education Authority, 1991) gives insight into how different communities discuss sex and whether they felt they were at risk of HIV/AIDS. In this study who gave the information was important. For example receiving information from a doctor or at school made it more acceptable and valued. Again the value of leaflets was questioned and problems with understanding mass media ads were highlighted. There was a plea for clearer messages which didn't need extensive knowledge of English language and culture for interpretation. These studies point to the need to make existing materials more culturally sensitive.

Making links

New initiatives targeted at black and minority ethnic groups are being developed in many settings: hospitals, primary care and the community. Lessons learned in each will provide valuable resources and ideas for other settings. At a local level there may be ways to share the results of these efforts. An overview of initiatives could provide contacts, or being more ambitious, a conference or occasional interest group could enable health professionals and other workers to share ideas and resources.

As both disease-specific programmes, for example on hypertension with the Afro-Caribbean community or diabetes and heart disease with the Asian community, develop, the resources and experiences should be shared with health promoters in primary care team, community groups and hospital. There will also be a need to bring together common themes emerging out of work with the separate groups.

CASE STUDIES

Case study 1

Jane is a practice nurse working as part of a primary care team in an inner city area. She is running a health promotion clinic focusing on the prevention of heart disease. Her third client at the clinic is Harold who has been diagnosed as hypertensive. The medication he is taking is acceptable and has lowered his blood pressure. The GP now wants him to consider changes in his health choices which could help improve the hypertension and generally reduce his risk of developing further heart disease. Harold has lived in England for 20 years and works as a bus driver. Before that he came from the West Indies. Many of his friends have hypertension and he is very concerned.

Jane asks questions which help Harold to discuss what he knows about hypertension and the treatment he is receiving. She gives information when he is unsure or has questions. He particularly wants to know why many of his Afro-Caribbean friends get hypertension. Together they discuss what changes Harold should make to help reduce the blood pressure and his risk of developing illnesses related to high blood pressure. Although Harold recognizes that smoking and weight are important issues for him to address, he decides he'd like to take more exercise. Jane supports this decision as a way to get started and knows she will return to the other risk factors at a follow-up visit. She explains their importance and answers Harold's questions but encourages him to focus on exercise. From her experience she knows that many patients find it difficult to make too many changes at once.

She begins by trying to understand Harold's views about exercise. The types of questions she uses include:

- What exercise do you get?
- How much exercise do you think people need to keep healthy?
- How do you feel about exercise?
- What do you think are the benefits of exercise?
- What do you think are the problems with exercise?

These help Harold to think through his feelings and experience. He decides he is going to start swimming at a local pool. Jane arranges to see him in a few weeks time to see how he is progressing. She gives him a booklet to read about hypertension, exercise and the other changes he may decide to make in the future.

Case study 2

Linda is a health visitor who is attached to a general practice which has a large number of Turkish patients. A Turkish-speaking mother arrives with her child for a child health clinic. Arrangements have been made for translation and advocacy support. Akgul joins the consultation and explains her role. She chats to the mother about both hers and the child's health. After the immunization has been given, the health visitor explains the next immunizations which will be needed. The mother says she has something else she would like to discuss. She is thinking of getting pregnant again and worries about the fact she is still smoking. Although she jokes about a smaller baby making for an easier delivery, she is worried that her smoking will harm the baby. She recently talked with a friend who had had a stillbirth.

Linda and Akgul welcome her interest in stopping smoking. They find out how long the woman has been smoking and how many she smokes a day. They discuss the times and situations it will be difficult to go without a cigarette and what she could do instead. The mother agrees to set a date to stop smoking and to try the suggestions that have been discussed. She says she has a friend who will help and she'll talk with her husband about stopping at the same time. The health visitor gives her a leaflet with other tips and arranges to see her again when Akgul is also available.

REFERENCES

Atun, R. and Jenkins, S. (1990) Health needs of the Turkish Community in Hackney: A Pilot Study of Child Health Clinic Attenders. (Unpublished)

Bahl, V. (1987) *Asian Mother and Baby Campaign*, DHSS, London.

Bhopal, R.S. and Samin, A.K. (1988) Immunisation Uptake of Glasgow Asian children. *Community Medicine*, **10**, 215–20.

Bloomsbury and Islington Health Promotion Department (1991) 'Getting Older, Keeping Well' (video).

City and Hackney Community Health Council (1991) *Experiments in Health Advocacy*, London.

Coronary Prevention Group and the Confederation of Indian Organisations (1991a) *Coronary Heart Disease and Asians in Britain* CO1.

Coronary Prevention Group and the Confederation of Indian Organisations (1991b) Action on Coronary Heart Disease in Asians. Health Education Authority, Department of Health, Coronary Prevention Group.

D'Aguilar, M. City and Hackney Health Authority. (Personal communication)

Farguhar, M. and Bowling, A. (1990) *Practice Nurses and Health Education –* Analysing Tape Recorded Consultations. City and Hackney Health Authority. (Unpublished)

Fuller, J. Lawson Practice. St. Leonard's, Nuttall Street, London N1 (personal communication).

Fuller, F.H.S. and Toon, P.D. (1988) *Medical Practice in a Multicultural Society*, Heinemann Medical Books, Oxford.

Haskey, J. (1991) The Ethnic Minority Populations Resident in Private Households. Estimates by County and Metropolitan District in England and Wales. *Population Trends*, **63**, 22–35.

Health Education Authority (1989a) *Smoking – helping people to Stop*. Putting Communication Skills into Practice. (Book and video.)

Health Education Authority (1989b) 'Teenage and Child Health and Lifestyles' (working title). Prepared for the HEA by MORI (unpublished).

Health Education Authority (1989c) 'Pregnancy Book Qualitative Review: Black and Minority Ethnic Groups', prepared for the HEA by Cities Research Unit. (Unpublished)

Health Education Authority (1990) 'A Qualitative Study of Smoking Among Black and Minority Ethnic groups: Developing a Health Education Resource', prepared for the HEA by Cities Research Unit. (Unpublished)

Health Education Authority (1991) Communicating With Ethnic Communities About AIDS, prepared for the HEA by Cities Research Unit. (Unpublished)

Health Education for Ethnic Minorities: A Resource List (1990) Health Education Authority, London.

Henley A. (1982) *Asians in Britain* (A series of three – Caring for Muslims and their Families, Caring for Sikhs and their Families, Caring for Hindus and their Families) Cambridge: DHSS/King Edward's College.

Hill, S.E. (1990) *More Rice Than Peas. Guidelines to Improve Food Provision for Black and Ethnic Minorities in Britain*, The Food Commission, London.

Learmonth, A. (1980) Asians' literacy in their Mother Tongue and English. *Nursing Times*, 28 February.

Lovell, S. (ed.) (1990) *Health in Any Language*, North East Thames Regional Health Authority, London.

MacLeod Clark, J., Haverty, S. and Kendall, S. (1990) Helping Patients and Clients to Stop Smoking. Phase 2. Assessing the effectiveness of the Nurse's Role. Final Report. Health Education Council, London.

McAvoy, B.R. and Raza, R. (1991) Can Health Education Increase Uptake of Cervical Smear testing Among Asian Women? *BMJ*, **302**, 833.

OPCS (1982) Population Trends no. 28, HMSO, London.

Potrykus, C. (1991) Tackling Racism Inside the NHS. *Health Visitor*, **64**, 104.

Rocheron, Y. (1991) Health Action and Race Project, Centre for Mass Communication Research, Leicester. (Unpublished)

Rocheron, Y. and Dickenson, R. (1990) The Asian Mother and Baby Campaign; A Way Forward in Health Promotion for Asian Women? *Health Education Journal*, **49**, 128.

FURTHER READING

Fuller, J.H.S. and Toon, P.D. (1988) *Medical Practice in a Multicultural Society*, Heinemann Medical Books, Oxford.

Mares, P., Henley, A. and Baxter, C. (1985) *Health Care in Multiracial Britain*, Health Education Council/National Extension College, Cambridge.

Mares, P., Larbie, J. and Baxter, C. (1987) *Trainers Handbook for Multiracial Health Care*, National Extension College for Training in Health and Race, Cambridge.

Mares, P., Larbie, J. and Baxter, C. (1989) *Entitled to be Healthy*, Health Visitors Association, London.

McNaught, A. (1987) *Health Action and Ethnic Minorities*, Bedford Square Press, London.

Cruickshank, J.K. and Beevers, D.G. (1989) *Ethnic Factors in Health and Disease*, Wright, London.

CHAPTER 11

Helping people with communication disorders

Jayne Comins

INTRODUCTION

In the UK, 2.3 million people have some form of language or speech disorder:

- 1.5 million have a defect that impairs communication;
- 800 000 people have difficulty in being understood at all.

Communication problems can afflict anyone of any age and they may be part of a physical, psychological or cognitive disorder. In humans, communication involves:

- articulation (involving tongue, lip, mouth, nose and palate);
- language (involving thought processes, grammar, meaning and memory);
- voice (involving breathing muscles and vocal cords);
- fluency (involving speed and co-ordination of the above);
- non-verbal communication (involving body language such as eye contact, posture and facial expressions).

Generally when 'speech' problems are talked about by the lay person and indeed by many health professionals, it can mean that the communication problem is a difficulty in articulation, language, voice or fluency.

The following sections outline the range of problems encountered in this most highly complex area of human skill. People in the health care professions and the general public will encounter those with communication disorders on a regular or occasional basis.

CHILDREN

The acquisition of language is a most remarkable accomplishment in children. A one-year-old child may only say one or two words, but by the age of three may have a vocabulary of up to a thousand words. Knowing the meaning of words is one thing but listening to, pronouncing words and putting words into sentences needs more skill. Exactly how language is learned is still not clear, but parents and anyone else in contact with the child are in the important position of being able to influence a child's development in this respect.

> It is not surprising that in homes where children are spoken to rarely, language development is hampered. And, conversely, in homes where parents talk interestedly to their children about where they are, what they are doing and how they are feeling, verbal development flows. (Marzollo and Lloyd, 1986)

Most children happily develop communication skills without any problems at all. Where there is a delay in language or speech development, advice may be sought from a speech and language therapist. Many therapists can arrange talks at local health clinics if requested and some districts run 'drop-in' and counselling sessions which advise parents on how to encourage language development.

Problems in childhood

Acquired childhood aphasia   Acquired childhood aphasia is a language disorder caused by cerebral dysfunction in childhood. This condition can appear after a period of normal language development.

Cerebral dysfunction   Head injury and some conditions of unknown cause can be responsible for childhood dysphasia; the language patterns of these children differ from the expected profile of children of the same age. Their sound system, grammar, the meaning they attach to words and their use of language may all be affected, so that the child is disadvantaged in communication. A speech and language therapist considers the child's medical background and can assess and review the child as appropriate. Planned intervention with a team approach is essential and advice and counselling of parents and carers is valuable. The areas assessed may include:

- speech understanding;
- word-finding;
- jargon words or other unusual patterns of speech.

Developmental speech and language problems

More commonly, there are children who have developmental speech and language problems affecting speaking and writing. Some of these problems may include:

- difficulty understanding speech;
- problems in producing and sequencing the grammar;   ·
- difficulty in making the sounds and words that make up language;
- specific reading and writing difficulties.

The term 'delay' is usually given to cases where speech and language skills follow the usual sequence of development but at a slower than average rate. However, the term 'disorder' is usually applied when the child is not developing in the usual sequence.

Most children who are referred to a speech and language therapist are under the age of five years. Language development is generally held to be critical during the first five years.

Difficulties in motor control

Difficulties children have in talking may be due to lack of motor control, as for example in cerebral palsy. Structural abnormalities such as cleft palate, or a hearing or visual loss may also cause problems. As with the range of disorders found in adult life, more than one of these problems can occur in the same person.

Communication skills are inextricably linked with learning and are tested as part of the National Educational Curriculum. Any breakdown in speech or language can block educational achievements as well as social skills. The speech and language therapist can promote the child's communication skills in the following areas:

- expressing feelings;
- exchanging information;
- using language creatively;
- initiating and maintaining social communication.

They will also work with the child's parents, carers and nursery or education staff on helping the child to make practical use of the skills gained in therapy.

Speech and language therapists will also collate background information on a child to help build a picture of their abilities, interests and needs. This assessment is wide-ranging and may include assessment of play, social and listening skills.

There is basic advice that anyone can follow with children developing their speech and language:

Do's and don'ts

Do

- Talk to children from the moment they are born. Smiles, gurgling and babbling are all important parts of language development and bed-time stories and nursery rhymes should be encouraged.

- Get children to talk about everyday activities such as shopping, eating and bathing to practise their newly aquired speech and language skills.
- Bear in mind that children usually understand speech more than they can speak themselves.
- Where the child has brothers and sisters, ensure that there are times when an individual child can get one-to-one undivided attention in a calm environment.
- Avoid making comparisons with others. There will always be other children who can say more or say less than this particular child.
- Encourage the child to talk for him/herself, rather than always speaking for them, and give them enough time to talk.
- Ensure that the child can hear and is listening.

Don't

- Correct pronunciation in the early stages of development. It is more important for the child to learn words and start forming sentences than to pronounce everything correctly.
- Show obvious concern about the child's communication: children can sense anxiety. It may be worthwhile consulting a speech and language therapist and there is no need to feel 'bad' or 'guilty' about referring a child as advice may be all that is needed. This is where an advisory/'drop-in' type service can be useful.

How parents can help with speech and language therapy

- Attend appointments with the child.
- Do not feel embarrassed about asking questions.
- Try to ensure the child attends regularly. Most children enjoy their visits to the speech and language therapist. Therapy takes the form of games and activities, and should be fun.
- Try to follow any advice the therapist gives, so that activities can be carried out and practised between appointments.

There are some excellent books giving encouragement to parents on how best to help children develop language. In addition, magazines aimed at parents often publish articles on the subject. Parents' classes at health centres and in nurseries and playgroups are sometimes arranged and, with increasing public awareness of the importance of language, more of these could be organized.

Cleft lip and palate abnormalities

Feeding and speaking are closely related. It is generally recognized that encouraging eating, chewing, sucking and swallowing assists in the development of talking.

Many babies with a cleft lip and palate do not have major feeding difficulties, but some do. Whilst sometimes the baby might choke and milk comes down the nose before it is swallowed, this usually occurs occasionally as a result of feeding too quickly.

Hospital staff should be able to advise on how best to manage the baby, though as each child is different it is not possible to lay down rules and often the mother is the best person to decide on the easiest way of feeding the baby. It is important that she should take her time and find the best position for the baby when feeding it.

Some districts have a feeding specialist who can advise on breast and bottle-feeding and on the various feeding aids such as specially designed teats and dental plates. Advice on feeding also needs to be tailored to the individual child and reviewed before and after lip and/or palate operations.

A specialist speech and language therapist in the cleft lip and palate team at the hospital may be able to help with problems in developing articulation and the correct nasal air-flow for speech. Regular reviews of the child's speech and language development will help to identify particular problems such as sounds being made too far back in the mouth during speech. Detailed examination of the condition of the palate using special equipment can also help in deciding what treatment to give. The results of speech assessments and the doctor's examination may be discussed in a team, since there are many different treatment options available, including speech therapy. Alternatively, it may be decided that the child is better off without treatment.

After the child is 10 years old, any further help from, for example, the dentist or speech and language therapist should be co-ordinated so that any speech therapy can be timed with orthodontic treatment.

HEARING IMPAIRMENT

Children

Many children have problems with mild hearing loss in their formative years. Middle ear fluid is the usual cause of hearing loss associated with a cold and catarrh. The 'glue' interferes with the conduction of sound to the inner ear. Often this is called 'conductive deafness'. There can be difficulties in judging the degree of hearing loss involved as it may vary from day to day.

It is important to be aware that this type of deafness is not a serious medical problem and that much can be done to help it. Learning difficulties and behavioural problems may arise from not being able to hear and these can be minimized by appropriate management.

The following information should be borne in mind:

- behaviour may be difficult because the child feels insecure and confused, especially as what is heard may vary on a daily basis;
- learning to speak might be slower;
- speech may at times be unclear;
- dealing with background noise and conversation might be a problem and therefore information may be missed.

How to help

Every effort should be made to enable the child to make the best use of their hearing.

- Speak clearly, but do not shout;
- get the child's attention first;
- avoid exaggerating lip movements;
- find out if the child has a 'good' ear and speak on that side of the child;
- allow the child to see your face and lip movements: note how people without their glasses say, 'I can't hear you without my glasses on'. Normal listeners fill in the gaps in sentences without realizing that they are doing so.

Recognizing behavioural difficulties, if they do occur, is also important. The child may become unusually talkative and have problems in taking turns in conversation: this may be due to anxiety about missing out on conversation if someone else speaks. Alternatively, the opposite may occur, and the child may opt out of conversations. Some children may get so frustrated at their failure to understand properly that they become disruptive or have temper tantrums.

If you are concerned about a child's language and speech development refer them to a speech and language therapist for assessment. This will normally include a detailed case history and assessment of the child's understanding, expressive language and speech sounds.

Children from deaf families may use British Sign Language at home, which should be recognized in the same way as other minority languages. Some other deaf children are more comfortable using manual communication if they have the opportunity to do so. Every deaf child should have access to a language environment in school which complements the language environment of that child's home and optimizes their ability to learn and to develop socially. Children, most especially deaf children, who have a restricted language environment develop restricted language.

Parents of children newly diagnosed as deaf can also be very vulnerable, and will need information which is appropriate, accurate and timely and given in a sensitive manner. They will also need unbiased information about the different teaching methods and resources available. A choice of different communication approaches should be available such as oral/aural, bilingual or total communication approaches, taking into account children's needs and the language used at home.

Adults

Adults who have been deaf from an early age sometimes lack confidence in communicating. Speech and language therapists help their ability to understand and make themselves understood.

Some of the features common in people with hearing disorders are:

- reduced precision of speech sounds, both consonants and vowels;
- lengthening of consonant and vowel sounds;
- deterioration in the quality of voice, e.g. may lack nasal tone;
- poor volume control; may talk too loudly or quietly;
- reduced pitch range and monotonous speech;
- alterations in rate of speech; speaking too fast or too slowly;
- excessive stress on words and syllables;
- problems in turn-taking and other non-verbal communication;
- withdrawal, avoidance of human contact and other changes in behaviour.

Many of these problems in communication may be eased by good posture and tone and proper breathing and voice use.

Bio-feedback machines such as Visispeech, Laryngograph and Speech Viewer can enable clients to see on a screen what kind of speech they are producing. Therapists can also provide training in voice projection and presentation and social skills.

Hearing therapists also rehabilitate people who are hearing-impaired. They will counsel people and their families to enable deaf or deafened people to come to terms with the effects of hearing loss. They play an important part in rehabilitation, reviewing a person's progress and providing ongoing therapy as necessary. They can also help with the use of hearing aids, teach lipreading and give practical help to people with tinnitus.

How to help

- Attract the person's attention before launching into a conversation so that they do not miss the beginning.
- Avoid using gestures which obscure lip movements.
- Speak clearly, but do not exaggerate your lip movements: this can make it hard for them to lip read.
- Have paper and pen handy to write important information down if necessary.
- Do not talk when walking away from the deaf person.
- Try to indicate that you are about to change the subject, rather than

launching into something new without warning, as this can be confusing.

- Rephrase sentences using different words if the deaf person has not understood what you say.
- If a client has trouble understanding a particular word or phrase, repeat it in context rather than in isolation.
- Avoid standing with your back to a window or bright light, otherwise your face will be in shadow and lipreading will be difficult.
- Keep your face visible and avoid wearing sunglasses or shaded lenses when talking – your eyes are also very important in communication.
- Remember that hearing aids amplify background noise as well as speech.
- Allow more time for conversation so that the person is not under pressure.
- Remember that lipreading and listening with hearing aids (or without them) is tiring and that fatigue affects memory.
- Check that the person has understood any information that is particularly important. If in doubt, write it down.

INTELLECTUAL DISABILITY

Intellectual problems may be caused by depression, head injury or other neurological or psychiatric conditions. Dementia is another condition which affects thought processes, which is why careful assessment is so necessary in order to be clear about the person's abilities and difficulties. Problems in intellectual skills may affect how information is received and acted upon: it may be difficult to ascertain how well a patient is able to deal with information. Dementia is most commonly found in the elderly population, and is therefore increasing now that people are living longer. Dementia may have a variety of causes, of which the two most common types are multi-infarct dementia and Alzheimer-type dementia. The first is caused by impaired cerebral blood supply, and the latter by a primary degeneration of brain tissue. In younger people other forms of dementia may occur, such as Pick's disease.

Recognizing the problems

- Memory, especially for recent events, may deteriorate;
- personality may change in subtle ways;
- the person may be disoriented in time and possibly place;
- the person may seem to 'ramble' in speech;
- the person may appear depressed, or inappropriately suspicious;
- a person with dementia may avoid looking at us when we are

talking to, or about them. Little gestural and other or non-verbal feedback is produced in conversational situations.
- The affected person may misjudge what is a comfortable physical distance during conversation, coming too close, so that the other person may feel uncomfortable and want to move away.

Managing the problems

- Encourage a regular routine of care and activity;
- help with orientation by reminders and visual displays of information, if you know the person can read it;
- ensure hearing and vision are optimal;
- in initiating conversation make sure that their attention is gained, for example by touching their arm or saying their name;
- encourage them to look at you when talking, but not to get too close (if that is a problem);
- give time to respond to questions and information given;
- reduce background noise to help concentration;
- use short utterances to present one idea or question at a time, but do not 'talk down' to the person affected;
- if the person rambles, try to bring them back on course with a tactful question or a reminder;
- find different ways to say the same thing if the person appears not to understand, but do not shout or use exaggerated oral movements.
- remember that if the person is ill or under the weather, their intellectual problems may be worse;
- resume a conversation at a later stage if speech is disoriented or meaningless. Avoid distressing the person by 'prodding';
- encourage visitors, but singly rather than in groups;
- encourage some organized activities;
- provide a calm atmosphere;
- gently discourage inappropriate behaviour.

As in any type of disorder, it is important that families understand the nature of dementia and are given information and support to help handle it.

LEARNING DIFFICULTIES

The full range of communication problems may occur within this client group. However, people with learning difficulties will obviously require a different approach to therapy as good communication skills are particularly important if they are to live an independent life.

To identify those who may benefit from developing their communication or eating and drinking skills, screening programmes should be available based on the needs relating to the client's environment and circumstances.

Good communication amongst all those trying to assist the client helps to clarify problems and objectives, whilst also encouraging progress. Specific training can be given to carers and other professionals and counselling and support can be made available to families and carers as well.

It is also argued that those in contact with a person with learning difficulties should be aware that the way they themselves speak can impede communication. It is possible that those in authority may use language more appropriate to young children, so that power relationships come into play and distort the potential for a healthy relationship between two adults.

Assessment of the client's communication skills and needs would include the following information:

- basic social skills;
- understanding of language;
- verbal expression;
- use made of augmentative communication such as Makaton Vocabulary;
- purposes communication is used for;
- intelligibility;
- fluency of speech.

Therapy aims at improving communication in real-life situations relevant to the client, and being able to employ the best strategies for learning. A communication programme can take many forms, including individual programmes, group learning and work skills.

Autism

Any professional dealing with people who have a learning difficulty (or mental handicap depending on which term is used) will undoubtedly meet those who have autistic features. The problems of people who have this condition will vary in degrees of severity. Problems may be marked or mild and may even affect those who appear to have normal or superior intelligence. This spectrum of problems can make it difficult for the professional to recognize. As with any of the charitable bodies mentioned thoughout the text, the National Autistic Society is keen to promote awareness of the disorder and how to recognize it.

Autism may include the following features:

- seeming not to be aware that they belong to the human species;
- intuitive understanding, thoughts, feelings and needs of others may not be considered or may be responded to inappropriately;
- indifference to other people;

- impaired verbal and non-verbal communication;
- slow learning;
- poor adaptation to situations;
- limited, repetitive and stereotyped behaviour;
- difficulties in social relationships;
- limited play and imagination;
- difficulty in changing routines;
- ability to perform tasks that do not require social skills but difficulty with those that do;
- bizarre behaviour;
- joins in activities only if cajoled.

The range of communication problems found in other client groups may apply to autistic people and communication may need to be pitched at a basic level. Basic social skills may need to be taught and encouraged and work on the verbal understanding and expression. In some cases a non-speech system such as Makaton Vocabulary may be helpful. This method involves developing the use of signs. Abstract reasoning can be a real problem which is why more concrete, real-life approaches are important.

In the absence of any clear diagnosis carers will try to find ways of coping with the difficulties described. Parents or carers may benefit from counselling and this may be provided by the GP practice, hospital or voluntary agency.

NEUROLOGICAL DISORDERS

Head injury, strokes or neurological conditions such as multiple sclerosis, Parkinson's disease and motor neurone disease can impair pathways responsible for communication, which may lead to confusion.

Dysarthria

Dysarthria is the name given to speech caused by a disturbance of muscular control. In its more severe forms dysarthria may also include weak facial and eating muscles. Speech may sound slurred, monotonous and low in volume and breathing for speech may be affected.

Carers and professionals involved with people who have dysarthria can help by:

- ensuring good posture for efficient breathing;
- ensuring dentures fit properly, if worn;
- not pretending speech is understood when it has not been;
- listening and checking out information rather than pretending to follow what is said – a word or alphabet chart may be useful at this point;

- encouraging them to use gesture or any other means of communication apart from speech;
- providing a quiet environment and minimizing background noise;
- recognizing that the emotional content and expression of speech can alter the intelligibility of what the client is saying, for example, the person may be particularly difficult to understand if they are excited;
- encouraging them to practise reading aloud. The use of a mirror and a tape recorder may help to give the patient feedback about their own speech but there is a risk of this causing distress unless handled sensitively.

Dysphasia

When language breaks down, the resulting disorder is called aphasia or dysphasia. There may be a partial or near total loss of language, speech, reading ability (acquired dyslexia) and writing (dysgraphia). It is important to realize that the disorder is one of communication, not intelligence. Many people with this problem say they experience the feeling that words are on the tip of their tongue: 'I know what I want to say but I can't say it'. A patient's speech may be jumbled, disjointed or even incoherent and this is very distressing for them, their family and friends. It is sad that few people know about dysphasia and may therefore assume because the person is talking about what appears to be nonsense that their intellect is not disturbed.

The dysphasic or aphasic person (the words are interchangeable), may lose track of what is being said, forget a name at a particular moment, or struggle to find the right words. They may use completely the wrong word or they may choose a word that is similar in sound or meaning.

There are four main types of dysphasia.

1. 'Telegrammatic' speech which consists of key words such as the nouns and verbs needed to convey a message. Sentences sound stilted and unconnected and the patient struggles to find the correct words to say: 'Go home, bed'; 'Hurt leg doctor'.
2. Alternatively, the patient may have more fluent speech but again there may be word-finding difficulties. They may use inappropriate words or make grammatical errors. As in all speech and language disorders anxiety and stress may make the problem worse. Patients may understand others' speech and be aware of their own speech errors, but unable to correct them. One patient wanted to explain a series of operations she had undergone and in explaining how she had stitches said that she had 'lots of ambulances' all over her body. Clearly, stitches and ambulances belonged to the category 'hospitals' and so the error was related to the word she wanted to say.

3. Patients who seem to speak very fluently may in fact convey very little as many essential words are missing. Their ability to take in spoken information may be very limited. 'Verbal diarrhoea' and 'jargon dysphasia' are two expressions commonly used to describe this type of speech. Another patient told a doctor at a case history interview that he had had 'Semolinafinafight' and had lost lots of weight. Eventually a relative was asked what this meant. She could only think it to mean salmonella poisoning, which he had suffered during the war years.

4. Some patients have virtually no speech at all and any speech they attempt may consist of repetitive and sterotyped phrases.

The following are some real-life examples of dysphasic speech:

- 'my name is Spain' ('my name is Jane');
- 'me got it' ('I have got it');
- 'I want an apple' ('I want a pear');
- 'yes, please' (with shaking head), ('no thank you').

If a dysphasic person is wrongly considered demented, schizophrenic, deaf or unintelligent this may mean that they do not receive the appropriate help. It is important not to discourage the patient or their family but to be positive and to be aware about any likelihood of improvement. In an effort to be kind, people are often tempted to make over-optimistic predictions which can cause all sorts of problems if the expected progress is not made in the time predicted.

Bill was a successful playwright, with a string of West End plays to his credit. Aged 49 and at the peak of his career, he suffered a stroke. Overnight he was reduced to struggling to utter a few simple words, which made him angry both with himself and the people around him who could barely understand anything he was trying to say. But he was very determined, and this and a successful course of speech therapy helped to recover much of his speech. One of the biggest problems he had to overcome along the way was others' perception that strokes were incurable. Once a well-meaning colleague suggested that he took up a hobby, such as gardening, to take his mind off the fact that he might never be able to write again. Fortunately this remark only increased his determination, and two years later he had resumed his interrupted career. The only sign that he had ever had a stroke was a problem he had never suffered before – a severe inability to spell.

Clearly, stories of this kind do not always have a happy ending, but Bill's case illustrates the importance of being positive and encouraging.

How to help when there are problems in understanding

The aphasic listener may find that they cannot quite catch what is said. When the problem is severe, speech and written material may resemble a foreign language. Nursing staff, doctors and family may fail to understand the extent of problems with verbal understanding; for example, if a nurse approaches the patient with a cup of tea, it would be reasonably appropriate for the dysphasic person to reach out with their hand and say 'thank you' without having understood the words, 'would you like a cup of tea?' Contextual cues help our understanding enormously; having aphasia can be like suddenly waking in a strange, unfamiliar country. Because people with this 'receptive language' problem may appear to understand what is said to them more than they really do, they may be handled wrongly because an inappropriate assumption has been made about their level of understanding.

Suggested ways of enabling communication to be more successful:

- Keep language short, simple and to the point, without presenting too much information or too many ideas all at once.
- Try speaking a little slower if you are a naturally fast speaker.
- Try to speak clearly, but not to the extent that it seems artificial and condescending. It is important not to feel embarrassed or to embarrass the listener.
- If comprehension is not too badly affected, providing opportunities to watch TV and listen to the radio can be most helpful. Books, magazines and newspapers may also be useful in helping the patient to maintain a sense of reality and immersing them in normal language.
- If necessary try alerting the person to the fact that they are being spoken to by touching them on the arm or by gaining attention by calling them by name.
- Ensure that the patient does not have a problem with hearing, or if they are wearing a hearing aid that it is working properly.
- Ensure that the patient does not become tired or anxious.
- Rather than persist in trying to understand unclear speech, it may be wise to suggest to the client that you return to the topic later.
- Make sure that your facial expressions and lip patterns are visible to help understanding.
- Avoid sudden changes of topic.
- Avoid talking to the dysphasic person at the same time as someone else or against competition from the radio or television.
- Try to establish a daily routine, but not one that is too regimented. This will help the person keep track of what is going on.
- Keep in mind that the dysphasic person has 'good' and 'not-so-good' days which may affect their communication skills.
- The more relaxed the client, the easier they will find communication, though their speech may be particularly clear when they are angry.
- Try to be as encouraging as possible as the client's self-esteem may be low.
- Encourage the dysphasic person to take part in activities they would

have been involved in before the disorder began so that it has the minimum of impact on their lifestyle.

- Try to find easier ways to converse with the person. Speech and language therapists can help with this, and various voluntary bodies publish leaflets on the subject (see Appendix).
- Consider using pen and paper, drawing and gestures to encourage non-verbal communication, but bear in mind that the ability to use these may also be affected.
- Avoid appearing annoyed or upset if the person swears inappropriately. This is likely to be uncontrollable and is sometimes the first speech to come back; the person may have used swear words before the onset of dysphasia, but only within a limited circle of people. (It can also be a means of expressing frustration.)
- Sometimes singing can be used as a form of therapy. For example, one patient who was only able to use half a dozen words in speech could sing the tunes of several well-known songs, such as the National Anthem and 'She Loves You' by the Beatles. This helped him to feel able to be fluent at least occasionally.

There is a wealth of material available through voluntary bodies such as Action for Dysphasic Adults, the Chest, Heart and Stroke Association and from many speech and language therapy departments. Demonstrations and talks to educate staff and the general public in understanding the nature of this condition can be arranged as well as talks on how to deal with the loss and loneliness associated with it. Many people take the ability to communicate for granted and only when it is lost through illness do we appreciate this most complex of human skills.

Communication charts, sign systems and communication aids can also be very useful and specialists can provide advice on how to use them. A total communication approach aims to encourage any means of communicating, be it a sign, a facial expression or a gesture, and non-verbal communication may be well-preserved. Understanding the message rather than insisting on the correct words being used is the best approach and patience is needed by both parties.

How speech and language therapists can help

- Providing a carefully planned therapy programme of exercises and activities;
- arranging demonstrations and talks;
- advising on communication charts, sign systems and communication aids, and ways of communicating with patients;
- providing support to carers and families;
- explaining what therapy is for and what it aims to achieve;

- organizing stroke groups to enable sufferers to share their problems;
- providing counselling to help patients and carers come to terms with the loss of language.

If the person is having therapy, relatives should feel able to find out what the therapist is doing and be given advice. It is often a good idea for relatives and carers to be involved in a treatment session. Stroke groups can provide social activities to reinforce therapy. Meeting similarly affected people can be helpful to alleviate isolation and provide group support. Clubs often have their own committee and social programme which may include talks by professionals (doctors, health visitors, physiotherapists, occupational therapists) on problems related to the patients. The club may arrange entertainment, outings and other events to restore patients' confidence and enjoyment.

STAMMERING

It is thought that one person in every hundred stammers. Stammering is a pattern of speech which may include one or more of a range of speech behaviours such as:

- repetitions of syllables, sounds, words or phrases;
- silent pauses called 'blocks';
- physical struggles to speak;
- unusual breathing sounds;
- prolonging sounds;
- avoiding words and situations.

The terms 'stammering' and 'stuttering' are interchangeable. All of us stammer sometimes, but in some cases stammering can be severe enough to affect a large part of a person's everyday life. At its worst, stammering is an enormous hurdle to be overcome. A person stammering may try to use physical gestures to replace words. In adults particularly, stammering can also influence self-perception.

In children

It is very common for all children to hesitate or have some repetitions, especially when they are unsure of what to say, are tired, upset, nervous or excited, but these are normal dysfluencies and the child will usually be unaware of them. The development of stammering is not uniform, but differs from child to child and adult to adult.

The causes of stammering are not clear. The Association for Research into Childhood Stammering was set up to explore this area from a background of research and to develop successful therapy. It is known that more males than females stammer and that people of all intelligence levels and personality types are affected. There is some evidence that it can run in families, although it can also occur where there has been no family history of stammering. It seems that the pattern of developing language is inherited, rather than the stammer itself. The current thinking is that there is no single cause of stammering, and that several factors coming together at the same time within the person may be the trigger. These influences may be physical or emotional, and can be affected by family, friends and school.

There are several things that are important in working with the dysfluent child. The first is to involve the whole family, and the second is to seek early advice from a speech and language therapist. However there are also some simple ways in which anyone can help reduce communication pressures on young children and therefore encourage them to enjoy talking.

Do's and don'ts

Don't

- Draw attention to the stammer;
- complete remarks for them;
- speak for the child – 'No, he doesn't take sugar';
- mimic them;
- bribe them to speak better;
- insist on making them speak when they do not want to;
- talk about their problem in front of them – 'She has such an awful stammer – don't you darling?';
- compare them with others – 'Your friend Johnny doesn't stammer – why do you?';
- tell them to start speaking all over again;
- interrupt them;
- hurry them along – 'come on, we haven't got all day';
- lose eye contact – this may convey boredom or impatience;
- punish them for poor speech;
- highlight the problem by making them read aloud. A child who stammers can often feel more comfortable about reading with someone else in unison; gradually, they may progress to reading on their own.

Do

- Listen carefully to the child – concentrate on what the child is saying rather than how they are saying it;
- slow down your own rate of talking and ensure that you use a level of language that they understand;
- remain calm when you are speaking – if you are anxious, the child will pick this up, making things harder for you both;

- try to have a fairly relaxed lifestyle, with a regular routine at school and at home, so the child can feel relaxed and more sure of himself;
- give the child periods of regular uninterrupted time such as story-time and when they come in from school. This will help to prevent them feeling that they always get left out of conversation.
- talk about their speech if they want to;
- avoid messages which convey a feeling that dysfluency is wrong or shameful;
- listen with interest, full attention and in a relaxed atmosphere;
- speak in a relaxed way – don't talk too quickly or ask too many questions;
- allow the child to feel that they will not be interrupted while they are speaking;
- encourage people to take their turn in talking (especially in a family). This will allow the child to feel they will not be interrupted if they are struggling to talk;
- try to speak to a child on a similar physical level. For example, it may be less intimidating for the child if the adult sits down with them rather than towering over them;
- look at the child while they are talking and when you are talking to them;
- take the focus away from speech sometimes so that the child is doing things rather than talking, perhaps by giving them a toy to play with;
- give praise when the child is doing well, to help build their confidence.

Older children

As the child becomes older, it may be quite clear that they are stammering rather than being normally dysfluent. If this is the case, there are a number of ways in which you can help.

- Check with the teacher, parents or speech and language therapist about the approach that is being taken with the child. This will ensure that everyone involved is acting consistently.
- It may be useful to bring up the subject of stammering with the child to give them the chance to express any anxieties they may have.
- If the child only stammers in a particular situation, for example when talking about what they have been doing at school, consider finding out whether there is anything bothering him or her in the situation concerned. Let the child know that their speech difficulties can be discussed and that someone will understand.
- If a child is teased about their stammer, take the culprits to one side and explain that teasing can make the stammer worse just as any other kind of teasing causes pain and discomfort.

- Remember each child is an individual, so there are no hard and fast rules about how to respond to them. If you keep the above advice in mind, you will go a long way to helping the child.

How to help the adolescent or adult

Much of the advice on talking to child stammerers also applies to older people. But these are perhaps the three most important things to remember:

- Keep communications calm and unhurried

    I find that if people harass or hurry me it's harder to express myself fluently and my stammering is often worse.

- Maintain eye contact with the stammerer. React in the same way as you would with a fluent person

    I often can't get a single word out if I sense someone looking away when I'm trying to speak to them.

- Don't finish off sentences for a stammerer – it reduces self-confidence and increases frustration

    It's really irritating having someone finish sentences for you. I feel like a child.

Some adults may not have had any therapy or advice for a long period of time and may need an opportunity to find out about new therapies available. Being allowed to experiment with a stammer in a comfortable and supportive environment can also be important, which is one way in which speech therapy can help. The Association for Stammerers may also be able to provide valuable information on self-help groups and other subjects.

There are no 'miracle' cures and a stammer frequently has to be managed rather than cured. Unfortunately, this area of health promotion tends to attract practitioners who claim to have the perfect answer, but speech and language therapists will usually be able to advise on the likelihood of success of particular treatments. The Association for Stammerers also has a panel of advisers who can be helpful in explaining different treatment approaches, which may include speech control techniques, exploring and altering attitudes towards speech, and looking at communication skills in general.

Speech and language therapy

Refer to a speech and language therapist for specific advice. Teachers should allow teenagers time out of school to attend sessions with the therapist and provide support for any technique used: therapists are able to discuss classroom management with the teacher. Therapy may take place on an individual basis or in a group, on a weekly basis or as part of an intensive course according to the requirements of the client and the availability of speech therapy.

Adults who stammer

Many adults who stammer have to deal with other people's ignorance about stammering. People who stammer do not, as a group, have higher or lower intelligence than everyone else; nor are they emotionally damaged. Obviously, anyone experiencing difficulty in speaking is likely to be frustrated at the effort involved and some find their stammer sufficiently annoying to warrant therapy. However, many people with this problem do not seek help and have come to terms with it. Stammering does not have to get in the way of relationships and job opportunities. The social skills of a dysfluent adult can influence the success, or not, of an interaction.

Tony had stammered for as long as he could remember. He thinks he had some help with it as a child but doesn't know what kind. The frustrating part for him was that he only stammered occasionally, but always when he wanted to impress people, usually people he met for the first time or those in authority. Learning a fluency technique and some social skills helped his confidence considerably, as did coming to terms with the fact that all life's problems couldn't be blamed on his stammer.

VOICE DISORDERS

Of all forms of communication disorders, voice problems are probably the most easily preventable. A large proportion of them are caused by:

- smoking and excessive alcohol;
- vocal misuse, such as straining the voice by shouting and talking above background noise;
- stress factors which involve a conflict in talking about a problem.

'Dysphonia' is the term given to describe a voice disorder. 'Aphonia' describes the absence of any voice, such as in whispered voice, often a psychological problem or following the result of surgical removal of the larynx due to cancer.

Many voice disorders can be avoided by vocal hygiene and proper training in effective use of the voice. The British Voice Association can put enquirers in touch with trainers who can run workshops on 'Voice Care and Development for Schoolteachers', which aim to promote vocal hygiene for professional voice users. This latter group includes teachers, preachers, singers, actors, telephonists, salespeople or indeed anyone who depends on their voice to earn a living. Most professional voice users are not taught how to look after their voices. Even with proper training the effects of stressful life events cannot be under-estimated. Typical voice problems may include:

- loss of voice for no apparent reason but with normal looking vocal cords;
- laryngitis where there is virus to explain it;
- vocal nodule(s) where small swellings appear on the cords due to excessive demands on the voice, inadequate voice production and misuse of the voice.

How to care for the voice

Avoid:

- vocal cord irritants such as cigarettes, smoke, chalk dust, sprays and fumes;
- sudden changes of temperature and very hot food and drink;
- spicy foods and alcohol during the acute phase of laryngitis;
- going to bed dehydrated – alcohol is dehydrating and can make the throat feel very dry;
- excessive caffeinated drinks;
- unprescribed medicines and inhalers;
- aerosols, unless a prescribed drug;
- excessive, loud and vigorous gargling (the vocal cords may come together too forcefully);
- antibiotics in the absence of acute inflammation;
- working for lengthy periods in dry, dusty or hot environments – humidify surroundings with bowls of water and plants and keep rooms well ventilated;
- violent or habitually coughing and clearing the throat. This may have started off as a way of clearing mucus during a cough and cold, but may only make the irritation worse so that the coughing becomes a habit;
- talking above background noise, especially in smoky atmospheres. Teachers may need to use devices: bells, whistles or microphones instead of shouting;
- calling to people in another room; it is better to walk over to them than shout;
- poor slouching posture when sitting, standing or using the phone;
- mouth breathing, as this means cooler, unfiltered air is inhaled;
- talking forcefully or excessively when having laryngitis – it is better to have time off work or rest the voice;

- whispering instead of using the voice. There is no evidence that this is helpful, as the vocal cords still have to come together. It is better to rest the voice completely and do 'warm-up' exercises under supervision, gently proceeding to normal voice use;
- remedies may well be helpful but the possible benefits are not scientifically proved and so this is a controversial area. Some experts say that lozenges are helpful, while others believe they are irritants. Patients vary in what they say they find useful;
- neglecting to deal with issues of loss, anger, sadness, anxiety and other feelings, which may be contributing to the voice problem. Emotional problems may be reflected in the voice, as we use the voice for communication.

Often people are unconcerned about their voice and are more worried about any pain or discomfort. Very often voice and throat discomfort are related.

CASE STUDIES

Case study 1

Susan had been teaching for two years before she developed frequent discomfort in her throat and a hoarse voice which would sometimes disappear altogether. She rarely had time off from work and her GP had prescribed her several courses of antibiotics which occasionally helped for a short time, but then the problem returned. An ear, nose and throat (ENT) examination at the local hospital revealed that she had benign nodules on her vocal cords. A course of voice therapy from the speech and language therapist (SLT) helped Susan to understand how she was misusing her voice, and advice on vocal hygiene helped her discover how her voice was being affected by smoking and persistent throat clearing. She was also given relaxation exercises and shown how to increase the resonance and raise the pitch of her voice. Her boyfriend had encouraged her to use a deeper, husky voice as he found it 'sexy'. Often therapists have to explore the image voices have before helping with change. By reducing unnecessary vocal effort and following guidelines on vocal hygiene, Susan's nodules disappeared by the time she attended her ENT appointment six weeks later.

In addition to voice problems, some people say they have a 'lump' in the throat (globus pharyngeus). This may be related to an underlying disorder and would need further investigation. Alternatively, it may simply be caused by neck tension. Tension may be the combination of physical and emotional causes and these may need exploring in therapy. Trauma such as the death of a spouse may be sufficient to bring these problems to the attention of an SLT. Counselling is frequently used in therapy to enable the client to explore the nature of voice problems and how these link with feelings.

Case study 2

Michelle was referred to an SLT specializing in voice, who had also trained as a counsellor. She was complaining of feeling a lump in her throat and her GP referred her to the ENT department at her general hospital. ENT investigations, including assessment of her swallowing, revealed no abnormalities. The patient was referred to the SLT who established that the onset of the problem coincided with the death of Michelle's husband a year before. The therapist discovered during the case history interview on Michelle's first visit, that her husband, who had been dying of cancer, had asked her not to cry after his death but 'to be happy' and 'carry on living'. Michelle had longed to express her grief fully through tears, but had denied herself the experience of this important process and had 'bottled up' her feelings. Eventually, she began to believe that the lump in her throat was cancer. Only after fully acknowledging her grief and being given support in expressing her feelings did the 'globus' symptoms disappear.

Case study 3

Mary had a weak, breathy voice which her husband found appealing. However, her voice was not effective for classroom use as a teacher. Voice training enabled Mary to project a more powerful voice which had the effect of making those around her 'sit up and listen'. Sadly, she could not carry off her new assertive image and needed counselling in order to deal with the change.

ACKNOWLEDGEMENTS

VOCAL member charities and The College of Speech and Language Therapists' advisers.

REFERENCE

Marzollo, J. and Lloyd, J. (1972) *Learning through Play*, Unwin Paperbacks, London.

CHAPTER 12

Health education for people with physical disabilities

Christine M. Dowding

Health education and health promotion are just as relevant for people with physical disabilities as they are for able-bodied people.

It has been estimated that there are at least 6 million adults in the UK with at least one disability (Martin *et al.*, 1988). This is almost certainly an under-estimate as disability tends to be under-reported. Health promotion may be even more important for disabled people since they are dependent on maintaining what DeJong and Hughes (1982) have termed their 'thinner margin of health'.

Unfortunately a number of barriers to health promotion for disabled people have been identified (Stuifbergen *et al.*, 1990). These include structural barriers such as time, distance, availability of services and discrimination. Individual characteristics such as age, education, personal attitudes and cultural factors were also identified as potential barriers. Health care professionals, who focus so heavily on the individual's disability that they overlook other factors, were also cited as possible barriers to successful health promotion.

This chapter will focus on the additional needs of this client group which will be illustrated by case histories where appropriate.

Before discussing disability it is useful to differentiate between impairment, disability and handicap as defined by the World Health Organization (1980). These terms are often used interchangeably when strictly speaking they have quite different meanings.

Impairment: in the context of health experience, an impairment is any loss or abnormality of psychological, physiological or anatomical structure or function.

Disability: in the context of health experience, a disability is any restriction or lack (resulting from an impairment) of ability to perform an activity in the manner or within the range considered normal for a human being.

Handicap: in the context of health experience, a handicap is a disadvantage for a given individual, resulting from an impairment or a disability, that limits or prevents the fulfilment of a role that is normal (depending on age, sex and social and cultural factors) for that individual.

The following examples are offered in order to clarify the range of problems that may result from an impairment.

	TEACHER	CONCERT PIANIST
Impairment	Loss of a finger	Loss of a finger
Disability	Minimal	Unable to play piano to previous standard
Handicap	None	End of career

There are many ways to categorize types of disability but for the purpose of this chapter the most simple method is probably to look at the cause and the progress of the condition.

CONGENITAL	ACQUIRED
e.g. Spina bifida	e.g. Spinal injury
e.g. Down's syndrome	e.g. Heart disease
TEMPORARY	PERMANENT
e.g. Colles' fracture	e.g. Amputation of leg
e.g. Temporary colostomy	e.g. Diabetes
RELAPSING/REMITTING	PROGRESSIVE
e.g. Multiple sclerosis	e.g. Parkinson's disease
e.g. Some cancers	e.g. Alzheimer's disease

Congenital disabilities

This subject has already been discussed in Chapter 7. However, such disabilities can produce different problems in adolescence and adulthood. The progression from dependent child to independent adult is often a difficult time for both children and parents. Children who are disabled by a congenital condition may find this transition more difficult to achieve for a variety of reasons. The impact and ramifications of the disability may become more apparent as the adolescent grows both physically and emotionally. This can be illustrated by considering a girl who has sustained burns of the chest, often as a result of a nightdress catching fire, who discovers that her breasts cannot grow symmetrically as a result of scar tissue. Thankfully this type of injury is much less common due to public education and legislation relating to the flammability of children's nightwear. Another example is of an adolescent boy with spina bifida who discovers that he will not be able to enjoy a full sexual relationship.

Case history

Mary (Brown) aged 22, spina bifida

Mary developed pressure sores over both ischial tuberosities due to sitting in a wheelchair for prolonged periods without relieving the pressure. She was admitted to hospital for assessment and treatment. Assessment revealed that she had seen the sores developing but had been reluctant to seek medical help as she feared that sick-leave might jeopardize her job. An important part of Mary's treatment, following surgery, was to help her establish a routine whereby she would examine all her pressure areas on a regular basis using a mirror. She also received help and guidance from an occupational therapist on ways to improve her working environment, and advice from a physiotherapist on the best way to maintain a good position in her wheelchair and in other chairs she used regularly.

In order to help young people with congenital disabilities to develop in a positive way, some of the following strategies may be useful.

1. Further detailed explanation about their disability using material available from a wide range of organizations, some of which are listed (see Appendix A).
2. Sex education from a specialist counsellor.
   The Association to Aid the Sexual and Personal Relationships of the Disabled (SPOD) employ trained counsellors who can give advice and help. A useful booklet entitled 'Sex for Young People with Spina Bifida or Cerebral Palsy' is available from the Association for Spina Bifida and Hydrocephalus (ASBAH).
3. Career guidance.
4. Opportunities for gaining confidence and independence away from the family, e.g. Winged Fellowship Holidays. Parents may need help and guidance in how best to help the child to gain some independence, however severe his disability. Many people gain advice and support from the numerous self-help groups that exist.

ACQUIRED DISABILITY

A disability may be acquired at any time during a person's life and may result from illness, an injury or surgery. The severity of the disability is usually the main factor in deciding the effect on the individual. In some cases, however, the cause of the disability may result in a psychological handicap which is more devastating than the physical disability. A woman who has had successful surgery to remove breast cancer may be so upset by the scars that she is unable to return to her normal life.

This may lead to the break-up of her marriage unless help is available and she is willing to accept it. A person who has been involved in a road traffic accident (RTA) and suffered facial lacerations may find it difficult to put the memory of the accident behind him as they are faced with the scars every time they look into a mirror. Another factor which will affect how an individual copes with an acquired disability is their age. As people get older they often become less flexible in their attitudes and may find it takes longer to learn new skills.

Case history

John Smith, age 19, RTA resulting in paraplegia

John was involved in an accident while travelling to college on his motorcycle. He sustained a fracture dislocation between lumbar vertebrae L3 and L4 resulting in a complete paraplegia. He was treated in a Spinal Injuries Unit where he had the benefit of a tailor-made rehabilitation programme. A considerable proportion of such programmes is concerned with various aspects of patient education and health promotion. Some of the most important features are detailed below:

- prevention of pressure sores;
- prevention of urinary tract infections;
- weight control;
- recognition of autonomic dysreflexia;
- sexual relationships;
- returning to work.

In the past many people felt that there was too much emphasis on Activities of Daily Living (ADL) and the physical side of rehabilitation. A changing view of the rehabilitation of spinal injured people has been put forward by Trieschmann (1980) as follows:

> Basically the rehabilitation should shift from physical functioning to psycho-social integration into the community. The latter entails the former, but the reverse is not true.

One of the main ways of helping spinal injured people to achieve this aim is by ensuring that they fully understand their injury and the potential problems which they face. One of the consequences of this approach is that the person may know more about his condition than some of the health care professionals who may be involved in his care, particularly after his discharge from the specialist unit.

Where they exist, the community liaison nurse should ensure that the GP and other health care professionals are conversant with caring for a person who has been spinal injured. This should help to defuse any problems which might arise.

The Spinal Injuries Association is a very active body with local groups around the country. They have a range of publications and offer help and support in a variety of ways.

TEMPORARY DISABILITIES

Temporary disabilities may not at first seem to be so serious but much can be done to promote good health and prevent or reduce complications. A temporary disability is often the result of an accident or an acute illness for which the person had no preparation. This can be illustrated by comparing the experience of a person who has undergone a planned laryngectomy and tracheostomy with someone who regains consciousness after an accident to find that he has undergone an emergency tracheostomy. The first person will have received a full explanation of the procedure to which he will have given his consent. He may also have met someone from the Laryngectomee Club and have gained some insight into the effects of the procedure. The second person will have received no preparation and may be extremely concerned and frightened about the future, despite being assured that it is a temporary measure.

Case history

Mrs Brown, age 70, right Colles' fracture

Mrs Brown slipped on an icy pavement and in an effort to save herself fractured her right wrist. She was taken to her local Casualty Unit where the fracture was reduced and the joint immobilized. She was kept in hospital overnight and discharged to her daughter's care the next day. The following strategy would have been discussed and explained to her before discharge:

- correct positioning of arm and use of sling;
- shoulder exercises;
- advice on ADL using one hand;
- advice on prevention of further falls, e.g. non-slip shoes, walking stick, etc.

When elderly people are admitted to hospital, particularly with relatively minor injuries, it is very important that they are encouraged to maintain their independence. They can sometimes lose their independence by the ministrations of over-zealous staff. It is often in the elderly person's best interests if they can be treated as a day case and returned to their own environment as quickly as possible.

PERMANENT DISABILITIES

Some permanent disabilities come from planned surgery as previously mentioned. This gives an opportunity for the individual to meet some-one who has successfully adapted to a change in their body and lifestyle. There are many self-help organizations who are very willing to perform this useful service, e.g. the Mastectomy Association and the Ileostomy Association. Other disabilities may develop through illness or an accident when there is no opportunity to provide support and education prior to the event. In some instances an individual may find that he adapts to his new circumstances fairly quickly. A young man who has a leg amputated after a road traffic accident (RTA) can usually learn to walk with a prosthesis without much difficulty. He should be able to return to work or if necessary retrain for a new job. He may need an adapted car but it is unlikely that he would need adaptations to his home. An older person who had a similar accident may be in a very different position. He may be suffering from arthritis or some other degenerative illness which would hinder his progress with a prosthesis. Another potential problem for older people is the risk of developing pressure sores on the stump of their limb. Once this has happened many people give up using the prosthesis all together. Careful observation of the stump should alert staff to act quickly should a problem arise.

Case history

Jane White, age 28, diabetes

A routine medical examination revealed that Jane had developed dia-betes. She was referred to her local hospital and seen at the Diabetic Clinic which co-ordinated the various services that she might require. It is vital that all diabetic people fully understand their condition and if at all possible are able to control their own treatment. She was advised on various aspects of her condition by medical staff, dietitian and the diabetic liaison nurse. They would have covered some of the following points:

- the importance of regular follow-up;
- the need to carry some form of identification, i.e. Medical Alert bracelet;
- how to use a blood glucose monitor;
- dietary advice;
- how to administer insulin;
- how to recognize hypoglycaemia and hyperglycaemia;
- the need for regular eye examinations;

- the need for daily feet examination;
- the local British Diabetic Association (BDA) contact.

While most of the above measures would be similar for an older person, it should be remembered that they may find it harder to adapt their lifestyle. Problems such as poor eyesight and reduced manual dexterity may mean than an older diabetic could not manage their regime without help.

The BDA provides a range of services to both diabetic people and health care professionals. This includes educational holidays for children and adults, a newsletter and over 300 local branches throughout the UK. It also has an educational section and publishes a range of very useful material.

RELAPSING/REMITTING DISABILITIES

Some people have a disability which alternates between a period of remission followed by a relapse. This can cause problems as it is usually difficult to predict the course of the disability. People with some types of cancer may be able to predict a remission between courses of treatment, but in many cases this is not possible. The uncertainty of this type of disability can put a great strain on an individual and their family. Holding down a job can be difficult if the person cannot work during a relapse. The problems that cancer sufferers encounter at work have been addressed in Chapter 13 but it should be emphasized that similar problems exist for people with other conditions such as multiple sclerosis. As with so many aspects of employment, much depends on the type of work that the disabled person is engaged in. It is often easier for professional people to take time off work or to work from home if their condition is relapsed. Employment is an important part of most people's lives and provides much more than an income. Some of the positive benefits of employment are listed below:

- giving structure to the day;
- providing company and friendship;
- enhancement of self-worth and self-esteem;
- sports and other recreational facilities may be available;
- health screening and health promotion may also be available.

Case history

Anne Smith, age 36, multiple sclerosis

Anne was cooking lunch for her family when a pan of boiling water fell onto her legs. She was unable to get out of her wheelchair and so the water soaked into her clothes, causing severe scalds to both her legs. She was admitted to the Regional Burns Unit for routine burn therapy. Some areas of her legs needed grafting and this was carried out successfully. Assessment by the multidisciplinary team revealed that Anne was having extreme difficulty in looking after her two small children and running her home. She had been very reluctant in the past to accept any form of help. She explained that she had not wanted to admit to herself that her condition was relapsing. After her accident she agreed that a full ADL assessment by the occupational therapist would be a good idea, and that it could incorporate a home visit so that adaptations could be carried out before her return. This decision was welcomed by her husband, who had found his suggestions ignored in the past. Anne received intensive physiotherapy and found that she was better able to cope with the spasticity in her legs which had been a long-standing problem. Another important aspect of Anne's care was the counselling sessions with the unit psychologist which helped her to accept the nature of her disability. Anne was transferred back to the care of the community nurses, having agreed to a range of services which would enable her to continue in her role as housewife and mother.

Relapsing and remitting disabilities can cause a variety of problems not least of which is the psychological effects of hope followed by a depression when a relapse occurs.

People with multiple sclerosis are often disadvantaged when compared to people who have suffered a spinal injury. Many people who suffer a sudden injury or serious illness will receive rehabilitation as a matter of course. A person with a slow onset condition such as MS may find that assessment and provision of aids, adaptions and services are unlikely to be planned. Such action may not be taken until the person needs a wheelchair or presents with a serious problem such as incontinence. Whenever an MS sufferer is in contact with any health agency, an opportunity exists to help improve this situation.

PROGRESSIVE DISABILITIES

People with progressive disabilities share some of the characteristics of people with relapsing and remitting disabilities. It is often difficult for people to accept the changes that a disability brings when the future is so uncertain. Most progressive disabilities have a very gradual onset which can make it difficult to find the right time to provide rehabilitation and support services. Parkinson's disease is a relatively common condition which can cause severe disability. McLellan (1988) stressed the importance of beginning treatment at the time of diagnosis by giving a full explanation of the nature and prognosis of the disease. This is also a good opportunity to provide literature from self-help organizations such as the Parkinson's Disease Society.

Case history

Peter Black, age 55, Alzheimer's disease

Over a period of several months, Peter's wife had noticed that he seemed to be having difficulty with his memory. A diagnosis of Alzheimer's disease came as a great shock to her as she thought the problem was going to be temporary. She received a great deal of help and support from the Alzheimer's Disease Society. As Peter's condition deteriorated, their daughter moved back into the family home to help care for her father. The family also received support from various members of the primary health care team although the brunt of the burden fell on Peter's wife.

People who care for someone with a progressive disability can easily find that they become trapped in an ever-expanding committment. It is essential for the mental and physical well-being of carers that they are able to take a break. A variety of options such as respite care, day care and Care Attendant Schemes are described in the booklet *Taking a Break* (Health Education Authority, 1987). Some people with progressive disabilities may require residential care when their condition deteriorates. A Young Chronic Sick Unit or a Cheshire Home can provide a suitable setting where a certain amount of independence and autonomy can be preserved.

The task of promoting health and preventing disease and disability has never been an easy one. When one considers people who already have a disability, the task can appear to be even more challenging. Health promotion is generally divided into three areas: primary, secondary and tertiary prevention. Primary and secondary prevention should be available to disabled people in just the same way as they are available to everyone else. Unfortunately this is not always the case and reasons for this will be discussed later. Warren (1986) identified three major difficulties in developing tertiary prevention. The first was the difficulty in co-ordinating the various people and organizations who might be responding to the perceived problems of each disabled person. The second difficulty was to find acceptable ways of maintaining surveillance without unwelcome intrusion. This can sometimes be achieved by using various registers and may improve as more GP practices computerize their records. The third difficulty concerned the number of people who could be helped by services already available but who are either unaware of their existence or unwilling to use them.

It is important that disabled people have all the information available so that they can make informed choices for themselves. Particularly vulnerable people who are unable to make such choices should be monitored by the primary health care team so that they do not become further disadvantaged.

This raises the question of personal freedom and choice versus the health of a group of people. This dilemma can be seen when one considers such issues as random checking of drivers to measure blood alcohol, the use of seat-belts and the fluoridation of drinking water. A positive way to approach these dilemmas is by making sure that preventative measures are subjected to rigorous evaluation. Unfortunately, reports of such evaluation in the media are not always helpful, as they tend to dwell on one particular aspect of what is usually a complex issue. Some of the publicity surrounding breast screening has been contradictory, which is not helpful when one is trying to promote screening as being beneficial.

Most disabled people have had some contact with rehabilitation services and some will have undertaken a full rehabilitation programme. It has been reported by Teague *et al.* (1990) that health promotion is not generally a part of most rehabilitation programmes. One of the reasons for this may be that rehabilitation generally has been described by Beardshaw (1988) as fragmented and piecemeal, with most disabled people receiving little practical help. A health promotion philosophy could and should be incorporated into all rehabilitation programmes.

Health maintenance is a term used to describe the two complementary and overlapping networks of health promotion and health recovery. It is the second network, that of health recovery, which focuses on people with disabilities. Teague *et al.* (1990) identified four health enhancement domains as follows:

1. physical health;
2. psychological health;
3. social health;
4. spiritual health.

As discussed earlier, focus is too often on physical health with less attention given to the other factors. The two main objectives of health maintenance are to teach the disabled person to become personally responsible for his own health and to co-manage his own rehabilitation programme. The first objective is gaining wider acceptance having been standard practice in Spinal Injury Units for quite some time. It is unfortunate that some health care professionals still feel threatened by a person who has more than superficial knowledge of his own condition. The second objective is slowly being met as more individuals are encouraged to take part in care planning. There is still, however, a great difference between areas which hold open case conferences involving the disabled person and those where discussion of a person's progress is held behind closed doors. Changes in attitudes must also be supported by increased resources. Chamberlain (1985) argued that treating people partially and imperfectly was not the best way of using scarce resources. She stated that while most people living in Britain could expect at least five decades of good health, the limitation of this success was the poor health maintenance for older and disabled people. It is to be hoped that new initiatives in Community Care (Secretaries of State for Health and Social Security, 1989) will help redress the balance.

It is usual for rehabilitation programmes to finish when a disabled person returns to work and/or achieves independent living. One of the ways in which an individual can maintain his health is by participating in a wellness programme. Rehabilitation can be said to encompass five phases:

1. assessment;
2. planning;
3. provision;
4. placement;
5. follow-up.

A wellness programme can form a useful link between hospital and community in the follow-up phase. The components of a Wellness Lifestyle Programme described by Abood and Burkhead (1988) are summarized below:

- self-awareness
  e.g. values, attitudes, capabilities, expectations;
- health awareness
  e.g. health risks, physical fitness, nutritional awareness, emotional awareness;
- wellness skills
  e.g. problem solving, self-care, decision making;
- wellness resources
  e.g. personal resources, social support, community.

The potential benefits of a wellness programme for a disabled person are many and varied. If the individual can progress from a position of just coping with his disability to an increase in psychological, spiritual and physical growth as suggested by Abood and Burkhead (1988) this would be very worthwhile.

A survey by Stuifbergen *et al.* (1990) examined the barriers to health promotion for disabled people. They interviewed 135 disabled adults who reported a wide range of disabilities. Some of the most frequently cited barriers were lack of money, feeling too tired, lack of time and lack of transport. Another finding of the study was anecdotal evidence that negative attitudes of health care providers could sometimes undermine health promotion services. Both Warren (1986) and Stuifbergen *et al.* (1990) suggest that an increase in health promotion for disabled people might reduce the ultimate cost of health care for this client group. While the financial implications of health promotion are important, of greater importance is improving people's quality of life.

The Prince of Wales Advisory Group on Disability (1985) published some very useful guidelines for anyone who is planning services for people with severe disabilities. The key principles are:

- choice;
- consultation;
- information;
- participation;
- recognition;
- autonomy.

These principles can be applied to almost any setting in which one is involved in health promotion and health education. The principle was utilized by Johnson and Cedrone (1990), who took a group of severely disabled people on holiday in order to teach them how to travel safely, efficiently and enjoyably. Evaluation of the experiment was very positive. The participants had acquired many new skills and since their return they considered travel to be within their range of ability.

The ability to make choices is clearly linked to the amount of information available to disabled people. Many self-help organizations provide written information which can be referred to over a period of time. When information is given verbally, there is rarely an opportunity to refer back to the source.

An important part of life for people with disabilities is being able to share activities with able-bodied people. PHAB clubs (Physically Handicapped and Able-Bodied) provide a venue for people to mix and enjoy sports and social events.

Health education and health promotion should be available to all disabled people and should be an integral part of all rehabilitation programmes. The Royal College of Physicians (1986) highlighted the need for a major expansion of research in the services provided for disabled people, particularly rehabilitation techniques and different ways of providing care. Improvements in these services, together with an increase in health, should result in a better quality of life for all disabled people.

REFERENCES

Abood, D.A. and Burkhead, E.J. (1988) Wellness: A Valuable Resource for Persons with Disabilities. *Health Education*, **19**(2), 21–5.

Beardshaw, V. (1988) *Last on the List: Community Services for People with Disabilities*, King's Fund Institute, London.

Chamberlain, M.A. (1985) Prospects in Rehabilitation. *British Medical Journal*, **290**, 1449–50.

DeJong, G. and Hughes, J. (1982) Independent Living: Methodology for Measuring Long-term Outcomes. *Arch. Phys. Med. Rehabil.*, **63**, 68–73.

Health Education Authority (1987) *Taking a Break*, London.

Johnson, J.R. and Cedrone, S. (1990) Enabling Disabled Travellers. *Rehabilitation Nursing*, **15**(2), 92–4.

McLellan, D.L. (1988) in *Rehabilitation of the Physically Disabled Adult* (eds. C.J. Goodwill and M.A. Chamberlain), Croom Helm, London.

Martin, J., Meltzewr, H. and Elliott, D. (1988) *The Prevalence of Disability Among Adults*, O.P.S.C. Surveys of Disability in GP Report 1, HMSO, London.

Secretaries of State for Health and Social Security (1989) *Caring for People: Community Care in the next decade and beyond*, CM. 849, HMSO, London.

Stuifbergen, A.K., Becker, H. and Sands, D. (1990) Barriers to Health Promotion for Individuals with Disabilities. *Family and Community Health*, **13**(1), 11–22.

Teague, M.L., Cipriano, R.E. and McGhee, V.L. (1990) Health Promotion as a Rehabilitation Service for People with Disabilities. *Journal of Rehabilitation*, Jan–March, **56**(1), 52–6.

Treischmann, R.B. (1980) *Spinal Cord Injuries – Psychological, Social and Vocational Adjustment*, Pergamon Press, New York.

The Prince of Wales Advisory Group on Rehabilitation (1985) *Living Options*. Prince of Wales Advisory Group on Disability, Room 142, 222 Marylebone Road, London NW1 6JJ.

The Royal College of Physicians (1986) Physical Disability in 1986 and Beyond. *Journal of the Royal College of Physicians*, **20**(3), 160–94.

Warren, M.D. (1986) Promoting Health and Preventing Disease and Disability: an Introduction to Concepts, Opportunities and Practices – Part 2. *Physiotherapy Practice*, **2**(1), 3–10.

World Health Organization (1980) *International Classification of Impairments, Disabilities and Handicaps*, HMSO, London.

CHAPTER 13

Helping those with chronic or life-threatening illness

Gill Oliver

The promotion of health in those with chronic or life-threatening illness may sound like a contradiction in terms: this is far from the truth. The health of a woman with chronic breast cancer for example can be significantly enhanced if her educational and informational needs are identified and met (Maguire, 1980; Hayward, 1975). She can be helped to minimize further complications from her disease and to reach her fullest potential for health. Similarly patient education and promotion of healthy attitudes and lifestyle can ensure that a young man brain damaged in an accident is enabled to take his rightful place in society.

Individuals are increasingly being encouraged to accept responsibility for their own health and well-being currently and for their future. The rapid pace of developments within the National Health Service (HMSO, 1990) is allowing patients a higher degree of choice, a right of autonomy and a greater participation in decision making. True involvement for patients and clients will not happen without strategies that ensure understanding, information and advice not only about their disease and its implications but about how these may be modified by changes in attitude, behaviour and lifestyle. The increasing assertiveness that our current culture encourages requires levels of knowledge and skill still broadly lacking. Patients, their families and friends do not always have the knowledge and information that is necessary for them to make informed choices and decisions about adapting to altered function, responding to changed circumstances or to the management of their disease and its effects. Carers do not always have the communication or teaching skills that are an integral part of the enabling process.

Health care in the UK has moved from the paternalistic pattern of earlier generations when doctor knew best and patients did as they were told, to a culture in which the patient is seen as a rightful partner in the planning and decision-making process, and the involvement of family and friends is an essential, not an option.

A clinical view of health cannot simply be defined as the absence of disease. People with chronic or life-threatening illness still have a potential for health or wellness. Health is better defined as the ability to perform one's own role or to realize one's potential (Stromberg, 1989). This concept of health is, therefore, quite compatible with a diagnosis of cancer, brain damage or cardiac disease. Health is seen as an entity separate from illness. Individuals can be at any stage of health, and at any stage of illness at the same time.

This chapter aims to define the client groups that can be described as chronically ill, to identify their needs relative to achieving their potential for health and describing ways in which these needs might be met. A chronic disease is one which is lingering or lasting but not necessarily one which is life-threatening. Chronic illness may be punctuated by acute episodes which obviously affect the course of the underlying illness. There is a tendency to assume that chronic illness is associated with a diagnosis of malignancy but there are many instances where cancer is not chronic for example, and where chronic illness is caused by a disease other than cancer.

A life-threatening illness is one which is expected to cause the death of the individual either imminently or after a period of gradual deterioration. It follows then that there are many illnesses falling into the above category. Each will have differing implications for the patient, his family and the carers. For example, chronic arthritis will cause mobility problems, a diagnosis of cancer may lead to emotional difficulties, and major surgery resulting in altered body image and changed function can create difficulties in social and family relationships. In each case the individual concerned will need help, support and information to ensure that he is enabled to take an active part in his care.

CANCER

This is probably the disease to which most people would refer when discussing chronic or life-threatening illness. Malignant disease is a huge problem. It is estimated that one in three of the population will develop the disease. One of the principal risk factors for cancer is ageing and it is acknowledged that the numbers of elderly in our population will rise dramatically. This means that helping people to live with cancer must be set in the context of helping elderly people to live with cancer – people whose function is decreasing as a result of ageing, people who are less mobile, whose body mass is less, whose immune systems are less efficient and whose lung and liver function is reduced (Fentiman, 1990). Cancer is a disease that can be characterized by exacerbations and remissions with treatment that can be severe and toxic. The implications of cancer are felt not only by the patient but by his family too. The implications of cancer therapies cannot be ignored. Cancer can affect the physical, emotional, social and spiritual status of the patient. Following diagnosis patients report obvious changes in the ways people relate to them. Myths and misconceptions sadly are still widespread (Eardley, 1986): the fear of contagion and contamination; the embarrassment of not knowing what to say; the very real possibility of being refused a mortgage, life insurance or a job.

MOTOR NEURONE DISEASE

Over the past few years a much greater public awareness of the devastating effects of this disease has become apparent. With the publicity surrounding well-known individuals suffering from the disease the insidious deterioration in function that is associated with the disease is becoming more widely understood. As ability becomes less and less individuals will require greater support in practical, physical and emotional terms. The necessity to maximize whatever potential exists for self-help and self-care must be paramount.

MULTIPLE SCLEROSIS

Again a disease that has achieved a much higher public awareness over recent years. It is a chronic disease characterized by relapses separated by often long remissions during which the sufferer may remain well. This is a disease that has the ability to affect almost any part or system of the body: the senses may be compromised, for example, with disturbances of speech or sight. While not life threatening in itself, as a progressively degenerative disease the incapacity that it produces may ultimately lead the patient to an increasing dependence on others for help with the most basic activities of daily living.

CHRONIC OBSTRUCTIVE AIRWAYS DISEASE (COAD)

This group of diseases affects a huge number of our population to varying degrees. The ability to breathe freely is one of the most basic and critical functions and if bronchitis or emphysema, for example, have compromised this function, the body's ability to oxygenate its tissues is impaired, breathlessness and dyspnoea impede movement and even conversation. Mobility is lost and with it some of the individual's ability to function in society. Deterioration may be rapid or gradual, leading to increasing dependence on others. COAD, like cancer, may be punctuated by acute infective episodes requiring a significantly higher level of support from health carers. After each such episode a residual loss of function may be expected. Ultimately the extent of the disease will be such that life cannot be sustained.

CHRONIC CARDIAC DISEASE

Many people live long and full lives with some degree of cardiac insufficiency or dysfunction. Whatever the cause, the effects on an individual may be such that his quality of life is significantly reduced. His mobility may be restricted, his exercise tolerance severely limited. Ineffective oxygenation may lead to tissue damage requiring long-term management of venous ulcers for example. Breathlessness restricts movement and conversation. Chronic cardiac disease can often be progressive, leading to increased dependency and increased demands on informal carers, health professionals and statutory organizations.

ARTHRITIS

Both rheumatoid and severe osteo-arthritis can be considered as chronic illness and both have the potential for severely restricting mobility. Associated pain which can be difficult to control affects the quality of the individual's life, impinging on his relationships, activities and socialization. The emotional effects of long-term, chronic painful disease can be profound, the prescribed medication itself creating additional problems with side-effects such as fluid retention, indigestion and allergic responses in the form of rashes and swelling.

The joint pain and loss of movement associated with osteo-arthritis tends to be progressive and while not life-threatening in the accepted sense of the word can significantly change the lifestyle to which a sufferer has previously been accustomed.

Rheumatoid arthritis, again a disease of exacerbations and remissions, is severely restrictive. A lady who had previously been able to get up and dressed in the morning in half an hour may find, for example, that during acute phases of her disease these activities can take up to two hours as the stiffness and immobility in fingers and wrists makes normal movement almost impossible. The implications for someone who has been used to exercising some degree of control over her life will be severe. It may become impossible to work, for example, or to run the home, and the loss of self-esteem and of role calls for major readjustments alongside the specific physical ramifications of the disease.

CONGENITAL ABNORMALITIES

This heading covers an enormous range of illnesses and conditions most of which, though, are found in very small numbers. From the rare disorders of metabolism such as Hunter-Hurler syndrome or phenylketonuria to physical defects such as spina bifida, these diseases produce a variety of problems. In severe cases the abnormalities are incompatible with more than a very brief life, and care and support are directed to the comfort of the child and the emotional and practical support of carers and parents. In other cases however the illness becomes chronic. It is compatible with life but compromises activity or development in a number of ways. Where a high level of long-term care is required the demand on resources both human and practical may be immense. The effects on relationships and families can have severe and long-lasting sequelae. The strain of caring for a heavily dependent relative can lead to emotional and psycho-social difficulties, practical problems with housing and employment and financial constraints in meeting the increasing needs of the patient.

WHERE ARE THE PATIENTS?

Throughout the course of their disease the chronically ill will receive care in a variety of settings and from a wide range of both formal and informal carers. The exacerbations and remissions which are characteristic of this client group mean that needs will be changing continually and must therefore be continually re-assessed. In response to changing needs referral to different members of the health care team may be required; for example a physiotherapy opinion, or a request for financial advice from the relevant member of the Social Work Department.

People suffering from chronic illness, depending on the degree of incapacity, may receive the bulk of their care in residential long-term accommodation or in the community. However, acute episodes will require short-term admission to a specialist in-patient unit for control of symptoms or management of advancing disease.

When care is provided principally in the community, access to respite beds in local nursing homes or hospitals can be a positive help by allowing informal carers to have some 'time off' thus ultimately extending the length of time that the patient may remain at home.

Those with chronic illness benefit significantly from day care too which may be provided by voluntary or charitable organizations or within the National Health Service. Day care not only provides a breathing space for families but also allows the patient access to professionals offering the patient a wide range of supportive services such as physiotherapy, occupational therapy, skilled nursing care, complementary therapies and perhaps most importantly a supportive social environment which enables patients to meet with others sharing similar problems.

It is common to find people suffering from chronic illness in any health care setting. If their needs are to be effectively met the initial assessment must include details of their understanding of the disease and its implications, but more importantly an understanding of how they themselves may take part in increasing their own health and well-being by learning about altering behaviours and habits, and changing, for example, patterns of eating, drinking or exercise.

WHAT ARE THE PROBLEMS?

The difficulties and problems experienced by those with chronic illness are legion, and will differ quite significantly from one person to another even though the diagnosis may be the same. For the purposes of this section the problems have been categorized under a number of broad headings, although this is neither the only nor necessarily the best approach. Again what may be a problem for one family, for example dealing with large amounts of soiled linen, may not be so for another which had the advantage of a previously installed commercially sized washer/dryer.

Mobility

In the broadest sense mobility can include any movement from the basic ability to move an arm or leg to exercise on a treadmill or bicycle or take part in a programme of physical activity over and above normal living. Chronic illness and its treatments have the potential to affect movement at every level.

Brain damage from an accident, for example, may incapacitate an individual physically to the extent that he is no longer able to feed or dress himself. Severe dyspnoea and breathlessness can prevent a sufferer from chronic obstructive airways disease from moving more than a few steps at a time and may extend such activities as making a hot drink from a task of a few minutes to one of half an hour or more. Cancer that has metastasized to the bony skeleton, perhaps to the femur, not only causes pain but also the potential for pathological fracture. Mobility may be restricted, leaving a woman with advanced, metastatic breast cancer housebound and unable to walk the short distance to her local shops. Progressive diseases such as motor neurone disease or multiple sclerosis will also affect the amount of physical activity that the individual is able to undertake.

As exercise is restricted at whatever level there will be related difficulties. Severe immobility leads to problems of venous stasis, respiratory difficulties, and the potential for skin breakdown from pressure. Loss of ability to self-care by being unable to reach the bathroom or kitchen creates increasing dependence on other people, a loss of self-esteem and role. Difficulty with negotiating stairs may mean a patient is restricted to one level – where street access is only by stairs he becomes a virtual prisoner in his own house. This will affect relationships with friends and neighbours, deny access to social activities, shops and theatres.

If chronic illness has necessitated the use of a wheelchair, design of buildings can create problems and dependence on another person becomes a necessity. As illness and incapacity progress formal exercise programmes in which individuals have previously taken part may become inappropriate. Jogging may have to be replaced by static exercises for example. In a continually changing situation, assessment remains the principle which must precede the information and education necessary to enable the patient and carers to respond in the most positive way to the changed circumstances.

Self-actualization

According to Maslow (1954) this is classified as the highest level of human motivation. He sees it as addressed only when more basic motives such as food and safety are met or partially met. Rogers (1970) feels it is a basic force – 'a tendency toward fulfilment and enhancement of the organism'. This holds good whatever the state of an individual's health or illness. Self-actualization can be achieved by certain behaviours which include assuming responsibility and working towards defined objectives. Self-actualization in parallel with chronic illness means striving for the fullest potential in whatever area is being considered.

A woman whose cancer has required major surgery resulting in the raising of a stoma may find that it has severely disrupted her previously very active social life. Her goal may be to rejoin a theatre club for example and feel able to take part in visits without having to worry about access to toilets, lack of equipment, leaks or smells.

Someone whose normal dexterity has been compromised by progressive neurological deterioration may find himself unable to continue his previously overwhelming interest in model making. If finer movements have been lost, ways must be found of harnessing such movement and skill as remains and channelling this into activity that brings with it a sense of purpose.

If chronic illness and repeated hospital admissions disrupt social activity to the extent that friendships are broken and family relationships disrupted normal social networking can be destroyed, leading to isolation and depression. Loss of self-esteem, motivation and interest create a vicious circle of boredom leading to loss of involvement leading to more boredom.

Relationships

In health, individuals develop relationships with a wide variety of people at many different levels. In illness these change and new ones develop as a result of a dependency on others for tasks that were previously done without help. Altered function or loss of mobility means some relationships flounder and support is required from new sources. The emotional response to knowledge of disease, prognosis, treatment and its effects in turn create strains in family relationships and friendships.

A man who had been used to being the stronger partner both in a physical and supportive sense realizes his osteo-arthritis has become chronic and increasingly incapacitating and he sees his role being eroded. From being the partner who provided support he finds he is now having to ask for it. He is no longer able to drive and the increasing pain he experiences is making him short tempered. The analgesics make him drowsy and unable to concentrate for more than a short period of time.

A diagnosis of cancer has devastating effects on the individual concerned but these reverberate through the family too. Recurrent disease is another critical time when support systems are particularly vital (Northouse, 1981). It is still difficult for some people to articulate the word cancer – it is not easy to offer help and support to a friend if you can't bring yourself to say the name of the disease. It may be easier to make excuses, pretend you're busy or that you didn't see the patient's husband as he passed you in the street.

For most of us our friends, families and partners are a vital part of our existence and we grow used to a comfortable relationship with them, interspersed perhaps with some turbulence from time to time. Chronic illness or the knowledge of a diagnosis of a life-threatening disease has the ability to turn these relationships on their heads, to sow seeds of anger, mistrust, doubt and fear. Where once communication was open and free it becomes guarded. The truth is kept back in the belief that it is best for the patient. Carers make decisions paying little attention to his rights for the truth and for autonomy to make his own decisions. Professional carers may be asked to walk a tight-rope between a couple who both know the 'truth' about a diagnosis but in the pretence of protecting each other will not enter into any discussion.

As illness encroaches further into health the levels of personal support that the client and his family require will increase proportionately.

Health responsibility

It was stated earlier that health and illness are best seen as separate entities rather than at opposite ends of a continuum. In this case the maintenance of the state of health alongside chronic illness is of critical importance.

In the UK two major health screening programmes have been established – breast screening and cervical screening. There is no reason why a woman who has rheumatoid arthritis should be excluded from either of these programmes although there is anecdotal evidence to suggest that in some places chronic illness precludes the invitation for screening. Likewise the regular checks on blood pressure for example that are carried out by GPs should be considered equally important for the chronically ill. A woman with chronic breast cancer is as likely to develop a maturity onset hypertension as her neighbour who is currently well.

The chronically ill are potentially liable to exclusion from programmes of health promotion and disease prevention. Any plan of care must therefore make explicit the essential nature and importance of activities such as screening, healthy lifestyle programmes and monitoring such as is available in well-woman or well-man clinics.

Nutrition

There are various studies that suggest dietary factors may have some link in the causation of disease and also some that suggest dietary alterations may affect the course or outcome of a disease process (Doll, 1979). The high public awareness of the Bristol Cancer Centre's dietary programme has led many people to embrace its recommendations, allowing them to regain some control over a part of their life.

Chronic illness can affect nutritional status in many ways. Disease toxicity, particularly in the case of malignancy, leads to anorexia, weight loss and cachexia. There can be physical reasons such as an inability to chew or swallow. Problems of metabolism may mean that ingested food cannot be utilized. Reactions to disease or treatment causing nausea, vomiting and constipation also lead to weight loss. Nutritional difficulties are not solely related to loss of appetite and weight. The opposite can be experienced when restricted activity, coupled with an inappropriate diet, can cause significant weight gain with subsequent related problems of movement.

The provision of food may be a problem for the chronically ill. The patient may have to depend on others for his shopping; the items of food which he needs or is able to eat may be more expensive than his budget allows; physical difficulties may mean that food has to be provided in a liquidized or fluid form. In some cases when the oral route is not possible, nutritional needs may have to be met parentally with an intravenous infusion, nasogastric tube or gastrotomy, for example.

Human beings normally derive great pleasure from eating and meals have developed a social value over and above the basic requirement for food. Chronic illness by isolating the patient or altering his function removes him from this social activity, with resulting increased levels of dejection and despair.

Stress and strain

Alongside the physical, practical and emotional problems of chronic disease are those with an emotional or psychological dimension. As each person is an individual with his own methods of coping, so each person will react and respond differently to the realization that he is in fact suffering from a chronic disease or one which sooner or later will threaten his life.

Anxiety and distress are common, and anger, resentment and frustration may be seen as incapacity overtakes ability and simple tasks such as cleaning one's own teeth become first difficult and then impossible. Those closest to the patient, his partner or principal carer often bear the brunt of the worst of the patient's anger. Visitors may see a clean and tidy lady sitting in bed, chatting happily about her recent visitors, how she managed a trip to the local shops in her wheelchair and met some friends for coffee. Once the front door is closed behind the visitors the veneer is stripped away and the frustration at being unable to walk to the toilet is vented on the carer. If this is mentioned outside the house visitors find difficulty in believing such a radical personality change from their own experience and may question the skills and abilities of the carer.

Chronic illness creates stresses and strains not only in the sufferer and his partner, family and friends but in the professional carers too. Highly dependent patients whose requirement is for total care are a huge drain on practical resources but on human resources too, a fact which needs to be recognized when rotas and workloads are planned.

Practical problems

The chronically sick will spend a large proportion of their lives cared for in a community setting where practical problems will increase with the progression of the disease. Acute episodes may require additional equipment and support with referral to such services as District Laundry and special refuse collection. Alterations to the house may be needed to enable the patient to make the most of any potential he has for movement or activity. Equipment such as humidifiers, suction apparatus, special lifting equipment, beds and chairs may be required, in turn needing extra space, power and water supplies. As the level of support is increased so the cost and resource implications rise too – a problem for both informal and statutory carers. In community care practical problems extend beyond management of the disease and the patient and encompass seemingly mundane areas such as housework, decorating and gardening. Where a disease has a finite life – a hip replacement for example or recovery from a myocardial infarction – most people would be prepared to let the dust lay and the grass grow. With a progressive disease such as multiple sclerosis, which may run a course of many years, another solution must be found.

Seemingly unrelated practical problems can crop up too – how to hold a children's party when Mum's bed is in the sitting room; how to get Dad to a family wedding when the Registry Office has no easy access for wheelchairs; how to have a family holiday without making Grandma, who has Parkinson's disease, feel that she is being neglected and abandoned.

HOW TO HELP

Increasingly, patient education and health promotion are seen as integral to the acute and continuing care planned and provided for all patients (Webb, 1988). For this to achieve its maximum effect the patient must be enabled to exercise autonomy and control. If it is his wish he must be involved in decisions that are made about his care – for example where will he be looked after – who will provide the care – how he will maintain his role as head of the household. A patient has an in-built right to this involvement if he wishes to exercise it but it will be a hollow activity without the facts on which to base decisions.

It must then be the responsibility of carers and health professionals to provide the information that is required at a level at which it can be understood at the time that it is needed. This in itself will demand that the provider of care has enhanced communication skills as well as a developed knowledge of the particular disease concerned.

SOURCES OF INFORMATION

Chronic illness suggests a pattern during which acute episodes may be treated, for example, in hospital. Not all illness at initial diagnosis can be described as chronic although some will fit into this category (for example motor neurone disease).

Initial diagnosis will almost always be given by the medical practitioner. This is a time of anxiety and stress particularly if the diagnosis is one of malignancy. There can be many blocks to communication. The language used may be technical and not understood; the doctor may use phrases and terms such as 'tumour' or 'growth' which can be ambiguous. The mention of the word cancer can mean that the subsequent part of the interview goes unheard or un-remembered. There are several possible solutions to this problem:

- a third person present;
- written back-up;
- tape recording of the interview;
- arrange a follow-up interview;
- provide contact name and number.

During an interview factual details of the disease must be discussed together with the proposed treatment and its implications.

Megan

Megan's breast cancer had been diagnosed some ten years previously and she had coped well with her mastectomy and subsequent radio-therapy, returning to work after a two-month break. Recent non-specific aches and pains in her back and legs were investigated by X-rays and then a bone scan revealed multiple metastases. The consultant explained as gently as possible to Megan that her disease had not only returned but was widespread throughout her body. She had many questions. How soon would she die? Would the pain become un-bearable? Should she give up work? What about her children? Why has it happened?

Informational needs

The urgent need was for the information which would allow Megan to make decisions about her future. This included:

- explanation of the disease recurrence;
- how radiotherapy would be used to control the pain;
- the side-effects associated with such treatment.

Once these immediate problems had been addressed there were others where further support was required and these included:

- possibility of pathological fracture and preventive surgical fixation
- the possibility of changing her job to one which required less walking and climbing stairs
- how she would discuss with her teenage children what was happen-ing in terms of her disease and its prognosis

Who provides the information

The responsibility for diagnosis and prescription rests with the medical practitioner and in most cases this will be the principal source of information. It is well recognized that much detail goes unheard or unremembered and it is always helpful to have a third person present, whether relative, friend or nurse. Initial information often elicits further anxieties and questions. Megan spent several sessions with the breast care specialist nurse, who was able to explain what was happening in terms that she could understand. The information was given so that Megan could use it to formulate her own thoughts and wishes rather than as explicit advice that she was encouraged to follow. In this way her autonomy and rights as an individual were respected but the knowledge and experience of the specialist nurse were made available to her. Although Megan had had radiotherapy in the past this course of treatment differed significantly:

- it was palliative rather than curative;
- the number of fractions (individual treatments) was 5 rather than 20;
- the expected side-effects were minimal;
- she would be able to continue working during her treatment.

These details were available to Megan from the therapy radiographer who gave her treatment and time was made available for advice and counselling.

Megan worked as a manageress in a busy department store and her job involved being on her feet for a large part of the day as well as frequent trips from one department to another. She was able to discuss possible changes in her working practice that would lessen the physical activity, and information on her employment rights was available to her from the Personnel and Occupational Health Departments of the company for whom she worked.

As a single parent who was now facing the prospect of a life-threatening disease Megan needed information on the future financial security of her teenage children. The medical social worker was able to provide details of help that might be available alongside the provision which she had already made.

Chronic disease must be managed on many levels. The help required by any individual must be aimed at preserving his autonomy while allowing optimum health. This cannot happen without an awareness of the implications of the disease. Information must be made available and in Megan's case a wide variety of health care professionals and lay people were available to provide it.

As an illness or disability becomes greater an individual's opportunity for positive health lessens and practical help and support are needed. It is still important that this is provided after full discussion with the patient, involving his family only if he wishes. As ability and mobility decrease dependence increases, often accompanied by feelings of frustration and despair at the loss of control. Knowledge, help and training must be offered for the patient to accept or reject as he chooses.

Karen

Karen, although only in her mid-thirties, has widespread carcinoma of the cervix. Previous radiotherapy and major surgery left her with a colostomy which she had managed herself until her recent deterioration. Latterly too renal problems had resulted in the need for an indwelling urinary catheter. Karen has become weak and lethargic. Her interest in her surroundings is minimal, she no longer seems to want to see her children and is becoming increasingly short tempered with her mother, who has moved in to enable Karen to remain at home rather than face admission to hospital which she had determinedly refused.

Mrs Grayson, Karen's mother, was fortunate in having a supportive GP and the involvement of the community nursing service had ensured that Karen's husband and mother understood the implications of the recent change in her condition. Many of Karen's problems stemmed from her own lack of awareness of what was happening to her and her fear of the future. An accurate assessment of her informational needs was urgently required and these were met by referral to the local Macmillan Nursing Service liaising closely with the Community Staff and GP. Karen and her family were helped to come to terms with the changing situation and together she and the carers began to plan. Moving about had become increasingly difficult and she had not been downstairs for over a week. This increased her feelings of isolation and uselessness and also made caring more difficult for her mother.

Arrangements were made to borrow a hospital type bed from Community Loans, which was installed in the front room downstairs. This achieved the dual objectives of returning Karen to the centre of family activity and the additional height of the bed enabled her to watch the activity in the road outside, regaining some sense of belonging to the community again.

Mrs Grayson was taught the practical skills of managing the bed and also the commode which had been acquired at the same time. She learned how to move her daughter so that neither she nor Karen were at risk from injury. Community and Macmillan staff co-operated jointly in this activity, and they were also able to provide booklets that included hints on caring for very sick people at home (Cancerlink). As Karen became progressively weaker a zimmer frame, Spenco mattress and sheepskin for the chair were also acquired. Changes in the patient's condition demanded the teaching and learning of new skills: special care of skin and pressure areas, a soft toothbrush and mouthwashes to maintain a fresh mouth, and the introduction of liquid supplements as Karen became increasingly anorexic.

Although initially unwilling to involve outsiders, Karen gradually came to realize the strain to which her mother was being put and decided to take advantage of some of the services which had been suggested to her:

- district linen service;
- special refuse collection;
- district stoma care specialist;
- clinical psychologist;
- social work department.

Mrs Grayson needed some practical help too with re-arranging the family dining room so that it became more suited to Karen's needs. The special skills of occupational therapists can be useful here. Some larger items of furniture were removed to make room for a high seated chair, stocks of linen, stoma appliances and equipment. Before any changes were made Karen was asked for her views and as far as possible these were respected. Feeling some returning sense of control Karen became more interested in her surroundings and spoke to several of her friends on the telephone, which had been resited to be within reach of her bed.

Although Karen's mother was determined to continue to care for her daughter for as long as it took both she and her son-in-law realized that some outside help would be essential. The options were discussed and Karen played her part in making the decision which was to take advantage of the variety of services that were available locally:

- Marie Curie Cancer Care (sitting/nursing service);
- Cancer Relief Macmillan Fund (financial aid);
- social service sitting service;
- day care at local hospice;
- crossroads or 'relief of carers' schemes.

EDUCATIONAL NEEDS

Educating for health is quite compatible with a diagnosis of chronic disease which may last for many years. In itself it may not necessarily be terminal in the accepted sense of the word. For example a significantly disabled person with chronic cardiac disease may live within the confines of the disease, dying ultimately from a malignancy, an accident or infection unrelated to the underlying disease.

The needs of such an individual are highlighted as people become more assertive and determined to make choices about what happens to them and to take part in their own care. Most health education can be included under these headings:

- eating habits;
- exercise;
- smoking;
- self-care;
- adaptation (to immobility for example).

Nutrition

Chronic or progressive illness is often accompanied by increasing loss of mobility. This can be made worse by being overweight, which will also make lifting more difficult for the carer. Dietary advice is available from medical and nursing sources and a suitable diet rich in protein and fibre but low in fat and carbohydrate not only reduces risk of obesity but may also lower the risk of further or future coronary artery or circulatory disease.

A balanced healthy diet also ensures that cellular growth and repair are maintained, at the same time preventing the problems which constipation can bring. Chronic disease may bring with it physical or emotional difficulties which compromise the intake of a normal diet. Soft or liquidized foods may be needed, with the provision of a mincer or food processor. Occasionally tube feeding, nasogastric or gastrostomy may be the only way of continuing to use the gastro-intestinal tract. Nutrition in extreme circumstances has to be maintained using total parenteral nutrition, with the additional practical difficulties this may bring.

Anxiety and distress, depression and frustration can all reduce appetite particularly in chronic disease and practical efforts are needed to overcome these. Seemingly unrelated agencies can actually have a marked effect on appetite and the desire for food:

- support groups;
- self-help groups;
- diversional therapies – visits, music, art.

Informal carers can manage tube or intravenous feeding regimes if they are provided with the required level of training and education. This allows the opportunity to maximize patient and family involvement, with professional intervention only as a last resort. The patient must always be involved when decisions are taken regarding his care and it is his wishes that must be taken into account. Practical help will be needed too relating to:

- obtaining and storing equipment;
- preparing feeds;

- cleaning equipment;
- obtaining drip stands, bags etc.;
- disposing of used equipment.

Exercise

Keeping fit has become an increasingly high profile activity in the late twentieth-century. This may range from simple arm and leg movements to running a marathon. For those people who are chronically ill an exercise or activity programme needs to be developed which takes into account their own wishes and desires as well as their physiological need for movement. Exercise must be tailored to ability and assessed and planned jointly with the patient. A man of 65 who has a right hemiparesis following a cerebrovascular accident for example will be encouraged to develop any residual movement on his right side together with physical activity that encourages deep breathing and sufficient activity to increase the heart rate. Exercise routines are best discussed and taught by a physiotherapist and then monitored and encouraged by family, friends and carers. As different movements are taught they must be practised and the rationale behind their use understood. Treadmills, rowing machines and exercise cycles can all be used in certain circumstances and may provide an individual with the scope for exercise which would otherwise be denied him. The strategic use of bags of flour or sugar in the home can take the place of weights and sandbags.

Maintaining an agreed level of exercise not only benefits respiratory and musculoskeletal systems but helps to prevent obesity and boredom too. For the chronic sick, as for anyone else, the setting of achievable goals is a useful prelude to any programme of exercise. A lady significantly disabled with arthritis for instance may find that with perseverance her exercise tolerance for walking increases from 50 to 500 yards over a period of time, allowing her to get to the local shop which had previously been beyond reach.

Where progressive immobility means that walking is no longer possible help with transport may be needed. For example:

- financial help to purchase a car;
- adapted car or van to accommodate a wheelchair;
- adapted controls for hand use only;
- provision of a charity transport minibus;
- local authority transport for the otherwise housebound;
- organized outings through local charities or support groups.

Tobacco use/misuse

A number of chronic diseases affecting large numbers of the population are directly attributable to the use of tobacco; for example, chronic obstructive airways disease (COAD), heart disease and lung cancer. There is increasing social pressure to reduce smoking and public areas are often designated as no-smoking areas. In the face of a diagnosis of cancer for example an individual may have great difficulty in reducing or stopping his use of cigarettes – the nicotine has become a necessity. A smoker and his family will first need to understand the basic facts about smoking and how it may compromise treatment, create further ill health, or affect non-smoking family members. The way in which this information is communicated is important and it is essential to ensure that it has been understood. Patients may not realize that there is evidence to suggest that radiotherapy is less effective if a patient continues to smoke and that side-effects are significantly worse. Not all people appreciate the dangers of passive smoking. Many districts now have smoking cessation programmes and there is often no reason why these should not be made accessible to the chronically sick. Smoking also affects appetite by causing taste and smell alterations and stopping smoking may actually improve appetite and appreciation of sur-roundings – the scent of flowers, for example.

As anyone who has tried will know, to stop smoking is not easy. The rationality of stopping and the future benefits may be well understood by the patient but smoking is a behaviour that is hard to change. Various tricks can be used such as:

- avoiding activities which were always associated with a cigarette;
- avoiding areas where people habitually smoke;
- finding something to occupy the hands – knitting, modelling.

A strategy for smoking cessation needs to be agreed with carers and family and most of all to have the commitment of the patient himself.

HEALTH PROMOTION

In spite of chronic illness there is still a place for people to become involved in national screening programmes. For example, a cervical smear may identify pre-cancerous changes in the cervix of a woman who is significantly incapacitated by chronic obstructive airways dis-ease. Early management of the dysplasia can prevent the development of invasive disease with all its attendant problems.

Hypertension may exist unsuspected for many years and the chroni-cally ill or disabled should not be excluded from health checks open and available to the population as a whole. Other national programmes include breast screening, well woman and well man checks, urinalysis and faecal occult blood tests as a screen for colonic cancer.

These health promotional activities, although widely available, are not always easily accessible and assessment of the needs of the chroni-cally sick should include investigation of their needs for such activity.

DENTAL AND SKIN HEALTH

Chronic illness can be debilitating and predispose to a wider variety of infections than would normally be expected. Part of the overall plan of care must therefore include the information and teaching necessary to prevent infection or tooth decay, for example, and to pick up the signs of skin breakdown or pressure as soon as it has occurred.

Radiotherapy to the mouth area, for example, can accelerate dental caries and may even in some cases predispose to bone necrosis. Regular mouth checks and visits to the dentist are an important part of management. Where sensation is impaired skin integrity may be damaged by heat, cold, pressure, friction or the constriction of tight clothing. Good health practices include frequent visual checks of skin surfaces and especially hands and feet. Organizations such as the Disabled Living Foundation can provide information and advice on clothing adapted for a range of disabilities and others, for example, can provide a wide range of chairs, cushions, back rests and aids to support people in positions that will prevent problems of pressure.

ENSURING SUCCESS

This chapter is entitled 'Helping those with chronic or life-threatening illness'. This help must be given in a non-paternalistic way and must not be seen as indoctrination. Its efficacy and the key to successful outcome depend upon an accurate assessment of the needs and wants of the individual and his desire for involvement in the decision-making process. (To the terminally ill these two words, 'needs' and 'wants', are not necessarily synonymous.)

As the concepts of multi-professional care are developed it will become increasingly important to identify a key worker who may represent one of a number of different disciplines. This alone will not ensure success however.

Continuity of care and support must be ensured as the patient moves from one care setting to another – moves which may occur many times during the course of chronic illness. When needs or wants are identified they must be documented and the information made available to all members of the team who are involved. This must include informal carers and friends and relatives as well as the patient himself. The plan of care must have stated objectives and a widely understood programme of activity to meet them. Within this plan, teaching for good health practices must be included together with the help required to correct poor ones. When a patient with chronic cardiac disease is cared for at home a diary style document can be used to which all carers have access and in which all details of care are recorded.

This can go with the patient to a clinic appointment, for example, or if he is admitted to hospital during an acute phase of his illness. It will be available for the patient, too, allowing him the opportunity for true partnership in his care.

Where encouragement is needed for good health practices an awareness of the plan will make sure everyone can provide the encouragement and support that the patient needs to help him adhere to the agreements.

For example:

- increasing protein and fibre in the diet;
- a visit outside the house at least each week;
- dental appointment every three months;
- exercise programme designed by a physiotherapist to be completed every day.

A huge variety of professional and lay people belonging to statutory, voluntary and charitable groups will be involved with the chronically sick and terminally ill. Accurate and up-to-date documentation is only one way of ensuring communication. Case conferences can be a vitally important way of ensuring that new problems, changing circumstances, altered needs or other issues are comprehensively addressed.

The promotion of health and the education not only of the patient but of his family are nowhere more important than when dealing with chronic illness. When disease or illness has progressed to a point where cure or containment is no longer a possibility the place for health promotion may decline but the need for involvement of patient and family becomes significantly greater. Several studies have revealed the extent to which families have a lack of knowledge of the facilities that may be available to them. (Such organizations are listed in the Appendix.) Because of the vast numbers of helping and caring agencies, particularly where cancer or HIV is concerned, it is important to co-ordinate activity. One family was totally overwhelmed as representatives from 14 different organizations called at the house to offer help. This example stresses the need for a key worker to prioritize needs and oversee the involvement of other carers.

The chronic sick in spite of their illness remain full members of our society, although instances where this is called into question are frequently reported. A recognition of this fact will be the first step to ensuring that this group of people with their specific and special needs are provided with the advice and help that they need. While people in wheelchairs are excluded from cinemas and theatres, while museums remain inaccessible to the disabled and while shops do not provide appropriate toilet facilities we cannot pretend to be providing an equitable service for this group of people. If the chronic sick are denied access to screening programmes, to the facilities available to their so-called 'well' neighbours or to the specialist help that they require they will not be able to maximize their own potential for health nor to achieve the degree of autonomy and involvement to which so much lip service is paid. The five-point plan must be:

- accurate assessment of needs and wants;
- carers with appropriate knowledge and information;
- carers with teaching and communication skills;
- a caring culture in which the chronic sick are enabled to play a full part to the extent of their changing abilities;
- a health care system that ensures the chronically sick achieve the highest level of health available to them.

REFERENCES

Cancerlink (1986) *Caring for the very sick person at home*, Cancerlink, London.

Doll, R. (1979) Nutrition and Cancer: A Review. *Nutrition and Cancer*, **1**.

Eardley, A. (1986) Radiotherapy: What do Patients need to know? *Nursing Times*, **82**(16), 24–6.

Fentiman, I.S., Utrelli, S.U. *et al.* (1990) Cancer in the Elderly: Why so badly treated. *The Lancet*, **1**, 1020.

Hayward, J.C. (1975) *Information: A prescription against pain*, Royal College of Nursing, London.

HMSO (1990) *Working for Patients*, HMSO, London.

Hogbin, B. and Fallowfield, L. (1989) Getting it taped: The 'bad-news' consultation with cancer patients. *British Journal of Hospital Medicine*, **14**, April, 30.

Maguire, G.P., Tait, A., Brooke, M. *et al.* (1980) Effects of counselling on the psychiatric morbidity associated with mastectomy. *British Medical Journal*, **281**, 1454–6.

Maslow, A.H. (1954) *Motivation and Personality*, Harper and Row, New York.

Northouse, L.L. (1981) Mastectomy Patients and the fear of cancer recurrence. *Cancer Nursing*, June, 213–19.

Rogers, C.R. (1970) *On becoming a person: A therapist's view of psychotherapy*, Houghton Mifflin-Sentry Edition, Boston.

Silberfarb, P.M. *et al.* (1980) Psychosocial aspects of neoplastic disease and functional status of breast cancer patients during different treatment regimens. *American Journal of Psychiatry*, **137**(4), 450–5.

Stromberg, M. (1989) in *Cancer Nursing: A Revolution in Care* (ed. A.P. Pritchard), Proceedings of Fifth International Conference on Cancer Nursing, Macmillan Press, London.

Webb, P. (1988) Teaching Patients and Relatives, in *Oncology for Nurses and Health Care Professionals*, Vol. 2 (ed. R. Tiffany), Harper and Row, Beaconsfield.

FURTHER READING

Cohen, D.R. and Henderson, J.B. (1988) *Health, Prevention and Economics*, Oxford Medical Publications, Oxford.

Coutts, L.C. and Hardy, L.K. (1985) *Teaching for Health. The Nurse as Health Educator*, Churchill Livingstone, Edinburgh.
Doxiadis, S. (ed.) (1990) *Ethics in Health Education*, John Wiley, Chichester.

CHAPTER 14

Helping individuals with mental handicap or emotional dependence

Brian Kay

Among the more vulnerable groups in society who may place specific demands on health care professionals in relation to health promotion are those individuals who are physically and/or emotionally dependent due to some degree of intellectual impairment or emotional immaturity. There are a variety of labels applied to this group, of which the most widely used currently are 'people with a mental handicap' or a 'learning difficulty/disability'. This handicap or disability may result from a number of factors which may have arisen before, during or not long after the birth of the individual (see Table 14.1). The most common of these are: intrauterine infections such as rubella, cytomegalovirus, toxoplasmosis or, less commonly now, syphilis; genetic abnormalities; trauma resulting from accidents; toxins in the maternal bloodstream or poor maternal health. Many of the conditions can be identified and often prevented by sound pre- and antenatal care. In addition a number of problems may arise as a result of environmental and social

Table 14.1 Causes of mental handicap

Prenatal	Perinatal	Postnatal
Intrauterine infections	Infections	Infections
Genetic factors	Structural problems of mother	Disease
Toxins in maternal bloodstream	Improper birth processes	Trauma
Trauma to mother	Incorrect delivery	Toxins and diet
Maternal illness	Trauma	Untreated genetic disorder
		Isolation

factors in childhood which may leave an individual with some degree of intellectual or emotional impairment.

However effective our antenatal and child health care may be it is inevitable that health care professionals will, from time to time, be confronted with an individual with a mental handicap who will need help and advice, either directly or through the offices of a relative or advocate, on self-care and health promotion.

In general the health care needs of the person with a mental handicap are much the same as those of any other member of society, although there may be a greater incidence of some specific conditions such as epilepsy and sensory impairments. The greatest challenge for the professional in this area is in helping the individual to recognize their health status and, in particular, to recognize when they are not well and to help identify their health needs and to plan out and maintain a healthy lifestyle. Much of this involves a sound educational strategy for this individual. How such needs are identified and met depends upon our understanding of the nature of mental handicap. The last three decades have seen a rapid and considerable change in our view of this client group. A composite view of this might help in determining an appropriate approach to meeting their needs. In general we can identify four models which have underpinned our approach to people with a mental handicap (Table 14.2). Up until the 1950s the general approach was based upon a medical model when mental handicap (mental subnormality, as it was called then) was seen to be a medical condition (disease) especially where specific syndromes, e.g. Down's syndrome, could be identified, and the approach was primarily custodial and was led by doctors, psychiatrists supported by asylum attendants, later to be replaced by nurses. When individuals remained out of institutional

Table 14.2 Models for understanding the nature of mental handicap

Model	Care leader	Change
Medical (custodial)	Doctor, psychiatrist Asylum attendant – nurse	Advances in psychiatry and treatment; Changing role of doctor and public expectations
Behavioural	Psychologist Nurse	Development of behavioural psychology; creation of a vacuum for a profession
Social	Residential social worker Nurse	Jay report Social services as lead agency
Educational	Teacher	Warnock report; falling rolls Status of teachers

care they received limited support from GPs and mental welfare officers.

There was often a failure by many to make a clear distinction between mental handicap and mental illness. By the late 1950s it became increasingly apparent that this model was not particularly effective.

Apart from a small number of specific disorders, e.g. phenylketonuria, congenital hypothyroidism (cretinism), medical treatment was not available for people with a mental handicap. This was highlighted as advances were made in the treatment of mental illness. The medical profession found mental handicap a less rewarding field in which to work. An alternative model was needed. This evolved in the 1960s with the advent and growth of behavioural psychology. The work of B.F. Skinner (Skinner, 1953) produced techniques which could be developed to replace inappropriate behaviours with more socially acceptable and appropriate ones. Thus the 'behavioural model' became paramount in care of people with a mental handicap. As a result mental handicap became very much associated with disturbed and bizarre patterns of behaviour, aggression, self-mutilation, screaming, temper tantrums, destructiveness and overt sexual behaviour. Clinical psychologists, who in mental handicap had spent the bulk of their time in IQ testing, moved into the professional vacuum created by the reduction of medical influence and occupied a key role in leading the care of people with a mental handicap, supported by mental handicap nurses who often implemented the behavioural programmes/interventions. However, this model was short lived for although it afforded more than had the medical model – for the first time for many families of people with a mental handicap a professional arrived who could offer a tangible change/improvement in the individual's condition – it also had obvious shortcomings. Just as few people with a mental handicap had definable medical condition/symptoms so, equally, it was only the minority of people who exhibited these violent, disturbed, or strongly antisocial behaviours. For the majority it was the lack of social skills which brought them to the attention of health care professionals. The fact that, even as adults, many people with a mental handicap required assistance with eating, dressing, personal hygiene, etc. was what made demands upon health and social services. In a sense it was not how the individual behaved, but how they did not behave that identified them. Thus by the mid-1970s we see the advent of the 'social model'. This model, much supported by the Jay Report (HMSO, 1979), saw people with a mental handicap as primarily needing social skills/training frequently using the behavioural techniques and the behavioural model to enable individuals to learn and acquire appropriate social skills.

Whilst it was suggested that residential social workers would be the profession most likely to lead in this model, in practice it was mental handicap nurses who took on this role. In fact this precipitated a fundamental change in the training of mental handicap nurses which resulted in the introduction of the 1982 Registered Nurse for the Mentally Handicapped Syllabus (National Boards for England and Wales, 1982). In parallel with this had been the steady realization that people with a mental handicap were not (as previously thought) ineducable. In 1970 legislation had been introduced to broaden statutory education to include children with a mental handicap (Education (Handicapped Children) Act, 1970).

This process continued apace and was much accelerated by the Warnock Report in 1978 (HMSO, 1978). This brought us to our fourth model – the 'educational model'. The rationale was that it could be recognized that some people with a mental handicap behave inappropriately or lack proper social skills, but what is the reason for this? The reason appeared to be that they learned inappropriate behaviour or failed to learn the appropriate skills because they have difficulty in learning; thus, the primary need becomes education and training. While some professionals will have a marked preference for a particular model it seems more practical to recognize that each model has much to commend it but is not self-contained and it is only by accepting a combination of these that we get a clear understanding of the needs of people with a mental handicap. The models give us one means of not only identifying some of the most relevant needs of people with a mental handicap in relation to health promotion but also of formulating strategies to meet these needs. Some people with a mental handicap who have specific needs related to their condition (such as problems resulting from their epilepsy, their sensory handicaps, particularly visual and auditory impairments, or complications related to respiratory, cardiovascular, gastrointestinal or neurological disorders) need help to learn how to recognize when such complications are affecting their well-being and what steps to take to prevent or alleviate these. This may range from recognizing an oncoming epileptic seizure and finding a safe environment, to maintaining appropriate diets and lifestyles.

Those people with a mental handicap who presented disturbed and challenging behaviours such as self-injurious behaviour, biting and scratching or hitting themselves or poking their eyes, or who damage their genital or anal areas, leave themselves vulnerable to infections and other complications and have an obvious need to understand the possible consequences and effects of their actions. Equally for those individuals who lack social skills the emphasis may need to be placed upon the importance of personal hygiene, environmental management and cleanliness and maintenance of an appropriate healthy diet. Equally some education and understanding may well be necessary in forming personal relationships and expressing sexuality. In terms of health promotion these last three models are clearly relevant in as much as some approaches will be medical, i.e. controlling epilepsy by the use of anti-epileptic medication and appropriate diet, the adherence to special diets in relation to some metabolic disorders and in knowing when to seek medical advice or treatment of respiratory infections and cardiovascular complications. On some occasions the replacement of inappropriate behaviour with more socially acceptable or appropriate behaviours may be the key components of promoting a healthy life-style. On other occasions it will be the teaching of appropriate social skills which will be the paramount factor – washing hands and face, cleaning teeth, care of hair, the appropriate use of the toilet, menstrual hygiene, the careful preparation of food, selecting a balanced diet, crossing roads safely, and appropriate precautions when engaging in sexual activities, are some examples. In most cases the role of the professional is going to be identifying and implementing a strategy of teaching the individual the personal skills and knowledge to cope with these potential difficulties. Two major challenges often prove to be the difficulty the individual may have in learning and, even more fundamentally, the difficulty the individual may have with communication, both receptive and expressive.

It is also necessary to recognize the context in which health promotion should be supported for people with a mental handicap. Whilst the current model of understanding mental handicap is based upon a concept of difficulty in learning the prevailing philosophy of care provision is drawn from the principle of normalization and the importance of social role valorization (Wolfensberger, 1972). This philosophy recognizes the right of people with a mental handicap to the same standards of living and access to the same services as any other citizen. It espouses the view that people with a mental handicap like any other citizen should occupy a valued role within society and should be able to function as autonomously as they can (Veatch, 1986). Much emphasis is therefore placed upon the right to be allowed to, and supported in, making informed choices about their lives and the right to take calculated risks as part of their growth and development. This may present some ethical dilemmas to health care professionals. In recognizing the autonomy of the individual, as with any other citizen, the person with a mental handicap must be allowed to make informed choices, which may mean they choose not to follow the recommended path, i.e. some people with a mental handicap may choose to smoke, may choose not to wear protective garments in relation to their epilepsy, may choose to eat unhealthy diets. In their desire to be paternalistic and to impose values and standards upon people with a mental handicap, some health care professionals find this difficult to manage, especially when their intent is clearly beneficent. For this reason it is necessary for some people with a mental handicap to have an advocate to speak for them and represent their views. This may be a relative, friend, volunteer, or appointed person. The problem may arise also where the professionals themselves are the advocates, i.e. nurses may be key workers. The important element is that, wherever possible, the individual makes the decision about his or her life based on the necessary information, and the health care professional must respect that decision. This is a key tenet of the Community Care Act 1989. The fact that a person has a mental handicap does not in itself negate their right or ability to make and enact decisions about their lives. There are, however, one or two ethical dilemmas which arise from this. The first and most difficult is in the area of informed consent. The ruling of the House of Lords in relation to Patient F makes it clear that no adult may give consent on behalf of another (National Health Service Management Executive, 1991). However, it is clear that people with a mental handicap may well need medical and nursing intervention in their lives, and gaining consent may be problematic. Some specific problems can be identified with this in relation to health promotion; for instance dilemmas encountered in screening for breast or scrotal carcinoma. This presents a dilemma which is double edged; if the health care professional (doctor or nurse) examines breasts or scrotum without clear consent they may be open to allegations of (sexual) assault; on the other hand, if they fail to detect developing carcinoma in a patient/client in their care, they are open to the criticism of negligence in their duty of care. The whole area of informed consent in relation to people with a mental handicap is fraught with potential pitfalls (Thorpe, 1989).

Many local health authority mental handicap services have sought to alleviate this problem somewhat, by developing carefully thought out risk taking or developmental care policies, which do much to define procedures and which offer some degree of protection to both the individual with a mental handicap and to the health care professional (South Lincolnshire Health Authority, 1988; McMillan, 1990).

The second ethical dilemma, which is in a way also related to informed choice, is the provision of adequate health care and advice to the individual who is profoundly handicapped or whose intellectual impairment is such that it renders them incapable of making decisions about their life and health. As previously stated, this individual should have an identified advocate who is responsible for representing the views and needs of this individual. Ideally this person should be independent of the service-providing agencies, and, in the case of an adult client, may be independent of the individual's relatives (some relatives may not always be objective enough to represent the best interests of the individual, especially where these may conflict with the aspirations or needs of the family).

There are a number of other ethical issues which may need to be explored – for example, the status of the person with a mental handicap, how competence should be assessed and regarded, the accountability of the professional, and issues surrounding paternalism of carers and the autonomy of the individual, but we do not have the space to pursue these here.

Whichever model we take for devising strategies to help and support people with a mental handicap we still tend to encounter the same challenges when looking at the issue of health promotion for this client group. We can use a number of techniques or approaches to help people with a mental handicap to perform certain desired behaviours which will enhance their health and well-being. For instance, we can help them to learn how to maintain personal hygiene and how to take obvious precautions in respect of their safety, crossing the road, being wary of strangers and so on. The dilemma is not so much in teaching the behaviours as in ascertaining that the individual understands why this is relevant. People with a mental handicap, almost by definition, may have difficulties in a cognitive understanding of some of the more abstract concepts. As an example, it may be difficult for the individual with a mental handicap to recognize when they are ill. Making the link between sensations and physical symptoms and the concept of illness can be tenuous. This is exacerbated for the individual who has difficulties in communication. For many of the more severely handicapped, recognition of ill health depends upon the careful observation of those who care for them and know them well. Parents and relatives and close friends are obviously crucial in recognizing where there is a change in, or cause for concern about, a person's condition. Equally mental handicap nurses have a component in their training which specifically concentrates upon the recognition and pathology of adverse health conditions in people with a mental handicap. The obvious signs, such as lethargy, loss of appetite, a general miserableness in a normally placid person, an increase in the incidence of epileptic seizures and obvious changes in mood, may be noticeable in this context.

Health promotion becomes difficult for the individual who has little concept of either health or illness. Some communication can be established with the non-verbally communicating person using symbols or cards. The individual can indicate where the pain symbol should be placed either on the diagram of their body or actually on their own body. Those individuals using recognized systems of communication such as Makaton or Bliss Symbols will have some ability to express themselves in this context and to describe their illness. However, there will always remain a number of individuals who will be dependent upon others to recognize their needs, either friends, relatives or advocates who know them well or skilled professionals who can observe patterns of behaviour and other symptoms and interpret them accurately. In the forefront of these will be the mental handicap nurse.

There is a wide range of professionals who may be called upon to support people with a mental handicap in recognizing their health needs and in acquiring appropriate strategies and skills to meet them (Figure 14.2).

In many areas, there will be a community mental handicap team (Grant, 1986; Royal College of Nursing, 1985). This will usually comprise the community mental handicap nurse, the social worker, the

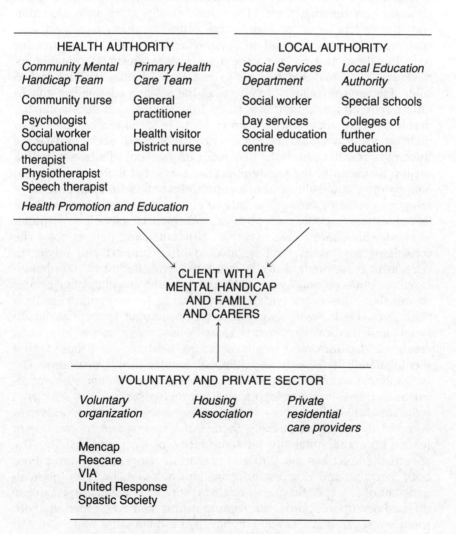

Figure 14.1   Support for those with mental handicap.

consultant psychiatrist, the clinical psychologist, the occupational therapist and should also include or have access to, the physiotherapist, the speech therapist and the dietician/nutritionist and to the primary health care team – general practitioner, health visitor, district nurse, practice nurse and other health care professionals in their professional relationships with people with a mental handicap and their families.

The community mental handicap nurse will be able to offer training and support to the person with a mental handicap and their family in acquiring personal social skills, in maintaining healthy lifestyles and in developing personal relationships. They will be able to identify many of the health needs of the individual and will be able to suggest strategies for meeting these. They will be able, often in conjunction with the psychologist, to identify the causes of many anti-social and challenging behaviours and to suggest and to apply techniques for reducing these and replacing them with more socially acceptable behaviours. They may have access to respite residential facilities and to some day service facilities. In addition, the psychologist will be able to offer advice and treatment in relation to emotional and developmental problems. They may, in conjunction with the social worker, be able to offer advice and skilled intervention to problems of social and family dynamics, resulting from the behaviour or presence of a person with a mental handicap in the family or home. The social worker will also be able to offer counselling, therapeutic intervention and support for a range of problems, as well as advice and information upon available resources and support both physical and financial as well as spiritual. They may also have access to respite, residential and day services. The consultant psychiatrist will be able to offer support and advice in relation to those medical needs associated with the individual's handicapping condition and associated problems such as epilepsy or genetic or metabolic disorders and will have access to appropriate medical colleagues. He/she will also be able to recommend appropriate medication and medical treatments. He may also have access to specific residential facilities, and to advise on the treatment of people with a mental handicap who have additional mental health problems. The occupational therapist will be able to offer a range of advice on appropriate strategies for developing and improving social skills associated with the activities of daily living, on available resources, aids and equipment and upon suitable therapeutic approaches to the use of leisure time and suitability for some forms of work and activity. The speech therapist has a key role to play in developing communication, both receptive and expressive, verbal and non-verbal and in the management of any specific speech-related disorder. She will also be able to offer advice upon appropriate feeding/eating methods, especially with the more severely physically handicapped individual.

The physiotherapist will be able to offer advice and therapeutic intervention to increase and promote mobility, to alleviate pain and disability associated with muscular and with some neurological disorders and to improve articulation and muscle tone as well as the use of appropriate physical and mobility aids. He/she will often work with groups of patients in this context.

The primary health care team will provide the usual range of services which they provide to all citizens and in some areas there may be specialist health visitors who work with people with a mental handicap.

Among other professionals who may offer advice and support and services to people- with a mental handicap are teachers working in special schools and in further education colleges where life skills courses are offered and in adult education departments in social education centres and health service establishments. Local authorities, through their social services departments, may offer places at social education centres and day centres and also offer residential facilities such as hostels, group homes and respite services, where residential social workers will provide support in social skills training. Equally, health authorities may offer residential, day and respite services where mental handicap nurses will be available to offer a wide range of skills and training for people with a mental handicap and their carers.

In many areas there may also be services provided by housing associations, private companies and voluntary organizations and many of these employ health care professionals who can offer advice and support, although in some cases charges may be made. There are also a number of voluntary organizations who offer advice and practical support to individuals with a mental handicap and their families; among these are Mencap, Rescare, Sense (for people with a mental handicap and sensory impairment) and a variety of groups with expertise in specific associated conditions, brain damage, autism, cerebral palsy, spina bifida and hydrocephalus. Local branches for these can be located by way of the local library or Citizens' Advice Bureau where lists are available.

In recent times many professionals have come to recognize the benefits of some alternative therapies for people with a mental handicap, such as aromatherapy and massage, and local mental handicap services should be able to put clients in touch with appropriate therapists. Where people with a mental handicap approach local service providers, they should be offered an extensive multidisciplinary assessment of their needs and an individual programme of support and intervention, appropriate to their needs and wishes.

Health promotion and education will be a key element of this and local services such as health promotion/education and family planning, etc. will often be included in this.

In meeting all the health needs of people with a mental handicap and in enabling and empowering them to manage their own lives and achieve their potential and lead healthy and fulfilled lifestyles it is important that professionals, carers, service providers and relatives, friends and advocates work in active and equal partnership with each other and the client/individual. It is on this basis of shared action planning that the most effective standards and approaches can be arrived at for helping people with a mental handicap to live valued and quality lifestyles.

Whenever possible, in promoting the health and well-being of the person with a mental handicap the emphasis should be placed upon enabling and empowering that individual to take charge of his/her own life, to make informed decisions and choices and to be as autonomous as possible. The role of the health care professional is to work in partnership with the individual and his or her carer to achieve this. Where individuals are likely to continue to be dependent on others for their health care needs, either due to their severe physical disabilities or their degree of intellectual impairment, the role of the professional is likely to play an active part in promoting and maintaining a healthy lifestyle for that individual and to advise and enable his or her carer and advocate to participate fully and skilfully in this process.

It might be helpful to look, now, at some examples in this respect. In order to do this we shall look at four case studies.

CASE STUDIES

Case study 1

Angela Stark is 46 years of age and is described as being moderately mentally handicapped. She was admitted to a mental handicap hospital at the age of 15 when it was discovered she was pregnant. The father of her baby was not known. Angela was in the care of her paternal grandmother who was unable to cope with her boisterous nature and the impending delivery of a child. Unfortunately the baby was still-born, but Angela remained in a mental handicap hospital where she was described as a moral defective with an IQ of below 70. She remained in the hospital until the age of 44 when in line with the development of community care she was placed in a small health service managed house for six people with a mental handicap. This house had 24-hour staff cover. After 2 years here Angela moved with 2 other people to a small house managed by a housing association. This house is unstaffed although Angela is a client of the local community mental handicap team and with her fellow householders receives regular visits from the community mental handicap nurse.

Angela maintains a reasonable standard of personal hygiene and as part of the household she helps in the cooking of the meals and the shopping. She is a trifle solitary and has difficulty occupying herself.

Unlike her fellow householders who have paid employment, Angela lost her job as a cleaner when her employer moved out of the area, and she spends much of her time at home. She is waiting for a place at the local Social Education Centre. She enjoys reasonable health although she is slightly overweight. She is believed to be sexually inactive and appears to be entering the early stages of the menopause.

In the case of Angela the professionals most likely to be involved in providing a service to her are the community mental handicap nurse, social worker, occupational therapist members and the community mental handicap team together with her GP when appropriate. She may eventually receive services from the Social Services and would in all probability benefit from attendance on the life skills course at the local further education college.

In terms of health promotion a number of needs can be identified in respect of Angela. Perhaps the four most significant would be the need to support her in planning and preparing meals, the need to address her excessive weight, her relative inactivity and lack of stimulation and her approaching menopause. Those health care professionals involved in her care together with Angela herself would look to undertaking a full assessment and developing with her an individualized plan of care and development for her – assuming that she consents to these interventions.

It would appear that there is linkage between her planning and cooking of meals (diet), her inactivity (exercise), understimulation and her being overweight. It would be desirable to help Angela recognize and understand this linkage and devise strategies for overcoming these collectively. The planning and preparation of meals, including the purchasing of food, may be a component of a local life skills course or may be covered in the Adult Education Department of the Social Education Centre. However, if Angela cannot access these it may fall to the community mental handicap nurse, community occupational therapist and the dietician to help her with this. The dietician would explain the basis of a healthy diet, presuming that Angela cannot read, this may be done by the use of a picture book approach. Angela would learn the importance of including the right amounts of nutrients, in particular carbohydrates, proteins and vitamins and minerals in a meal.

She could learn that foods fall into three main categories. She would be shown which categories foods fall into by the use of pictures and perhaps a colour coding, e.g. proteins (blue), meat, fish, dairy products, eggs and so on, carbohydrates (red), potatoes, bread, pastas; pictures can show these different forms, e.g. chips, mash, spaghetti, macaroni, rolls, toast, and minerals and vitamins (green), vegetables, fruit, milk, juices, etc. She can then learn that when planning a balanced meal she will need to have at least one item from each category. The planning of meals will have to be done in consultation with all those who are to eat the meal to ensure choice and variety. Identical picture cards could be taken by Angela when shopping to identify and purchase the items she needs. This part of the process would be helped by the community mental health nurse, occupational therapist and possibly the social worker. Likewise the cooking of the meal could be taught using recipe and instruction cards where the controls of the cooker can also be colour coded. In the case of Angela it may be of benefit to tape record some of the lessons so that she can use the tape in conjunction with her instruction cards rather like a 'talking book'. The emphasis would be on Angela achieving and maintaining these skills in order to develop more autonomy. Learning how to plan and prepare a well-balanced series of meals will do much to promote a healthier lifestyle for Angela and her fellow householders. In the process she will learn about safety in the kitchen and the importance of hygiene and the proper storage of food, etc. However, this is only one half of meeting her weight-related problem. She will also need to occupy herself more effectively to ensure adequate exercise and stimulation. Again Angela would first receive a comprehensive assessment which would look at her physical abilities, her interests and aptitudes and her level of intellectual functioning. A number of recreational and leisure activities could be identified and selected by Angela as examples of the way she would like to pass the time. They may well include sedentary activities like watching television or listening to the radio or music but should also include some physical exercise. In addition, Angela will need to identify those household activities which she has to undertake: making her bed, cleaning her room, washing, ironing, etc. Again, Angela can be helped to draw, paint or make cards or pictures which relate to these activities: washing, ironing, cooking, walking to the shops, going to the cinema, walking in the park, using her exercise bike/rowing machine, gardening; and then using a diary/ scrap book, she can plan out her daily activities. She can even plan several days in advance. If she cannot tell the time she can either have a clock drawn in the corner with the appropriate time for each activity or, alternatively, she can have a transparency with a clock or watch face (life size) drawn on it with the hands at the appropriate place which she then has to hold over the clock/watch face to identify the right time for each activity. Angela may also need to have optional activities with weather cards, i.e. sunshine – gardening; rain – painting, watching television, etc.

This activity plan may be relatively rigid at first but Angela will be encouraged to learn flexibility and should be praised for using initiative. A sensible, planned use of her time which includes appropriate exercise will also promote a healthier lifestyle for Angela, and in combination with her healthier diet may also ease her weight problem. Ideally, through the offices of the Disablement Resettlement Officer or Mencap

Pathways Scheme, Angela may be able to find gainful employment again.

The issue of Angela's approaching menopause will require a different approach. Again, a comprehensive assessment will be necessary. Angela may benefit from a visit to her general practitioner, perhaps accompanied by the community mental handicap nurse, and the menopause process will have to be explained to her to the level of her understanding. She will need to have the allied problems explained to her. She will need to recognize specific sensations such as pain, discomfort, flushes and dizzy spells which may be identified with this and to know what action to take, i.e. when she should rest, when she might benefit from some fresh air, when she should take analgesics and which would be most appropriate. Using her diary she can learn to recognize when her menstrual cycle is interrupted. She will need to be prepared for erratic and irregular menstruation. She will need to learn what symptoms are not related to her menopausal condition. She will need to recognize that at times her moods may change, that she may feel more emotional or upset or depressed and that this is likely to be part of her menopausal state; that this is normal. She will need to understand the importance of fluid balance and of obtaining medical advice, when appropriate. She will need to be able to make appointments to see her doctor. Again, some of this can be done using symbols, a diary or journal and through repeated discussion. Emphasis, in dealing with all these health needs, should be placed upon helping Angela to see the relationship and linkage between all these issues and her overall health and well-being and to recognize her ability to control and cope with these parts of her life. She should feel supported through this and should be a valued and equal partner in this process.

Case study 2

Roy Cooke is 24 years old and lives at home with his middle-aged parents. He is a tall, well-built young man who is very active and, at times, unpredictable. He is quite severely mentally handicapped and can present some difficult and challenging behaviours. During the day he attends the local social education centre where he is placed in the Special Care Unit because of his difficult behaviour. Once every two months he spends one week in a health authority managed residential unit which offers respite care to young people with challenging behaviours. Although Roy is often cheerful and likeable he is very active and can frighten other people by screaming very loudly, by running around pushing over furniture and occasionally other people, or he can upset people by inserting his fingers into his rectum.

This behaviour is restricting Roy's opportunities and access to social

activities and is proving increasingly difficult for his parents to cope
with.

A number of professionals are likely to be involved in meeting Roy's
needs. His hyperactivity and general behaviour may require advice
from the consultant psychiatrist and the dietician. It is essential that
the approach to Roy's care is co-ordinated and consistent, which will
require someone to link between Roy's home and parents, and the
social education centre and respite unit where Roy also spends time.
It is likely that either the social worker or, more appropriately, the
community mental handicap nurse will provide this link. The advice
and support of the clinical psychologist will be essential in meeting
Roy's needs. As with Angela, Roy will need a comprehensive assessment undertaking. Obviously, Roy has a wide range of needs and he
presents a number of challenges to his parents and service providers.
In terms of health promotion and Roy's health and well-being there
appear to be three main priorities: the management of his hyperactivity;
the replacement of his inappropriate behaviours – the screaming, and
destructiveness and his rectal manipulation; and the maintenance of
his personal hygiene in relation to the latter. In approaching Roy's
hyperactivity part of the assessment process would be to identify the
possible causes.

It is widely recognized now that some forms of hyperactivity may
result from allergic reactions and that dietary control may be beneficial.
A medical assessment for Roy may be arranged through either his
general practitioner or the consultant psychiatrist and the support of
a dietician sought where appropriate. Where necessary, it may be
advisable to help Roy to learn to avoid certain foods and for his parents
to be aware of this. In any event, a high rate of physical activity
in a young man like Roy will necessitate his having an adequate and
balanced diet and his parents and other carers will need to be aware of
this and the implications on the provision of meals. As a final resort, it
may be necessary for Roy's level of activity to be controlled by some
medication and the skilled intervention of the consultant psychiatrist
may be helpful here. In relation to Roy's challenging behaviours, his
screaming, the destruction of furniture, etc. and his rectal manipulation, a careful programme of management will be essential. The first
part of this will be a comprehensive assessment involving all those
who care for Roy. Each incident will need to be recorded in terms
of the time and duration of the occurrence, the actual nature of his
behaviour and a detailed record of what happened to Roy immediately
before and after his behaviour. This record should ideally be kept for
Roy at home, in the social education centre and the respite care unit.
This information should then be correlated and examined by all those
involved with Roy; probably, in this instance with the clinical psychologist taking the lead at this stage. The first objective will be to see

if there are any obvious features which regularly occur before or after Roy's antisocial behaviours – if something can be identified which either precipitates or triggers the behaviour (acts as a stimulus) or if some feature can be identified which reinforces or rewards Roy for his behaviour. In most cases, a factor or series of factors can be identified. Where this is the case a programme can be devised to break this cycle – either to remove the stimulus/precipitating factors or to remove the reinforcer. It is vital that such a programme is operated consistently by all who come into contact with Roy and that they understand the objectives and the process; one inconsistent individual can render the whole process ineffective. In some cases it may be necessary to seek advice on the ethical implications of such a programme – if a piece of behaviour is to be ignored or if it is decided to remove Roy from a particular situation for a short specified period (time out). Local agencies should provide a structure for considering the ethical dimensions of an intervention. All such decisions should be made in a setting where all those involved in Roy's care have the opportunity to discuss and accept the proposed programme. It should be remembered that decreasing or eliminating the undesirable behaviour is only half the solution to Roy's problem – this behaviour must be actively replaced with positive and acceptable appropriate behaviour. A programme of activities must be devised to occupy Roy, to engage his interest and to demonstrate to him that he is a valued member of society. These activities should be appropriate to his age, ability and interests. They should allow him to expend some of his energy appropriately. In the event that observation fails, in the first instance, to produce clear causes or reinforcers of his behaviour, further more detailed observation and assessment may be required together with a comprehensive physical assessment to eliminate any possible physiological or pathological causes (for example, thyroid-related conditions).

A significant part of the provision of care to Roy should be to enable him to acquire personal social skills. A range of priorities may be identified but in view of his tendency to rectal manipulation, perhaps washing his hands might be a valuable, high-priority skill. Again, after careful assessment of Roy's abilities and his interests (things he regards as rewarding and would be willing to work for – reinforcers) a training programme could be developed. This could be carried out in all three of Roy's life settings, or could be, in the first instance, undertaken by staff at the social education centre. The process of hand washing should be broken down into simple stages, e.g. collecting flannel/sponge, going to wash-basin, putting in plug, rolling up sleeves, turning on cold tap, turning on hot tap, and so on. An agreed instruction (prompt) should be identified for each of these stages, and also an appropriate reward for Roy when he completes the stage correctly. These prompts and rewards must be used consistently by everyone who is working with Roy. At first it may be necessary to physically take Roy to collect his flannel, to hold his hand over the tap etc., but as he learns to do this, these prompts can be faded out. Equally, as he performs the tasks successfully some of the rewards can be phased out. If he is not succeeding with a particular stage it may be necessary to examine this and break it down into even simpler stages, e.g. move hand towards the tap, place hand over the tap, grip tap, turn anti-clockwise – and so on. Much will have been achieved when Roy is able to go and wash his hands when is asked to. The ultimate achievement will be when Roy recognizes the need to wash his hands and goes to do so of his own volition and without the need of a reward. In the case of Roy, he should wash his hands when he has been manipulating his rectum. One area of caution would be to ensure that Roy does not regard washing his hands (playing with water) as a reward or rein-forcement of his rectal manipulation – in this case such an approach would have to be discontinued.

As can be seen, Roy presents a number of challenges to his parents and carers and a concerted effort would be needed to meet these. As with Angela, the most effective approach will be for parents, profes-sionals, carers and most importantly, Roy himself, to work in partner-ship to meet Roy's needs. A reduction of his antisocial behaviours, the acquisition of socially valued and acceptable behaviours and an improved level of personal hygiene would do much to start the process of ensuring that Roy leads a healthier lifestyle.

Case study 3

Barry Riley is 19 years of age and suffers from rubella syndrome. He is believed to be totally blind and extremely hard of hearing. He has marked spastic paralysis of all four limbs. He has some difficulty in swallowing and does not chew his food at all. He has a congenital heart defect and is prone to frequent respiratory infections. Until re-cently, Barry lived at home with his young, professional parents but his physical needs have made it hard to care for him and his three younger sisters. Consequently, Barry now lives with four other handi-capped people in a bungalow owned by Mencap Homes Foundation. He receives day care, three days per week, at a local health service day centre for people with a mental handicap. Barry receives regular visits and close support and love from his parents.

The health promotion needs for Barry present a very different diffi-culty from those of Angela and Roy. It is clear that Barry is highly dependent and is unlikely to be able to develop much autonomy for some considerable time. His physical handicaps and sensory impair-ment are such that it will be difficult to assess his level of intellectual functioning. Nevertheless, communication will be a critical factor in his development and an ability to communicate will allow him to express his needs and even to indicate when he feels unwell. A number of health care professionals would have a role to play in supporting Barry and those who care for and about him.

Two crucial professionals in Barry's care would be the speech therapist and the physiotherapist. Barry and his carers will need to develop a strategy for communication and the speech therapist would be best placed to participate in a comprehensive assessment of Barry's needs. She would, in conjunction with his parents and the staff at the home and day centre, help Barry to develop expressive and receptive communication, possibly using a signing system such as Makaton, depending upon how much movement and control Barry currently has in his fingers, hands and arms. Those who know Barry most intimately, his parents, carers and keyworker, should ensure that all his current patterns of behaviours are recognized and interpreted – does he cry when in pain etc.? A programme should also be identified for the best method of assisting Barry with eating – the most appropriate posture, the most suitable feeding aids and equipment, the ideal feeding techniques and the most suitable food consistencies and textures. The speech therapist will also be the key person in developing this programme and in assisting staff and carers to meet his needs. Encouragement of tongue movement will be essential to aid his swallowing and eventual speech, if this is possible. In line with this, careful assessment of Barry's hearing should be undertaken to ensure that maximum support is given.

Assessment will also be required of Barry's spasticity and as much as possible done to promote articulation and movement and to reduce pain, muscular wastage and atonicity. The physiotherapist will exercise a key role in this respect, using a range of techniques, including hydrotherapy. Barry must make optimum use of any movement he may have; he must also learn to relax and as well as the physiotherapist, professionals or therapists skilled in alternative therapies such as massage and aromatherapy may have much to offer Barry in this respect. Some medication both for his spasticity, his pain and his tension/anxiety may be part of a holistic approach to Barry's care. Careful attention to prevent respiratory infections, to prevent the excessive collection of fluid in his lungs and to ensure that his heart is not overtaxed will be required from all who care for him.

The primary approach to meeting Barry's health care needs and quality of life will be dependent upon the input of a range of health care professionals in supporting his parents and those who care for him at home and at the day centre. It will take a concerted effort by a team of carers to ensure that Barry leads a healthy lifestyle and the role of the health care professionals will be to support and facilitate that. Nevertheless, it should never be forgotten that the aim of any service

for a person with a mental handicap should be to promote independence and autonomy, and so as well as helping Barry to acquire skills
in communication so that he can express his needs, he should be
helped to learn to exercise control over his body to the maximum
ability, to use whatever motor ability he has. He should be helped to
learn to chew and to use his senses of smell, taste and touch. Through
the receiving of affection, dignity and love he should learn to value
himself and to develop a positive concept of himself as a valued
person. He should be helped to learn how to make choices about his
life. He should also be helped to learn how to occupy himself meaning-
fully and there are many modern approaches, using computers, which
can enhance this. Those caring for him will need to understand that
just because Barry is severely handicapped does not mean that he has
no concept of what is happening to him or no opportunity to give or
withhold consent to interventions. They will need to be responsive to
his behaviour, body language and movement and to recognize when
he is happy to co-operate and when he is resistive to interventions and
they should respond accordingly. The concept of a partnership of care
still applies, even with the most severely disabled individual. Nevertheless, the reality, in Barry's case, is that much of his health promotion
will be in the hands of others who will need to be enabled to recognize
and meet his varied and complex needs.

Case study 4

Melanie Watson is 22 years old. She is married and lives with her
unemployed husband in a council flat on a large urban estate. She
spends all her time caring for her 3-month-old baby and her husband. Melanie had lived at home since leaving special school at the
age of 19. She married Dave Watson eight months ago when she
discovered that she was pregnant. Her parents were not happy at her
marriage and wanted her to undergo an abortion. Since she chose to
ignore their wishes they have refused to have any contact with her.
Her husband has little contact with his widowed father. He spends
much of his time in the local public house or in the park playing
football with his friends. Melanie has no real friends on the estate and
she tries to care for her new son between watching television, making
up jigsaw puzzles and playing with a computerized games console.

In our fourth case study we find, in Melanie, a completely different
set of challenges. Whilst she may be of limited intellectual capacity, she
is unlikely to receive her services from those professionals who care for
people with a mental handicap. It is most likely that the health care
professionals involved with Melanie will be the GP, the health visitor,
the practice nurse and the local authority social worker. The primary health promotional needs for Melanie will be to acquire skills in

parentcraft, to learn, with her husband, the skills of managing and maintaining a home and to occupy herself appropriately. The health visitor will have much to offer Melanie in learning how to care for her baby – both physically, in terms of nutrition, hygiene and adequate warmth, and emotionally in terms of love, care and affection. Some local schools or colleges may offer courses in parentcraft and in some areas the National Society for the Prevention of Cruelty to Children may offer training units for family skills and parentcraft. Melanie will also need to learn how to care for herself, especially if she has been or is still breast-feeding her baby. The social worker may also be able to help Melanie and Dave in obtaining appropriate benefits and may also be able to endeavour to breach the gap between Melanie and her parents. Melanie's level of emotional immaturity may be a cause for concern and she will require guidance and help in recognizing and meeting her new responsibilities. In Melanie's case the general approach will probably be to teach her some of the skills she requires and to work alongside her as she develops and grows as a person. Yet again, an approach based upon respect for her autonomy, partnership and equality will be the most effective in enabling her to cope with the demands of her life. Some of the necessary advice and techniques required by the health visitor and social worker may be gained from their contact and liaison with the community mental handicap team.

Thus we can see that whilst, in many ways, people with a mental handicap or some degree of emotional dependence have similar health needs to any other member of society, they may require some specialized approaches to helping them to identify and meet their health needs. In the case of such individuals the emphasis for health care professionals should be upon empowering and enabling them to exercise as much autonomy as possible. They need to be given the dignity of acquiring the skills and understanding necessary to control their own lives, make their own decisions and choices and meet their own needs. Where the individual's level of impairment or disability is such that they cannot entirely manage their own affairs they should have an advocate to represent them and the role of the health care professional is to support that advocate and enable them to recognize the individual's health needs and play their part in ensuring that these are met.

People with a mental handicap are citizens of equal value in our society, entitled to the same provision of and access to services as any other member of society. The health care professional will recognize this both in terms of the services they provide and the way in which they provide them.

Working with and alongside people with a mental handicap is and should be a rewarding and inspiring experience for both professional and client alike.

REFERENCES

Education (Handicapped Children) Act. (1970) HMSO, London.

Grant, G. (1986) *Community Mental Handicap Team – Theory and Practice*, British Institute of Mental Handicap Conference Series, Birmingham.

HMSO Cmd 7212. *Special Educational Needs*: Report of the Committee of Enquiry into the Education of Handicapped Children & Young People, HMSO, London.

HMSO Cmd 74680 (1979) *Report of the Committee of Enquiry into Mental Handicap Nursing & Care*, HMSO, London.

McMillan, S. (1990) *The Risk Business*. Dissertation for Dip/MA Community Studies, University of Keele.

National Boards for England & Wales (1982) *Syllabus of Training. Professional Register – Part 5. Registered Nurse of the Mentally Handicapped*, Oxford, Bocardo Press.

The National Health Service & Community Care Act (1989) HMSO, London.

National Health Service Management Executive (1991) *A Guide to Consent for Examinations or Treatment*, NHSME, London.

Royal College of Nursing (1985) *The Role and Function of a Domiciliary Community Nurse for People with a Mental Handicap*, RCN, London.

Skinner, B.F. (1953) *Science and Human Behaviour*, Macmillan, New York.

South Lincolnshire Health Authority: Mental Handicap Services (1988) *Developmental Care Policy*, Pushsh.

Thorpe, L. (1989) Informed Decision Making. *Journal of Clinical Practice, Education & Management*, **3**(42), 16–19.

Veatch, R.M. (1986) *The Foundations of Justice*, Oxford University Press, Oxford.

Wolfensberger, W. (1972) *The Principles of Normalization in Human Services*, National Institute of Mental Retardation, Toronto.

FURTHER READING

Parrish, A. (1987) *Mental Handicap*, Macmillan, London.

Sines, D.T. (1988) *Towards Integration*, Lippincott Nursing Series, Harper & Row, London.

Thompson, A.R. and Mathias, P. (1992) *Standards and Mental Handicap: Keys to Competence*, Baillière Tindall, London.

Useful addresses

Action for Dysphasic Adults
Canterbury House,
Royal Street,
Lambeth,
London SE1 7LN

Action for Research into Multiple Sclerosis (ARMS)
4a Chapel Hill,
Stanstead,
Essex CM24 8AG

Amnesia Association (AMNASS)
St Charles Hospital,
Exmoor Street,
London W10 6DZ

The Arthritis and Rheumatism Council
41 Eagle Street,
London WC1R 4AR
Tel: 071-405 8572

Association to Aid the Sexual and Personal relationshops of the Disabled (SPOD)
286 Camden Road,
London N7 0BJ
Tel: 071-607 8851

Association for All Speech Impaired Children (AFASIC)
347 Central Markets,
Smithfield,
London EC1A 9NH

Association of Carers
Medway Homes,
Balfour Road,
Rochester,
Kent ME4 6QU
Tel: 0634 813981

Association of Disabled Professionals
The Stables,
73 Pond Road,
Banstead,
Surrey SM7 2HU
Tel: 07373 52366

ASH
5–11 Mortimer Street,
London W1N 7RN

The Association for Postnatal Illness
Institute of Obstetrics and Gynaecology,
Queen Charlotte's Maternity Hospital,
Goldhawk Road,
London W6

Association for Spina Bifida and Hydrocephalus
22 Upper Woburn Place,
London WC1H 0EP
Tel: 071-388 1382

Association for Stammerers (AFS)
St Margaret's House,
21 Old Ford Road,
London E2 9DL

Black HIV/AIDS Network (BHAN)
106–108 King Street,
London W6 0QU

British Association for Cancer United Patients (BACUP)
3 Bath Place, Rivington Street,
London EC2A 3JR
Tel: 071-613 2121/696 9000 or Freephone (0800) 181199

British Diabetic Association
10 Queen Anne Street,
London W1M 0BD
Tel: 071-323 1531

British Voice Association
77B Abbey Road,
London NW8 0AE

Cancerlink
17 Britannia Street,
London WC1X 9JN
Tel: 071-833 2451

Chest, Heart and Stroke Association
123–127 Whitecross Street,
London EC1Y 8JJ

Cleft Lip and Palate Association (CLAPA)
1 Eastwood Gardens,
Kenton,
Newcastle-upon-Tyne NE3 3DQ

Disabled Living Foundation
380 Harrow Road,
London W9 2HU
Tel: 071-289 6111

Down's Syndrome Association
133–155 Mitcham Road,
London SW17 9PG

Greater London Association for Disabled People
336 Brixton Road,
London SW9 7AA
Tel: 071-274 0107

Haemophilia Society
123 Westminster Bridge Road,
London
Tel: 071-928 2020

Headway, National Head Injuries Association
7 King Edward Court,
King Edward Street,
Nottingham NG1 1EW

Health Education Authority
Hamilton House,
Mabledon Place,
London WC1H 9TX

The Health Education Board for Scotland
Woodburn House
Canaan Lane
Edinburgh
EH10 4SG

Help for Health
Health Information Centre,
Grant Building,
Southampton General Hospital,
Southampton SO9 4XY
Tel: 0703 779091

Holiday Care Service
2 Old Bank Chambers,
Station Road,
Horley,
Surrey RH6 9HW
Tel: 0293 775137

Invalid Children's Aid Association (I CAN)
198 City Road,
London EC1V 2PH

Meet-a-Mum Association
c/o 2 Railway Terrace
Ponprilas
Hereford
HR2 0BH

Motor Neurone Disease Association
PO Box 246
Northampton NN1 2PR

Multiple Sclerosis Society
25 Effie Road,
Fulham,
London

National Association for Colitis and Crohn's Disease
98A London Road,
St Albans AL1 1NX
Tel: 0727 44296

National Association of Laryngectomee Clubs (NALC)
Ground Floor, 6 Ricket Street,
London SW6 1RU

National Autistic Society
276 Willesden Lane,
London NW2 5RB

National Childbirth Trust
9 Queensborough Terrace,
Bayswater,
London W2 3TB
Tel: 071-992 8637

National Council for One Parent Families
255 Kentish Town Road,
London NW5 2LK

National Deaf Children's Society
45 Hereford Road,
London W2 5AH

Parkinson's Disease Society
22 Upper Woburn Place,
London WC1H 0RA

Physically Handicapped and Able Bodied (PHAB)
Tavistock House North,
Tavistock Square,
London WC1H 9HX
Tel: 071-388 1963

Royal Association for Disability and Rehabilitation
25 Mortimer Street,
London W1N 8AB
Tel: 071-637 5400

Royal National Institute for the Deaf (RNID)
Nixon House,
321 Green Lanes,
Manor House,
London N4 2ES

Royal Society for Mentally Handicapped Children and Adults (Mencap)
123 Golden Lane,
London EC1Y 0RT

Spinal Injuries Association
Yeoman House,
76 St James' Lane,
London N10 3DF
Tel: 081-444 2121

The Terrence Higgins Trust
52–54 Grays Inn Road,
London WC1X 8JU
Tel: 071-831 0330; Helpline: 071-242 1010

Winged Fellowship Trust
20–32 Pentonville Road,
London N1 9XD
Tel: 071-833 2594

Index

Page numbers in **bold** refer to figures and those in *italics* refer to tables.